ULTRASONIC DIAGNOSIS OF CEREBROVASCULAR DISEASE

DEVELOPMENTS IN
CARDIOVASCULAR MEDICINE

Recent volumes

Hanrath P, Bleifeld W, Souquet, J. eds: Cardiovascular diagnosis by ultrasound. Transesophageal, computerized, contrast, Doppler echocardiography. 1982. ISBN 90-247-2692-1.

Roelandt J, ed: The practice of M-mode and two-dimensional echocardiography. 1983. ISBN 90-247-2745-6.

Meyer J, Schweizer P, Erbel R, eds: Advances in noninvasive cardiology. 1983. ISBN 0-89838-576-8.

Morganroth J, Moore EN, eds: Sudden cardiac death and congestive heart failure: Diagnosis and treatment. 1983. ISBN 0-89838-580-6.

Perry HM, ed: Lifelong management of hypertension. 1983. ISBN 0-89838-582-2.

Jaffe EA, ed: Biology of endothelial cells. 1984. ISBN 0-89838-587-3.

Surawicz B, Reddy CP, Prystowsky EN, eds: Tachycardias. 1984. ISBN 0-89838-588-1.

Spencer MP, ed: Cardiac Doppler diagnosis. 1983. ISBN 0-89838-591-1.

Villarreal H, Sambhi MP, eds: Topics in pathophysiology of hypertension. 1984. ISBN 0-89838-595-4.

Messerli FH, ed: Cardiovascular disease in the elderly. 1984. ISBN 0-89838-596-2.

Simoons ML, Reiber JHC, eds: Nuclear imaging in clinical cardiology. 1984. ISBN 0-89838-599-7.

Ter Keurs HEDJ, Schipperheyn JJ, eds: Cardiac left ventricular hypertrophy. 1983. ISBN 0-89838-612-8.

Sperelakis N, ed: Physiology and pathophysiology of the heart. 1984. ISBN 0-89838-615-2.

Messerli FH, ed: Kidney in essential hypertension. 1984. ISBN 0-89838-616-0.

Sambhi MP, ed: Fundamental fault in hypertension. 1984. ISBN 0-89838-638-1.

Marchesi C, ed: Ambulatory monitoring: Cardiovascular system and allied applications. 1984. ISBN 0-89838-642-X.

Kupper W, MacAlpin RN, Bleifeld W, eds: Coronary tone in ischemic heart disease. 1984. ISBN 0-89838-646-2.

Sperelakis N, Caulfield JB, eds: Calcium antagonists: Mechanisms of action on cardiac muscle and vascular smooth muscle. 1984. ISBN 0-89838-655-1.

Godfraind T, Herman AS, Wellens D, eds: Calcium entry blockers in cardiovascular and cerebral dysfunctions. 1984. ISBN 0-89838-658-6.

Morganroth J, Moore EN, eds: Interventions in the acute phase of myocardial infarction. 1984. ISBN 0-89838-659-4.

Abel FL, Newman WH, eds: Functional aspects of the normal, hypertrophied, and failing heart. 1984. ISBN 0-89838-665-9.

Sideman S, Beyar R, eds: Simulation and imaging of the cardiac system. 1985. ISBN 0-89838-687-X.

Van der Wall E, Lie KI, eds: Recent views on hypertrophic cardiomyopathy. 1985. ISBN 0-89838-694-2.

Beamish RE, Singal PK, Dhalla NS, eds: Stress and heart disease. 1985. ISBN 0-89838-709-4.

Beamish RE, Panagio V, Dhalla NS, eds: Pathogenesis of stress-induced heart disease. 1985. ISBN 0-89838-710-8.

Morganroth J, Moore EN, eds: Cardiac arrhythmias. 1985. ISBN 0-89838-716-7.

Mathes E, ed: Secondary prevention in coronary artery disease and myocardial infarction. 1985. ISBN 0-89838-736-1.

Lowell Stone H, Weglicki WB, eds: Pathology of cardiovascular injury. 1985. ISBN 0-89838-743-4.

Meyer J, Erbel R, Rupprecht HJ, eds: Improvement of myocardial perfusion. 1985. ISBN 0-89838-748-5.

Reiber JHC, Serruys PW, Slager CJ: Quantitative coronary and left ventricular cineangiography. 1986. ISBN 0-89838-760-4.

Fagard RH, Bekaert IE, eds: Sports cardiology. 1986. ISBN 0-89838-782-5.

Reiber JHC, Serruys PW, eds: State of the art in quantitative coronary arteriography. 1986. ISBN 0-89838-804-X.

Roelandt J, ed: Color Doppler Flow Imaging. 1986. ISBN 0-89838-806-6.

Van der Wall EE, ed: Noninvasive imaging of cardiac metabolism. 1986. ISBN 0-89838-812-0.

Liebman J, Plonsey R, Rudy Y, eds: Pediatric and fundamental electrocardiography. 1986. ISBN 0-89838-815-5.

Hilger HH, Hombach V, Rashkind WJ, eds: Invasive cardiovascular therapy. 1987. ISBN 0-89838-818-X

Serruys PW, Meester GT, eds: Coronary angioplasty: a controlled model for ischemia. 1986. ISBN 0-89838-819-8.

Tooke JE, Smaje LH: Clinical investigation of the microcirculation. 1986. ISBN 0-89838-819-8.

Van Dam RTh, Van Oosterom A, eds: Electrocardiographic body surface mapping. 1986. ISBN 0-89838-834-1.

Spencer MP, ed: Ultrasonic diagnosis of cerebrovascular disease. 1987. ISBN 0-89838-836-8.

Legato MJ, ed: The stressed heart. 1987. ISBN 0-89838-849-X.

ULTRASONIC DIAGNOSIS OF CEREBROVASCULAR DISEASE

Doppler Techniques and Pulse Echo Imaging

edited by

M.P. SPENCER M.D.

Institute of Applied Physiology and Medicine
Seattle WA 98122, U.S.A.

1987 **MARTINUS NIJHOFF PUBLISHERS**
a member of the KLUWER ACADEMIC PUBLISHERS GROUP
DORDRECHT / BOSTON / LANCASTER

Distributors

for the United States and Canada: Kluwer Academic Publishers, P.O. Box 358, Accord Station, Hingham, MA 02018-0358, USA
for the UK and Ireland: Kluwer Academic Publishers, MTP Press Limited, Falcon House, Queen Square, Lancaster LA1 1RN, UK
for all other countries: Kluwer Academic Publishers Group, Distribution Center, P.O. Box 322, 3300 AH Dordrecht, The Netherlands

Library of Congress Cataloging in Publication Data

```
Ultrasonic diagnosis of cerebrovascular disease.

   (Developments in cardiovascular medicine ; 61)
   Includes index.
   1. Cerebrovascular disease--Diagnosis.  2. Diagnosis,
Ultrasonic.  3. Doppler ultrasonography.  4. Transcranial
Doppler ultrasonography.  I. Spencer, Merrill P.,
1922-     ,  II. Series: Developments in cardiovascular
medicine ; v. 61.  [DNLM: 1. Cerebrovascular Disorders--
diagnosis.  2. Ultrasonic Diagnosis--methods.
W1 DE997VME v.61 / WL 355 U47]
RC388.5.U46  1986       616.8'107543       86-23465
```

ISBN-13: 978-94-010-8413-0   e-ISBN-13: 978-94-009-4305-6
DOI: 10.1007/978-94-009-4305-6

Copyright

Preface

This book is designed as a definitive report on current capabilities of ultrasound imaging and Doppler evaluation of the cerebral circulation, both extracranial and intracranial. The basic chapters are directed to the beginner in ultrasound and hemodynamics and for the expert in updating newly available modalities and techniques new to the field. The ultrasonic and hemodynamic principles are presented for physicians and vascular technologists in a practical way to avoid unnecessary mathematics. The aim is for maximum clinical utilization so that available equipment may be used more efficiently and provide more accurate diagnosis. The selection of authors represents a wide range of the expertise available in the world today.

M.P. Spencer

Preface

This book is designed as a definitive report on current capabilities in ultrasound imaging and Doppler ...

M.B.

Contents

Preface   V

Contributors   IX

1. Introduction   1
   Merrill P. Spencer, M.D.
2. Ultrasound physical concepts   7
   Merrill P. Spencer, M.D., Ronald E. Hileman, Ph.D., John M.
   Reid, Ph.D
3. Doppler instrumentation   29
   Robert S. Reneman, MD., Ph.D., A.P.G. Hoeks, Ph.D.
4. Normal anatomy, anatomical anomalies and collateral Pathways of
   the blood supply to the brain   43
   Robert Ackerstaff, M.D.
5. Normal blood flow in the arteries   57
   Merrill P. Spencer, M.D.
6. Normal physiology and pathophysiology of human cerebral blood
   flow   75
   P.C.M. Mosmans, M.D., E.J. Jonkman, M.D.
7. Cranial blood flow measurement by means of Doppler ultrasound   87
   H.R. Muller, M.D., E.W. Radue, M.D., M. Buser
8. Early carotid lesions and flow disturbances   103
   Robert S. Reneman, M.D., A.P.G. Hoeks, Ph.D.
9. Hemodynamics of arterial stenosis   117
   Merrill P. Spencer, M.D.
10. Vascular bruits   147
    Merrill P. Spencer, M.D.
11. Free hand Doppler techniques for examination of the extracranial
    arteries with continuous wave Doppler   157
    G.M. von Reutern, M.D.

12. Quantification of carotid stenosis using continuous wave Doppler
    and spectral analysis   179
    Ph. Arbeille, M.D., F. Lapierre, M.D., F. Patat, Ph.D., M.D.M.,
    M. Berson, Ph.D., D. Besse, Ph.D., L. Pourcelot, M.D., Ph.D.
13. Vertebral and basilar artery abnormalities   193
    G.M. von Reutern, M.D.
14. Doppler imaging   211
    Merrill P. Spencer, M.D.
15. Clinical application of real-time Doppler color flow mapping of the
    carotid artery   219
    Shinichi Takamoto, M.D., Ryozo Omoto, M.D.
16. Transcranial Doppler diagnosis   227
    Rune Aaslid, Ph.D.
17. Real-time B-mode imaging of the carotid bifurcation   241
    Anthony J. Comerota, M.D., Mira L. Katz, B.S., R.V.T., John V.
    White, M.D.
18. Clinical application of high resolution B-scan imaging with pulsed
    Doppler profiles (10 mHz)   257
    Michael Hennerici, M.D.
19. Intraoperative Doppler sonography   269
    J. Gilsbach, M.D., A. Harders, M.D.
20. Perioperative transcranial Doppler sonography   283
    A. Harders, M.D., J. Gilsbach, M.D.
21. Conclusion   291
    Merrill P. Spencer, M.D.

Credit and recognition list   301

Index   303

Contributors

Aaslid, R. Ph.D.
   Director of Cardiovascular Research Department, Institute of Applied Physiology and Medicine, 701 16th Avenue, Seattle, WA, USA
Ackerstaff, R., M.D.
   Department of Clinical Neurophysiology, St. Anthonions Hospital, Nieuwegein, The Netherlands
Arbeille, Ph., M.D.
   Service de Medecine Nucleaire et Ultrasons, CHR Bretonneau, 37044 Tours CEDEX, France
Berson, M., Ph.D.
   Service de Medecine Nucleaire et Ultrasons, C.H.R. Bretonneau, 37044, Tours CEDEX, France
Besse, B., Ph.D.
   Service de Medicine Nucleaire et Ultrasons, C.H.R. Bretonneau, 37044, Tours CEDEX, France
Buser, M.
   Kantonsspital Basel, Universitatskliniken, Neurologische Universitatsklinik, 4031 Basel, Petersgraben 4, Switzerland
Comerota, A.J., M.D.
   Chief, Section of Vascular Surgery, Department of Surgery, Temple University Hospital, 3401 North Broad Street, Philadelphia, Pennsylvania, USA
Gilsbach, J., M.D.
   Neurochirurgische Universitatsklinik, Universitat Freiburg, 7800 Freiburg I.BR., den, Hugstetter Strasse 55, Freiburg, West Germany
Harders, A., M.D.
   Neurochirurgische Universitatsklinik, Universitat Freiburg, 7800 Freiburg I.BR., den, Hugstetter Strasse 55, Freiburg West Germany
Hennerici, M., M.D.
   Neurologische Universitatsklinik, D-4000 Dusseldorf, Moorenstrasse 5, West Germany
Hileman, R.E., Ph.D.
   Vice President of Engineering, Carolina Medical Electronics, Inc., P.O. Box 307, King, North Carolina, USA
Hoeks, A.P.G., Ph.D.
   Rijksuniversiteit Limburg, Faculty of Medicine, Biophysics, P.O. Box 616, 6200 MD Maastricht, The Netherlands
Jonkman, E.J., M.D.
   Head Research Unit for Clinical Neuro-physiology, TNO Westinde Hospital, Lijnbaan 32, 2512 VA The Hague, The Netherlands

Katz, M., B.S., R.V.T.

Temple University Hospital, 3401 North Broad Street, Philadelphia, Pennsylvania, USA

Lapierre, F.

Service de Medecine Nucleaire et Ultrasons, C.H.R. Bretonneau, 37044, Tours CEDEX, France

Mosmans, P.C.M., M.D.

Clinical Neuro-physiology, TNO Westinde Hospital, Lijnbaan 32, 2512 VA The Hague, The Netherlands

Muller, H.R., M.D.

Kantonsspital Basel, Universitatskliniken, Neurologische Universitatsklinik, 4031 Basel, Petersgraben 4, Switzerland

Omoto, R., M.D.

Department of Surgery, Saitama Medical School, Moroyama-machi, Iruma-gun, Saitama, 350-04, Japan

Reid, J.M., Ph.D.

Biomedical Engineering and Science Institute, Drexel University, Philadelphia, Pennsylvania, USA

Patat, F., Ph.D. M.D.M.

Service de Medecine Nucleaire et Ultrasons, C.H.R. Bretonneau, 37044, Tours, CEDEX, France

Pourcelot, Le' A., M.D., Ph.D.

Universite Francois-Rabelais, Faculte De Medecine, 2 bis, Boulevard Tonnelle, 27032 Tours CEDEX, France

Radue, E.W., M.D.

Kantonsspital Basel, Universitatskliniken, Neurologische Universitatsklinik, 4031 Basel, Petersgraben 4, Switzerland

Reneman, R.S., M.D., Ph.D.

Department of Physiology, University of Limburg, P.O. Box 616, 6200 MD Maastricht, The Netherlands

Spencer, M.P., M.D.

Director, Institute of Applied Physiology and Medicine, 701 16th Avenue, Seattle, Washington, USA

Takamoto, S., M.D.

Department of surgery, Saitama Medical School, Moroyama-machi, Iruma-gun, Saitama, 350-04, Japan

Von Reutern, G.M., M.D., Ph.D.

Professor of Neurology, Klinikum Der Albert-Ludwigs-Universitat, Abteilung Klinische Neurologie und Neurophysiologie, 7800 Freiburg I.B.R., West Germany

White, J.V., M.D.

Department of Surgery, Temple University Hospital, 3401 North Broad Street, Philadelphia, Pennsylvania, USA

Introduction

M.P. Spencer

The major goal of ultrasonic techniques in cerebrovascular diagnosis is to provide noninvasive information which will point the way to stroke prevention. Each year in the USA, approximately 400,000 people suffer strokes; one third die within a month and two-thirds of the survivors have some degree of permanent disability [1]. Therapy is generally unsatisfactory and prevention is our major weapon. Ultrasound is a modality with much to offer in the crusade against stroke. Uses range widely from identifying and quantitating high-risk lesions for intervention therapy to eliminating the heart and arteries as the probable source of symptoms or following the progress of the lesions and studying the natural history of atherosclerosis. The diagnostic capabilities of ultrasound imaging and Doppler extend from the heart to the terminal cerebral arteries (Fig. 1).

Cardiac abnormalities may produce stroke by embolism to the brain [2]. This book does not explore the used of echocardiography but Table 1 lists the clinical types of patients whom should be explored and what lesions should be looked for.

Doppler Ultrasound has been recently extended transcranially into diagnosis of abnormalities in the basal arteries of the brain and for intraoperative guidance of vascular surgeons and neurosurgeons. This new modality is described in Chapter 16. Full utilization of the ultrasound modality can lead to solving many of the mysteries of stroke leading to prevention and improved treatment.

The stroke problem

Stroke is defined [3] as a clinical syndrome of neurological findings, sudden in onset, whose vascular origins are limited to occlusion or rupture of a cerebral artery. Occlusion is generally from primary intracranial thrombosis or by secondary embolism from an extracranial site producing regional ischemia and infarction. Arterial rupture produces intraparenchymal or subarachnoid hemorrhage producing ischemia by interrupting the regional blood supply from spasm or compression of local tissue. Stroke ranges in severity from the transient ischemia attack (TIA) which may resolve within a few minutes to more serious grades of permanent impairment, unconsciousness and death.

The classification of cerebrovascular accidents according to the Framingham Cardiovascular Disease Survey is a follows:

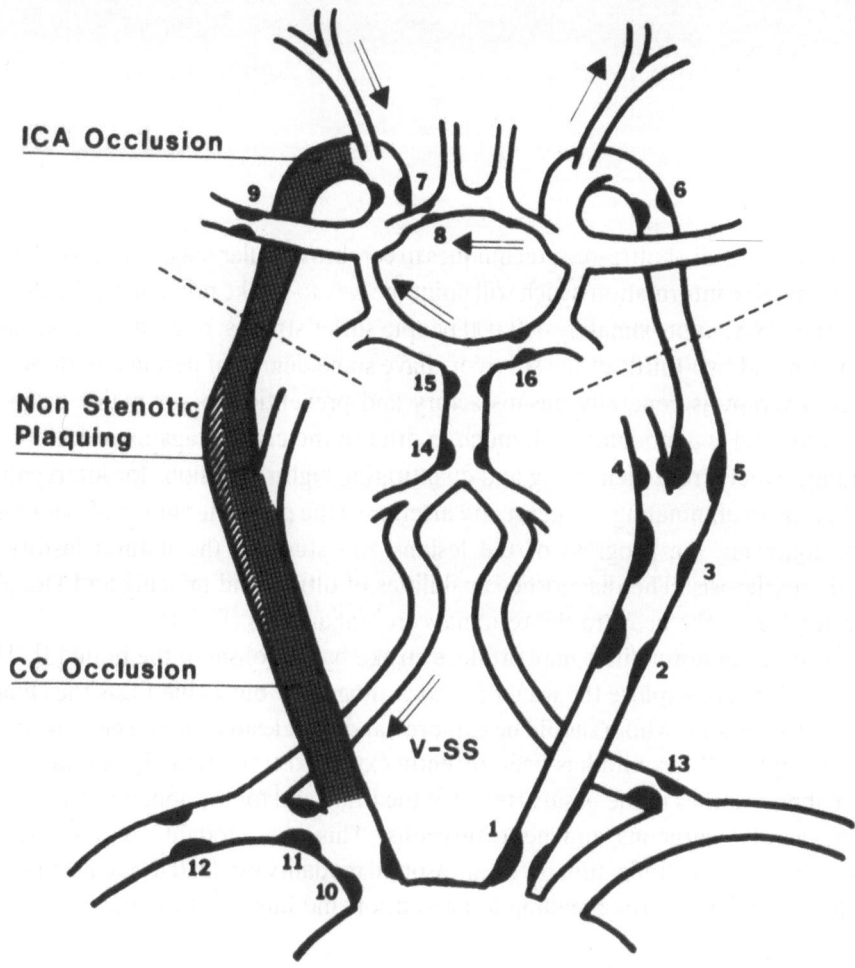

Figure 1. Diagnostic capabilities of Doppler and ultrasound imaging. On the left the limits of diagnosis for carotid disease severity range from nonstenotic plaquing (cross-hatching) to total occlusion of the common carotid and internal carotid arteries. The numbers represent diagnosable sites of stenosis and occlusion. 1, 2 & 3) represent stenosis at the origin, the middle and at the bifurcation of the common carotid; 4 & 5) represent stenosis at the origins of the external and internal carotid arteries; 6 & 7) stenoses of the parasellar and supraclinoid components of the carotid siphon; 8 & 9) stenosis of the anterior cerebral and middle cerebral arteries; 10, 11, 12) stenosis or occlusion of the innominate and subclavian arteries; 13) stenosis at the origin of the vertebral arteries; 14, 15, 16) stenosis at two levels of the basilar artery and posterior cerebral arteries. Collateral effects diagnosable are illustrated by means of the double shafted arrows. V-SS represents vertebral to subclavian steal.

ABI – Atherothrombotic brain infarction causing a localized neurological deficit with the absence of a known source of embolism or intracranial hemorrhage, hypercoagulabile states, or other diseases causes,

EM – Cerebral embolus with a clinical picture as for ABI but with a known cardiac source of embolism,

ICH – Intracerebral hemorrhage,

SAH – Subarchnoid hemorrhage, and

TIA – Transient ischemic attack.

Stroke from ABI is mostly a disease of the elderly increasing in risk rapidly after the age of 50 [4] (Fig. 2). In 1981, it was estimated in the U.S. alone that 164,000 died of stroke and there were 1.87 million disabled survivors. Besides the personal impact to the victim, family and community, the total cost of stroke in the U.S. in 1976, was estimated to be over seven billion dollars [5]. Though the numbers are diminishing somewhat, [6] stroke remains the third leading cause of death in the United States [7].

Fifty four percent of stroke (exclusive of TIAs) is produced by diseases of the major arteries [8, 9]. Carotid artery disease is responsible for almost half of infarctions due to atherosclerosis [8]. According to Fields [10] 40–50 percent of all strokes are secondary to atherosclerotic disease of the cervical carotid arteries. Gurdjian found 30 percent of strokes are associated with occlusion or stenosis of the cervical internal carotid artery. Theories for predisposition to atherosclerosis for this site are discussed in Chapter 5. Table II lists the pathological stages of plaque development and highlights those which are diagnosable by cerebrovascular ultrasound.

There is widespread agreement that TIAs are harbingers of major stroke [11, 12, 13, 14]. This has led to surgical removal of plaques found at the carotid

Table 1. Sources of embolism from the heart.

I. Explore TIA or stroke patients whom have
   – Hypertension
   – Previous myocardial infarction
   – Audible murmur
   – Arrythmia
   – Cardiomyopathy – congestive
II. Look for
   – Mural thrombi in left ventricle
   – Left ventricular aneurysm
   – Bacterial endocarditis
   – Atrial fibrillation – (Echo is not good in finding atrial thrombi)
   – Mitral stenosis – 10–25 percent of patients have left atrial thrombus
   – Mitral valve prolapse
   – Atrial myxoma
   – Aortic or mitral valve prostheses

4

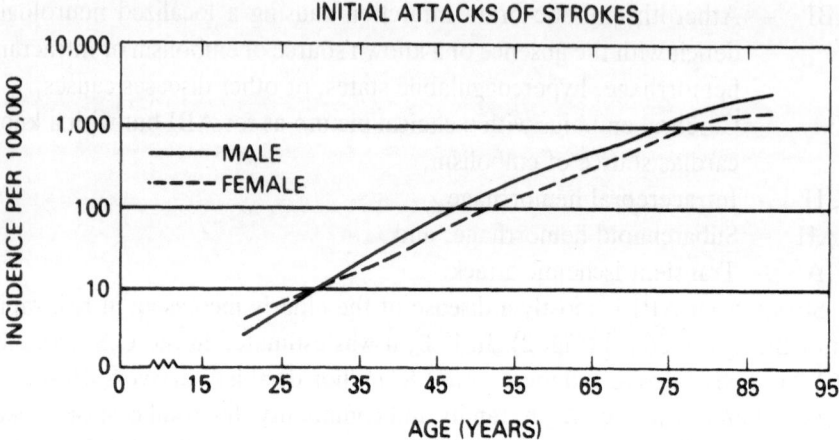

Figure 2. U.S. statistics on initial attacks of strokes. Stroke incidence increases with age with males leading females in age matched studies. From Robins and Baum [4].

bifurcation in the neck with the assumption that embolic mechanisms of stroke from this site are the cause of stroke and their removal will prevent stroke. Thus considerable effort is placed on determining if there is an atherosclerotic plaque in this surgically accessible site. This book explores all the current ultrasound techniques for diagnosis and qualitation of carotid plaques.

The ultrasonic opportunity

The growth of noninvasive techniques for diagnosis of disease of the extracranial arterial circulation has been questioned [15] on the basis that the physicians are

Table 2. Atherosclerotic plaque.

Morphology	Ultrasound detectability
Endothelial Damage	No
Platelet Deposits	No
Fibromuscular Growth	No
Endothelial Repair	No
Fatty Streaks	Yes – B-mode
Plaque Growth	Yes – Doppler
Necrosis	No
Calcium Deposits	Yes – B-mode
Intraplaque Hemorrhage	Yes – B-mode sometimes
Plaque Rupture	No
Crater Formation	Yes – B-mode if large
Thrombus	Yes – B-mode, occasionally
Occlusion	Yes – Doppler and B-mode

making management decisions on test results without knowing the answers to such important questions as whether or not surgery for extracranial vascular disease actually prevents stroke and because the clinical use of noninvasive studies depends on the bias of the physician; leading for example, to the recent expansion for surgery on the asymptomatic carotid stenosis. New information, of course, is not the cause of poor clinical decisions, rather our lack of understanding of the mechanisms of stroke is at fault. Because these decisions are sometimes difficult, the managing physician needs all available noninvasive diagnostic information in the campaign for preventing stroke and alleviating symptoms of cerebrovascular insufficiency. Meanwhile Doppler and ultrasonic imaging are making a contribution in understanding the natural history of atherosclerotic lesions and their relationship to stroke [16].

Two principal types of ultrasonic equipment presently marketed for extracranial vascular scanning are (1) Doppler with frequency spectral analysis and (2) two-dimensional, real time B-scan imaging. The diagnostician must make a decision about which equipment will be used and learn the skills of examination. To this end this book is considerably dedicated. The editor ventures his conclusions in the final chapter.

The interpretation of results must be made in the light of the patient's symptoms and the treatment options available to the referring physician. For the purposes of clinical management decisions and guidance of the ultrasound examinations, patients may be categorized according to the following clinical situations:

R Repeat follow-up patient examination for progress of a lesion or for postsurgical monitoring.
A The asymptomatic cervical bruit or head noises heard by the patient.
D Dizziness, syncope, headache or other nonlateralizing symptoms of possible cerebrovascular insufficiency.
V Symptoms suggestive of vertebral-basilar arterial insufficiency.
T Transient or minor focal lateralizing symptoms including minor transient speech defects not clearly a TIA.
F Focal and lateralizing symptoms meeting the clinical criteria of TIA or RIND.
S Stroke-lateralizing neurological symptoms which leave permanent disability.

The ultrasound examination and interpretation should keep in mind the following current concepts:

1. The highest priority for carotid endarterectomy is placed on patients with TIAs or RINDs who have very tight stenosis.
2. TIA patients with moderate degrees of plaquing and stenosis are often treated with antiplatelet medication in lieu of surgical intervention.
3. Carotid endarterectomy is often performed on patients with asymptomatic carotid artery stenosis if the carotid stenosis is severe.
4. Patients with minor completed strokes may be operated after 6 weeks if cervical carotid stenosis is found on the appropriate artery.

5. Endarterectomy is not performed on totally occluded carotid arteries.
6. Subclavian and vertebral abnormalities are usually not surgically recon-
    structed unless considerable evidence of symptomatic significance is estab-
    lished. Faced with a patient with symptoms of posterior circulation insuffi-
    ciency, preferential surgical attention is given to any carotid stenosis found.

In bilateral carotid artery stenosis, ultrasound can be of help in determining
which side is given operative priority. Generally, surgeons in Seattle will operate
the 'symptomatic side' first, but, if symptoms are minimal and the side opposite
demonstrates a greater degree of stenosis, it may be relieved first in order to
protect the symptomatic side when later operated. The use of Doppler to identify
intracranial collaterals may be of help in establishing this rationale. Further
discussion of clinical opinions is found in Chapter 20. To open up all the possibilities of ultrasound, one should understand many physical and physiologic
principles as well as examination techniques and interpretive skills.

References

1. Kerson LA, Olmos-Lau N: Review of ischemic cerebrovascular disease: Pathophysiology, clini-
    cal symptomatology, and their implications for therapy. Card. Rev. and Reports. Vol. 5: 3 pp.
    227–239, March 1984.
2. Kotler MN, Mintz GS, Segal BL: Two-dimensional echocardiography for stroke patients. Geri-
    atrics 38: 57, 1983.
3. Walker EA, Robins M and Weinfeld FD: Clinical Findings. The National Survey of Stroke
    (American Heart Assoc. Monograph # 75, Ch. 3, p I–13.
4. Robins M, Baum HM: The National Survey of Stroke Incidence. Stroke 12 (suppl 1): I-45, 1981.
5. Adleman MS: The National Survey of Stroke. Econ. Impact STROKE 12: I–69, 1981.
6. Saltero I, Kiang L, Cooper R, Stamler J, Garside G. Trends in mortality from cerebrovascular
    diseases in the United States, Stroke 9: 549, 1978.
7. Dyken et al.: Risk Factors in stroke. Special Report. Stroke 15, 1105, 1984.
8. Gillum RF, Fabsitz RR, Feinleib M, Wolf PA, Margolis JR and Brasch RC: Community
    surveillance for cerebrovascular disease: The Framingham Cardiovascular Disease Survey, Pub-
    lic Health Reports 93: 438, 1978.
9. Gurdjian ES: Critique of Occlusive Disease of the Carotid Artery and Stroke Syndrome.
    Neurology 11: 724, JAMA, 1961.
10. Fields WS, et al.: Joint study of extracranial arterial occlusion as a cause of stroke. I. Organization
    of study and survey of patient population. JAMA 203: 153, 1963.
11. Whisnant JP, et al.: Transient cerebral ischemic attacks in a community. Mayo Clin Proc 48: 194–
    198, 1973.
12. Ziegler DK, Hassanein RS: Prognosis in patients with transient ischemic attacks. STROKE 4:
    666–673, 1973.
13. Ostfeld AM, Shekelle RB, Klawans HL: Transient ischemic attacks and risk of stroke in an
    elderly poor population. STROKE, Vol. 4, November-December, 1973.
14. Toole JF, Yuson CP, Janeway R, Johnston F, Davis C, Cordell AR, Howard G. Transient
    ischemic attacks: A prospective study of 225 patients, Neurology 28: 746, 1978.
15. Sandok BA. Noninvasive techniques for diagnosis of carotid artery disease. (Editorial)
    STROKE, 9: 427, 1978.

Ultrasound physical concepts

M.P. Spencer, R.E. Hileman and J.M. Reid

Introduction

Ultrasound is a mechanical vibration which is bascially no different than audible sound waves. The limits of human hearing ability are between 20 and 20,000 Hertz (cycles per second) but the upper limit decreases with age. Middle-C on the piano is a note caused by vibrations of the piano string 262 times per second (262 Hz). This frequency of vibration is usually called the fundamental carrier *frequency* on which some higher frequencies (harmonics) may be superimposed. Each octave, on the piano, represents a doubling of the fundamental frequency as we go up the scale and higher frequencies have a higher pitch. Sound waves having frequencies higher than the human hearing are called ultrasound. Frequencies which are 100 times higher than those of the human hearing range 2–10 million Hertz or megahertz (MHz) are the most commonly used frequencies in medical diagnosis. The concepts summarized in this chapter are discussed in more detail in many available textbooks [1–11].

Basic properties of sound waves

Ultrasonic waves have a short wavelength and travel with properties which we usually associate with light rays rather than with sound. That is, ultrasonic waves can be formed into narrow beams instead of spreading out in all directions. The wavelength is a particular dimension of the wave which helps to define many of its properties. Fig. 1 shows a vibrating surface at the left in contact with a compressible material represented by the rows of dots. These dots can be thought of as molecules in the tissues of the body. As the source vibrates, it moves back and forth from left to right, pushing against and pulling apart the molecules. Each push moves the compressed region to the right. This series of compressions is a *wave* and the distance between the compressed regions is the *wavelength*. Fig. 2 introduces a concept of an omnidirectional transmitter and multiple receivers or

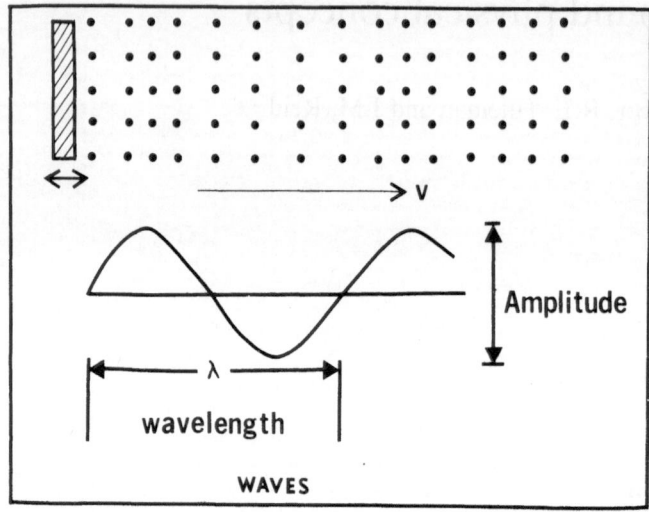

Figure 1. Definition of wavelength. The wavelength is the physical distance between corresponding points of a repetitive waveform. At the upper left a transducer face is shown alternately compressing and spreading out the molecules of the transmitting medium. The wave is propagated from left to right with velocity v.

detectors. If an ultrasonic transmitter is radiating waves throughout the space around it and is stationary with respect to receiving detectors, the frequency detected at receiving points is exactly the same as that of the transmitter. The waves are moving at a relatively constant velocity in all directions. The wavelength leaving the transmitter is equal to the wavelength at any one of the receivers. We therefore have the mathematical relationship shown in Fig. 2 between sound frequency, velocity, and the wavelength.

When ultrasound is formed into beams we find that the minimum width of the beam possible to attain is about one wavelength. Thus, a wavelength is an important parameter in setting the resolution of any diagnostic system using soundwaves. To form such beams it is necessary to use sources of sound which are large with respect to the wavelength. The probes, which are applied to the skin, are therefore usually one centimeter or greater in diameter.

Interaction of sound waves and tissues

The primary characteristics that affect the propagation of ultrasound within the body are the speed of sound in tissue, the magnitude of the ultrasonic attenuation coefficient, and the density of the tissue. For most ultrasonic imaging and measurement systems the speed of sound within body tissues is assumed to be a constant. This is only approximately true, with variations of 5% from the mean value being common [12]. Of particular interest for calculations related to the

SOUND WAVES

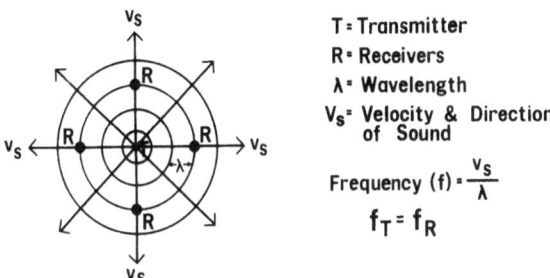

Figure 2. The relationship between a sound wave frequency, its velocity and wavelength. When the transmitter source and the receivers are stationary with respect to one another the frequency detected at the receiver is the same as that at the transmitter.

Doppler effect, is the speed of sound in blood at a normal body temperature of 37° C. The normal speed of sound in blood is reported to be from 1580 to 1585 m/sec with the speed of sound being slightly higher for males than females due to differences in percent hematocrit [13, 14]. These figures are for 44 percent hematocrit for men and 41 percent for women. For patients with a low hematocrit, the velocity of sound will be less by approximately 1 m/sec for each percent hematocrit.

The density of tissue within the body is also one of the prime determinants of ultrasonic propagation within the body. The acoustic impedance, z is defined by the equation

$$z = pC \qquad (1)$$

where p is the density and c is the speed of sound in tissue. Reflection of part of the ultrasonic wave occurs whenever the ultrasonic wave reaches a boundary where there is a change in acoustic impedance as defined above. Thus, either variations in the density of tissue or variations in the speed of sound within tissue, or both, can be responsible for the reflections which are the basis for ultrasonic B-Scan or sector-scan images.

As ultrasonic waves travel through the soft tissues of the body, they are absorbed, reflected or scattered. In most soft tissues, sound is absorbed to a degree which is proportional to the frequency. When travelling into the body by 1 cm and back again, the power in the sound wave is reduced by about one-half for every megahertz of frequency. For example, at a frequency of 5 MHz sound waves travelling 1 cm into and out of the tissue will be reduced in power to 1/32 of their original energy. Lower frequencies are, therefore, used for deeper penetration into the body (Fig. 3). Absorption figures in the body are about average for muscle; they are less for fat and considerably less for blood (about 1/10 of that for

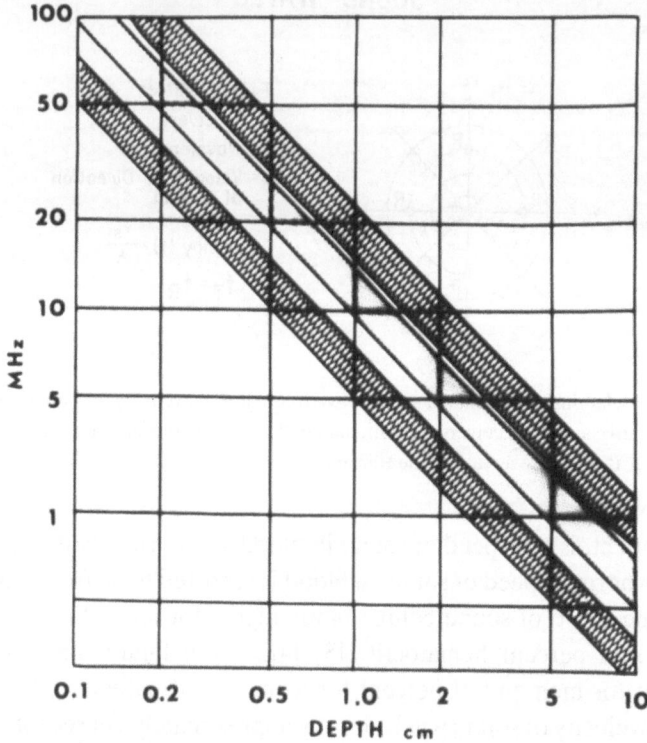

Figure 3. Chart of ultrasound frequency giving the maximum echo strength from small scatterers (red cells) theoretically determined for various depths of three intervening tissues.

muscle). Absorption is caused primarily by conversion of sound energy into heat.

Ultrasound waves can be bent or refracted when passing into tissues transmitting sound with greater or lesser velocity. The velocity in fat, for example, is approximately 10% lower than that of other tissues. The bending effect can be calculated from Snell's Law of Optics.

Scattering is a major process by which ultrasound radiation is deflected. The scattering of ultrasound is a much more pronounced and useful effect. The reflections which are sent back towards the examining ultrasonic probe from tissues in the body are used by a variety of medical ultrasonic diagnostic instruments.

The ultrasound transducer

The 'heart' of a transducer or the sensor which is placed against the body is a material which will change its dimensions when an electric field is applied to it or which will generate an electrical field when it is deformed by a vibration as

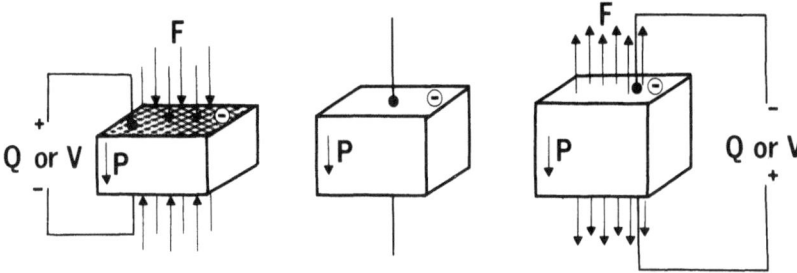

Figure 4. Diagram of the piezo electric effect. In the center is illustrated a biased ceramic material with electrodes on opposing faces. On the left application of a voltage results in a change in thickness. On the right application of a reversing voltage polarity produces an opposite change in thickness. Application of pressure on the material produces an electrical charge on the surfaces.

sketched in Fig. 4. This element called the crystal, is usually a single or poly-crystalline material in which the crystal structure is aligned suitably with the field produced by the electrodes and with the surfaces of the material. Practically all medical transducers use a poly-crystalline ceramic which has the property of being electrostrictive; that is, it will change its shape in response to an electrical field. These ceramics are a poly-crystalline, lead zirconate titanate. The components of the transducer (Fig. 5), including the ceramic, are placed in a protective case with suitable lead wires connecting it and the crystals to the electronic apparatus. Generally, a backing material is used for isolation to provide greater

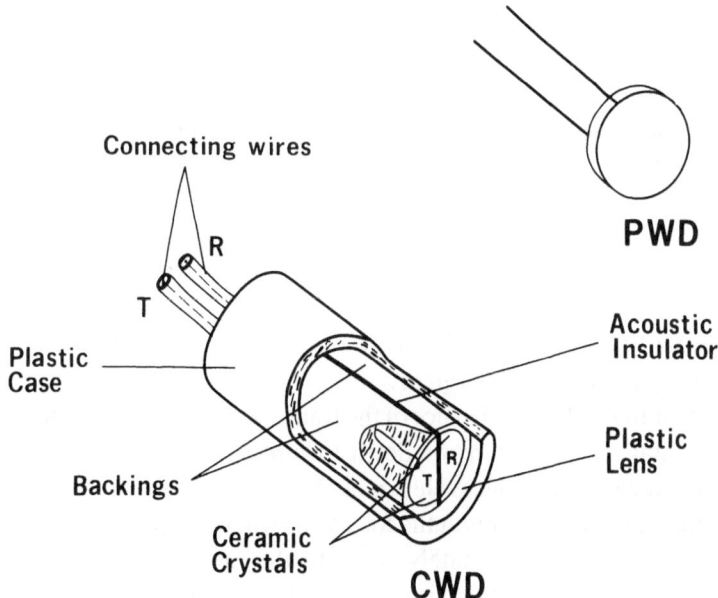

Figure 5. Cut-away view of ultrasound transducer. Two elements are shown for CWD operation but both may be used for pulsed echo operation. PWD crystal may be substituted for a more efficient pulsed Doppler operation.

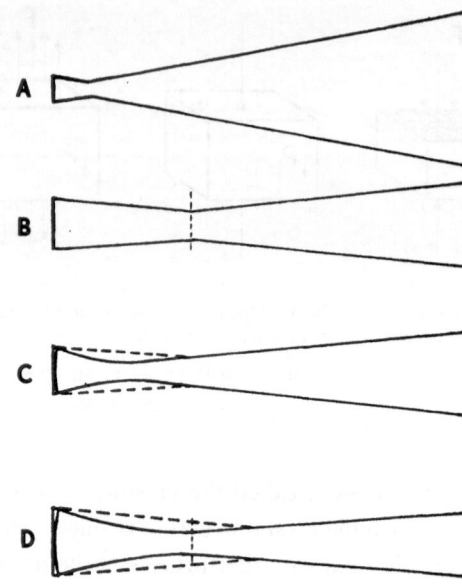

Figure 6. Outline of approximate field shape for focussed and unfocussed transducers. A-small unfocussed transducer, B-larger unfocussed transducer, C-transducer with focussing. The sound field can be narrowed only in the near field region. D-large transducer with focussing producing a smaller field at a greater range.

strength and to widen the bandwidth of the transducer. Various means of focuss-ing may be built into the continuous wave transducer.

The most sensitive frequency for operation of a ultrasound transducer is the fundamental resonant frequency inherent in the ceramic crystal element. The frequency at which the electronics operate the transducer is usually adjusted to coincide with the resonant frequency of the transducer.

Focussing

The natural focussing of an ultrasonic transducer may be illustrated in Fig. 6. Three major points are illustrated:

1) The near field, close to the face of the transducer is approximately the shape of the crystal itselt but narrows down towards a focal zone. The far field, at greater ranges, diverges as shown in Fig. 6.

2) The minimum field occurs at the focal zone where the near field changes to the far field and is approximately equal to the radius of the transducer. This narrowest focal point of the beam is found by dividing the square of the radius by the wavelength (Fig. 7).

3) In the near field, the width of the beam is directly proportional to the size of the transducer, while in the far field the width is inversely proportional to the

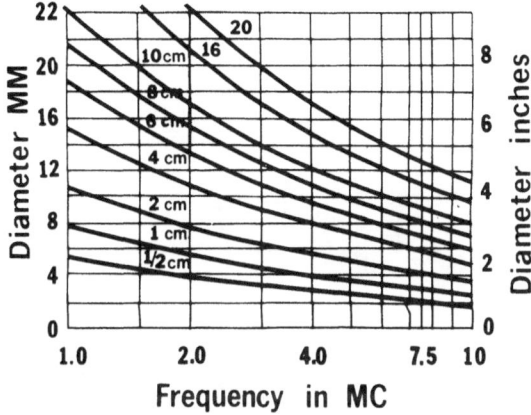

Figure 7. Chart of near-field extent as a function of transducer diameter and ultrasound frequency. Curves are numbered according to the near-field length.

size of the diameter of the transducer. The longer diameter focuses more sharply than the narrow diameter. In addition, the focal zone represents a region of sensitivity where the transmitter beam and the projected receiving 'beam' are usually made to overlap.

Figs. 5 and 6 also illustrate how additional focus to the sound beam can be provided by means of the lens placed over the transducer or using a spherical-shaped crystal element. The lens, as provided, is generally a concave shape because the velocity of sound in the lens material is higher than that of the coupling jel and body tissues. It is interesting to note that with light using glass lenses in air, a convex lens is necessary for focussing because the speed of light in the optical lenses is lower than the velocity in air.

The photographs of the actual focussed acoustic fields shown in Fig. 8 were taken with a Schlieren optical system, which makes the sound waves visible. For very strong focussing, the field is concentrated with a short focal zone, while for deeply focused transducers the focal zone is longer.

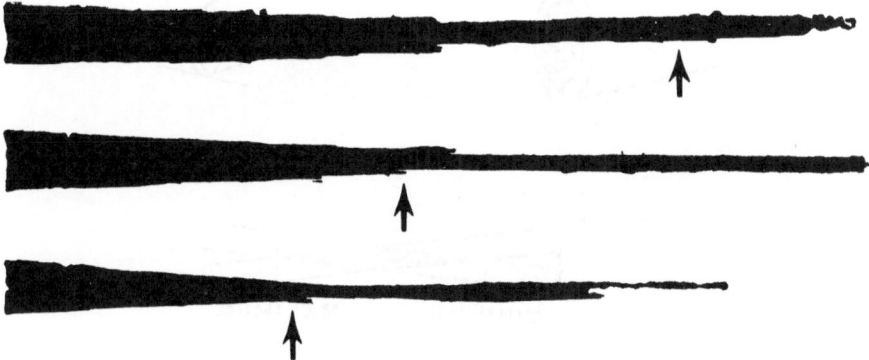

Figure 8. Schlieren photograph of an actual sound field shapes for three different lenses applied to the same diameter transducer. Arrows mark focal length.

14

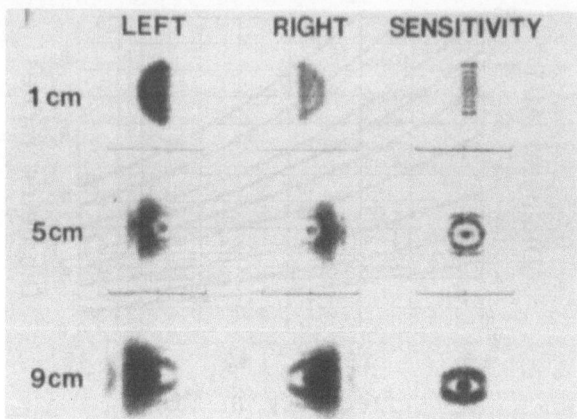

Figure 9. Ultrasonic beam field profiles of a continuous wave Doppler transducer. Individual fields of the left and right 'D' shaped crystals are shown individually at 1, 5, and 9 cm. The right-hand column represents the combined sensitivity produced by the overlap of transmit and receive fields. Courtesy of Dr. John Klepper, Institute of Applied Physiology and Medicine, Seattle, Washington.

CW Doppler transducers

The face of the transducer containing the elements of a continuous wave transducer is shown in Fig. 5. The continuous wave transducer is generally made by splitting a disc-shaped crystal resulting in a 'D' shaped cross-section of the sound field. The focal zone of a focussed continuous wave transducer is shown in Fig. 9. This oval shape results from the fact that there are basically two principal diameters of the 'D' shaped crystal. An additional method for focussing (available to continuous wave 'D' shaped transducers) is that of angling the two halves of the transducers in a fashion shown in Fig. 10.

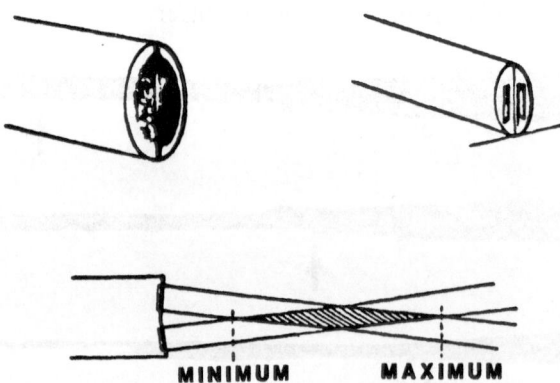

Figure 10. Method for focussing CW transducer by tilting the transmit and receive crystals to the desired focal zone.

Ultrasonic Pulse Train

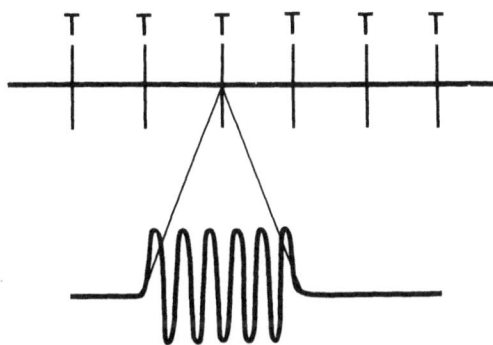

Figure 11. Diagram of an ultrasonic pulse train from typical transmitter. Below is an expansion of an individual pulse showing the sinusoidal ultrasonic waveform content.

Pulsed echo ultrasound and 2-D imagers

Rather than continuously energizing the transducer, a series of pulses may be applied by repeatedly switching the electrical energy to the transducer off and on in a pulse train. Generally, the duration of the pulse is considerably shorter than the interval between pulses (Fig. 11). The pulse repetition rate (PRF) represents the rate at which the pulses are applied, generally, around 1–2 kHz. The internal content of the pulse is an ultrasonic frequency itself of only a few oscillations. During the interval between pulses, when the transmitter is turned off, the crystal serves as a receiver and the receiving amplifiers are 'listening'. If the pulse is travelling through the tissues at a rate of approximately 1500 m/sec, an echo from considerable depth may be received before the next pulse is sent. By listening at any interval at a specific interval of time after each pulse, the reflections from a specific section of tissue can be examined. There is a limit to the depth in the tissues from which echoes can be detected before another pulse is transmitted. For deeper structures longer intervals between pulses must be used. This principle of echo ranging was developed for sonar and radar using sound and radio waves.

In echocardiography the echo display is termed the 'A' mode display, (Fig. 12). The time interval on the display is proportional to the distance between the transducer and each successive reflecting structure producing amplitudes. Because sound waves travel at such a high speed in soft tissues (approximately 1 mile/sec), they return in a rather short time. The time which elapses between transmission of a pulse and reception of an echo, from a structure 1 cm away, is 13.3 millionths of a second (microseconds). This short time interval also means that the transmitting pulse cannot last very long or it would occupy several

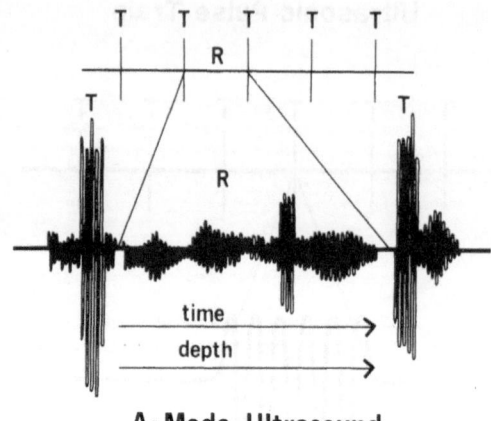

A - Mode Ultrasound

Figure 12. Upper section: transmitted pulse train. Lower section: amplified received signal of ultrasonic echoes between repeated pulses. The amplitude of the received signal is modulated according to the reflectivity of tissue interfaces. Time between pulses is calibrated in depth of tissue.

centimeters in space. Pulse lengths of the order of microseconds occupy distances in space in the order of millimeters.

Since one 'A' mode display is repeated for each pulse there are e.g. 2000 displays per second. This enormous data rate can be used to produce a two-dimensional image by use of 2-D transducers. Various means of sweeping the sound beam back and forth are used to spread the beam over a 2-D space. The amplitudes of the A-mode are used on a graded gray scale to produce an image of structures both static and moving (Fig. 13). Two-dimensional echocardiography is an example of this use. The resolution of the image is dependent on the shortness of the pulse but is generally higher along the line of the sound beam (range resolution) because focussing in depth is better by means of short pulses than is allowed by the attainable width of the sound beam.

There are two ways of displaying the high pulse repetion rate of ultrasonic A-mode pulse echoes. The 'T-M' or time motion mode (T-M) or (M-mode) moves the A-mode line at right angles to itself on an oscilloscope or strip of paper moving at a constant speed. The amplitude of the echo along the line modulates the intensity of the oscilloscope beam producing a grey scale display. This display is useful for quantitating changes in diameter or velocity of motion of a vascular structure.

Two-dimensional images may be made by sweeping the A-mode beam through a plane in the tissues and across an oscilloscope screen at the same time so that each position on the screen corresponds to a specific position in the tissues. The amplitude of reflection at each position in the tissue modulates the intensity of the oscilloscope beam to generate a grey scale in the 2-D image. Highly echogenic tissues such as a deposit of calcium in an artery wall produces a bright spot at its corresponding depth and position on the screen and may even produce a shadow.

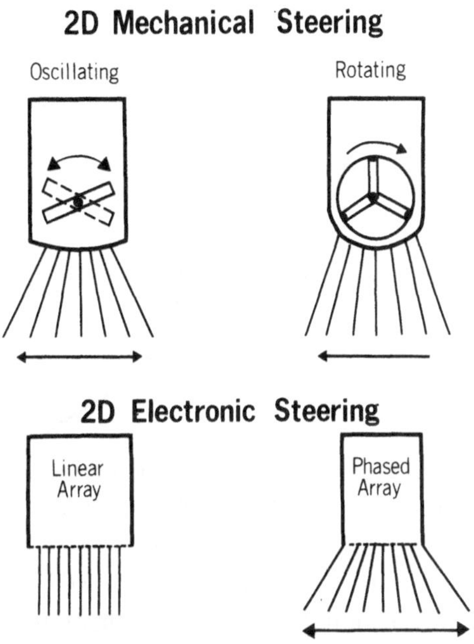

2D Mechanical Steering

Oscillating

Rotating

2D Electronic Steering

Linear
Array

Phased
Array

Figure 13. Diagram of four types of transducers for producing real time two-dimensional images. Upper left represents an oscillating ultrasonic mirror or transducer.

Blood is relatively echo free and therefore normal vessels appear as clear spaces between echogenic artery walls. Obviously blood is not completely echo free because the Doppler effect from moving red cells depends on some echogenicity. 2-D echo can, in fact, image blood if it is moving slowly so that the frame rate (rate at which a complete sweep through the tissue occurs) can 'catch' it. Present day ultrasound echo machines have frame rates generally 20–30 per second. Examples where blood motion can be seen are in the veins and in stagnant recirculating areas in the arteries such as in a large crater in an atherosclerotic plaque.

Transducers for 2-D ultrasound may be classified as mechanical or array. Mechanical transducers use a single crystal which is moved back and forth or along a line to produce a sector image (generally trapazoidal) or a square image (Fig. 14). An array of separate crystals may be placed in a straight or curved line and each crystal pulsed in sequence to produce an image of a square or trapazoi-. dal section of tissue (Fig. 15).

The ultrasonic frequency with which the transducer crystals are pulsed is important in determining the depth to which the tissues may be visualized as well as the resolution or detail which the image displays. 'Resolution' is a term defining the ability to separate in space, two closely spaced interfaces as illustrated in Chapter 17 on 'Real Time B-Mode Imaging of the Carotid Bifurcation'. Resolution is dependent upon the wavelength as well as signal-to-noise ratios. For depths of the carotid arteries in the neck up to 3–4 cm the ultrasound

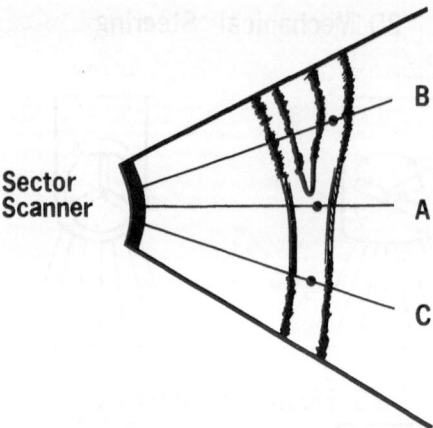

Figure 14. Diagram of sector scan angles showing how at 'A' the image is best but the Doppler angle is poor; at 'B' and 'C' the Doppler angles are improved but the image quality deteriorates.

frequency used in the transducer is between 5 and 10 MHz. The higher frequencies with their shorter wavelengths provide the best theoretical resolution but lose signal at depths especially beyond 3 cm. The lower frequencies provide less image resolution but penetrate deeper to represent more even representation of echogenicity. 5 MHz transducers such as manufactured by Carolina Medical Electronics and Advanced Technology Laboratories provide additional imaging of the subclavian and vertebral arteries because of the greater depth capability.

The relative imaging advantages of the 2-D sector scanner and the 2-D linear scanner are of importance. Fig. 14 illustrates how with the sector scanner the resolution falls off at the edges because the angle of incidence with the vessel wall becomes less advantageous for maximum range resolution. In contrast, the linear array permits more uniform quality between the center and the edge of the image (Fig. 15).

Recently equipment has been developed to provide a simultaneous B-mode grey scale image by a 2-D color Doppler image. The Doppler image is provided by

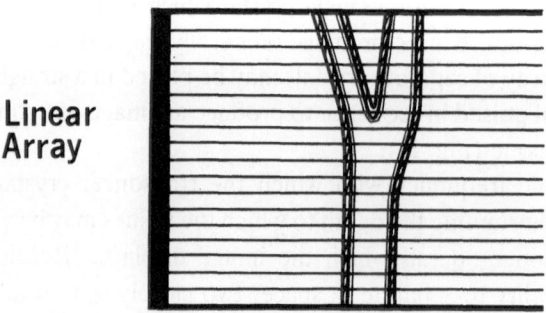

Figure 15. Diagram of a linear array of carotid arteries illustrating how image quality is uniform across the image plane.

means of circuitry called 'moving target indicator' which, subtracts echoes from tissues not in motion from each A-mode line leaving only a spatial representation of velocity along the normal Doppler A-mode line. This color-coded 2-D image of velocity is added back on top of the normal B-mode image. This technology is further discussed in Chapters 14 and 15.

The Doppler effect

Christian Doppler studied the frequency of light waves. His equation applies equally well to sound waves. The frequency appears to shift when a source of light or sound moves relative to a receiver. Doppler's equation relates the shift in frequency with the velocity. His equation is well-known to physicists to detect the movement of the stars 'the red shift'. With ultrasound it is used to detect the velocity of blood flow. The frequency of the ultrasound appears to shift when the ultrasound reflects off of moving blood cells. The blood cells move at different velocities, the display shows different frequency shifts.

Scattering is much stronger from other tissues than from erythrocytes or groups of erythrocytes in the blood because their diameter is small compared to the wavelength of the ultrasound. The wavelength of a 5 MHz ultrasound is 308 micra while the diameter of a red cell is between 7–8 micra. The scattered ultrasound is re-radiated in all directions. The scattering red cells vibrate at the same frequency as the incident wave. They may, therefore, be considered a multitude of small transmitters which are moving with the blood velocity. Since the velocity of sound in blood is constant (1560 m/s), the moving wavelength in front of the transmitter as the ultrasound is radiated, is shortened and behind the direction of movement, the wavelength is lengthened. A remote receiver will detect a frequency different from the frequency of the transmitter which difference is called the *Doppler effect*, (Fig. 16). The ratio between the velocity of the transmitter and the velocity of sound is equal to the ratio of the difference frequency and ultrasonic frequency of the transmitter. The Doppler effect is a common everyday observation, when the sound of a moving vehicle such as an automobile or train appears to emit frequencies greater when coming towards the observer than when moving away from the observer. The angle between the line of motion and the observer has an effect on the Doppler shift (Fig. 17). The difference in frequency (f) varies in direct proportion to the cosine of the angle between the direction of the moving particle and the direction of the receiver.

Two types of Doppler instruments are available. The continuous wave (CW) Doppler and the pulsed wave (PW) are distinguished by their continuous emission of ultrasound or in short pulses. These two types and their respective advantages are discussed in the chapter on Doppler instrumentation.

In a practical CW Doppler probe, the transmitter and receiver are incorporated side-by-side. This means that the angle between the transmitter beam and

THE DOPPLER EFFECT

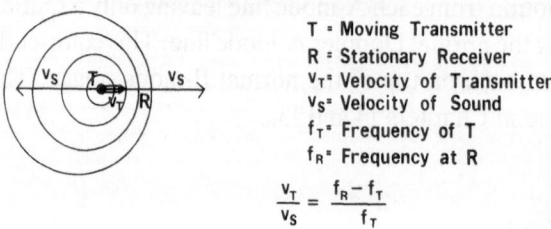

T = Moving Transmitter
R = Stationary Receiver
V_T = Velocity of Transmitter
V_S = Velocity of Sound
f_T = Frequency of T
f_R = Frequency at R

$$\frac{V_T}{V_S} = \frac{f_R - f_T}{f_T}$$

Figure 16. Principle of the Doppler effect produced when a transmitter (T) is moving toward a stationary received (R). When the Doppler shift (f_R-f_T) is measured and the frequency of the transmitter as well as the velocity of sound in the medium are known, the velocity of the transmitter can be calculated.

the receiver direction to and from moving blood cells is the same and, therefore, doubling the Doppler effect for any angle (Fig. 18). To make the calculations in the Doppler equation, the frequency units should be in the same units and the velocity units should be the same; i.e., Hz and m/sec.

Table 1 provides a convenient reference for several frequently used ultrasonic probe frequencies for various probe angles. It should be particularly noted that the frequencies evoked by the Doppler shift are directly proportional to the ultrasonic frequency; for example, a pitch provided by a 10 MHz flow meter is twice that produced by a 5 MHz flowmeter. The fortunate result of using ultrasound for blood velocity detection is that the Doppler shift frequency falls within the range of human hearing. Simply listening to the Doppler frequencies and using the discriminating abilities of the human ear and brain is a useful technique when interpreting many dynamic features of the blood flow in the arteries, veins, and heart. If the velocity is very high, as is often found in jets through constricting stenoses or valve regurgitations, the resulting pitch of the Doppler shift may be too high for some persons to hear. Zero crossing meters (discussed in the chapter

THE REMOTE TRANSMITTER
Doppler Effect vs Scattering Direction

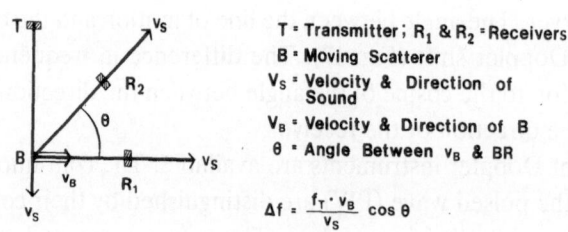

T = Transmitter; R_1 & R_2 = Receivers
B = Moving Scatterer
V_S = Velocity & Direction of Sound
V_B = Velocity & Direction of B
θ = Angle Between v_B & BR

$$\Delta f = \frac{f_T \cdot v_B}{v_S} \cos θ$$

Figure 17. A remote transmitter is used to produce scattering from a moving particle. The resultant Doppler frequency is dependent upon the angle between the direction of the moving particle and the direction between the particle and the receiver.

THE DOPPLER TRANSDUCER

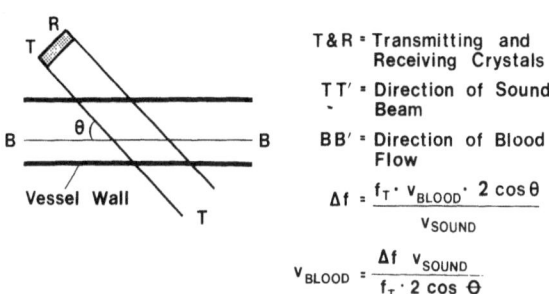

T & R = Transmitting and Receiving Crystals

T T' = Direction of Sound Beam

B B' = Direction of Blood Flow

$$\Delta f = \frac{f_T \cdot v_{BLOOD} \cdot 2 \cos \theta}{v_{SOUND}}$$

$$v_{BLOOD} = \frac{\Delta f \cdot v_{SOUND}}{f_T \cdot 2 \cos \theta}$$

Figure 18. The Doppler equation when both transmitter and receiver are at the same position in space remote from the moving scatterers. The effect of the angle between the direction of the scatterer and the direction of the sound is doubled i.e. 2 cos O.

on Doppler Instrumentation) or spectral analyses may be used to process the signal. Spectral analyzers which provide a visual display of the frequencies and amplitudes continuously with time, are therefore convenient for observation while listening to document the results of the examination and to teach the principles of Doppler ultrasound diagnosis.

Table 1.

Ultrasound Probe Frequency (MHz)	Angle of Sound Beam (Deg)											
	0		**10**		**20**		**30**		**45**		**60**	
2	2.56	0.39	2.53	0.40	2.41	0.42	2.22	0.45	1.81	0.55	1.28	0.78
2.25	2.88	0.35	2.84	0.35	2.71	0.37	2.5	0.40	2.04	0.49	1.44	0.69
2.50	3.21	0.31	3.16	0.32	3.01	0.33	2.78	0.36	2.27	0.44	1.6	0.62
3	3.85	0.26	3.79	0.26	3.61	0.28	3.33	0.30	2.72	0.37	1.92	0.52
3.5	4.49	0.22	4.42	0.23	4.22	0.24	3.89	0.26	3.17	0.32	2.24	0.45
5	6.41	0.16	6.31	0.16	6.02	0.17	5.55	0.18	4.53	0.22	3.21	0.31
6	7.69	0.13	7.58	0.13	7.23	0.14	6.66	0.15	5.44	0.18	3.85	0.26
7.5	9.62	0.10	9.47	0.11	9.04	0.11	8.33	0.12	6.8	0.15	4.81	0.21
10	12.82	0.08	12.63	0.08	12.05	0.08	11.10	0.09	9.07	0.11	6.41	0.16
COS	1		0.98		0.94		0.87		.71		.5	

Upper-left / lower-right cell key: KHz / m/s and m/s / KHz

$$f_D = \frac{v \cdot f_u \cdot 2 \cos \emptyset}{c}$$

f_D = Doppler-shifted frequency (Hz)

v = Velocity of blood (m/s)

u = Ultrasonic frequency (Hz)

$\emptyset$ = angle between soundbeam and flow direction

c = velocity of sound in blood (1560 m/s)

Frequency spectral analysis

The advent of real time spectral displays greatly increased the utility and utilization of Doppler ultrasound. The real time spectral display has the following advantages:
- Rapidly learning how to use Doppler ultrasound.
- Resolves velocity gradients in the sample volume, providing detailed information about circulatory diseases.
- Quantified measurements of parameters that may indicate disease, its extent and severity.

When the instrument detects the reflections from many cells, the reflections add up to a spectrum, the same way the sound of each string in a piano add up to a chord. The spectrum sounds more like noise than like a chord or a single note on the piano, because each flow stream of blood cells produces a note proportional to its velocity. A piano can produce only 88 notes. Cells can move at more than 88 different velocities. Thousands of blood cell groups can produce thousands of frequencies. Red blood cells group together in stacks. These stacks probably reflect more than each individual cell reflects. Although stacks are not individual cells, the distinction is not critical to explain frequency spectral displays.

Figs. 19A and 19B illustrate the idea of representing the distribution of blood velocity flow streams by a corresponding distribution of frequencies on a display of a Doppler frequency spectrum. This type of translation of velocity to frequency is most often provided by a Fast-Fourier Transform spectral analyzer. This display is derived from the concept of the Fourier series. It has been shown, mathematically, that any complex frequency such as any sound heard by the ear, can be described by a set of fundamental sinusoidal waveforms each with a specified amplitude and frequency at some multiple of the fundamental or lowest frequency of the sound wave (Fig. 20). The FFT provides a very practical updating of the frequencies as they occur (generally every 10 m sec). Each 10 m sec sample interval is first adjusted so that the beginning and ending of samples do not produce artificial frequencies (Fig. 21). Each sample can then be treated as a separate Fourier series and displayed every 10 m sec to provide an apparently continuous frequency analysis. This whole process may be thought of as passing the original sound wave in the form of an electrical signal through a set of band-pass filters and displaying the frequency range each filter represents on a vertical scale, while the amplitude of each frequency is represented as the density or brightness of each line representing the individual frequency sampled. This continuously running display can then be spread out on a time base as shown in the figures.

PARABOLIC PROFILE & DOPPLER SPECTRUM

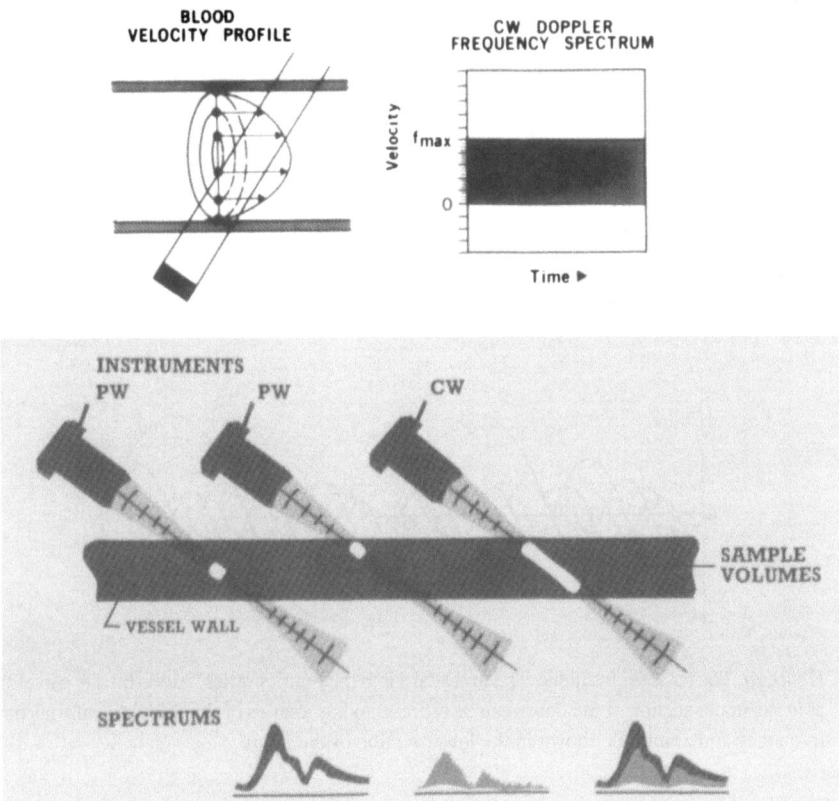

Figure 19A. Relationship between the blood velocity profile and the Doppler frequency spectrum produced by a continuous wave ultrasound beam covering the entire cross-section of a blood vessel. In the case of a parabolic laminar velocity profile of blood velocities, the resultant Doppler frequencies and energies are equally distributed across the frequency spectrum.

Figure 19B. Diagram of how the sample volume affects the frequency spectrum. A pulsed wave (PW) instrument with the sample centered in the vessel produces a narrow spectrum of high frequencies. A PW instrument with the sample near the wall of the vessel produces a broad spectrum that includes mostly low frequencies. A continuous wave (CW) instrument is sensitive across the entire vessel, producing a broad spectrum with both high and low frequencies.

Pulsed Doppler

Sample volume

The region where blood flow can be detected by a Doppler instrument is called the SAMPLE VOLUME. The width of the beam determines the lateral dimension of the sample volume. Whether the ultrasound is pulsed wave (PW) or

24

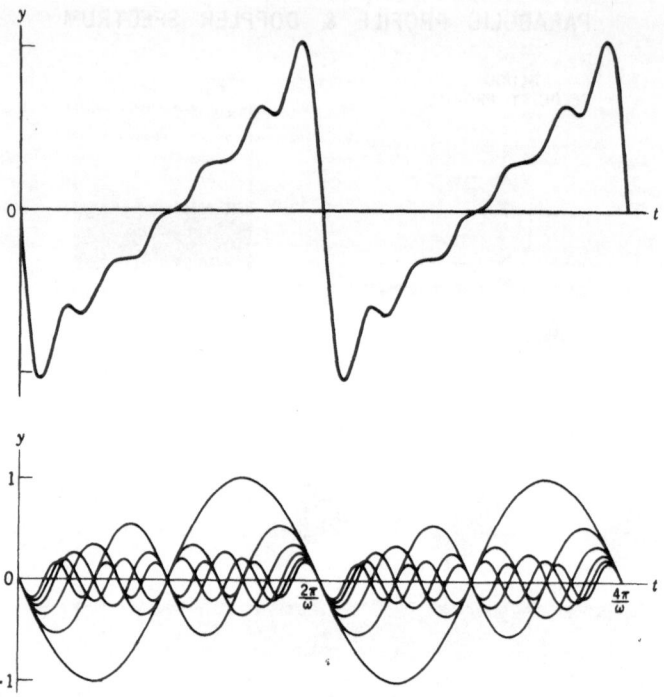

Figure 20. The basis for frequency spectral analysis in the Fourier series. Any arbitrary waveform such as in the upper section of the figure can be represented by a series of sinusoidal waveforms of varying frequency and amplitude shown in the lower section of the figure.

continuous wave (CW) determines the axial dimension (Fig. 19B). Pulsed wave (PW) ultrasound produces short sample volumes. Continuous wave (CW) ultrasound produces long sample volumes. The size of the sample volume will influence the spectrum. When a PW instrument samples the blood that flows in the center of the vessel, it detects cells moving at nearly the same velocity. The spectrum that results is very narrow. When a PW instrument samples tha blood that flows along the walls of the vessel, the spectrum that results has a lower peak frequency and is broad. The wall friction slows the blood cells, the blood cells move in a broad range of velocities, and the spectrum broadens. A CW instrument samples the blood in the center of the vessel and along the walls of the vessel. The sample volume is long. The spectrum that results shows both the well-defined peak and the broad part of the spectrum. It is sum of both of the PW spectrums from all ranges across the vessel. In addition to how the instrument influences the sample volume, disease can change the shape of the vessel wall and change patterns in blood flow. Stenosis causes localized increase in velocity and causes turbulence distal to the stenosis. Rough walls cause localized irregularities in velocity without increasing the peak velocity.

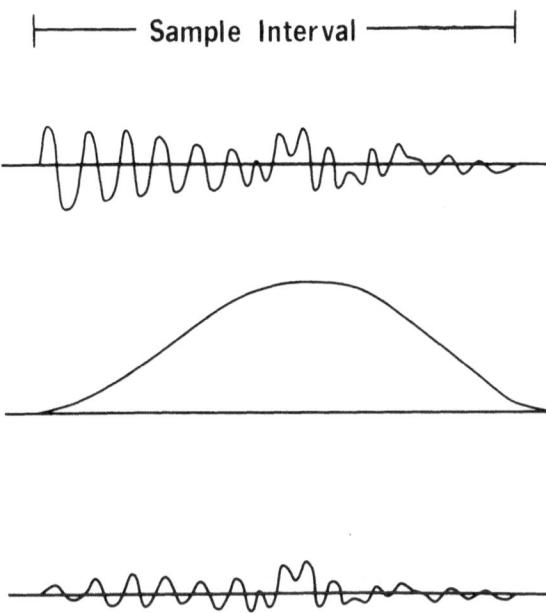

|——————— Sample Interval ———————|

Figure 21. Diagram of how Fourier analysis can be applied to a short pulse of sound wave shown in the upper section. The middle section illustrates the amplication function applied over the sample interval. The lower section illustrates how the amplication function eliminates the discontinuities at the beginning and ending of the sample interval.

Aliasing

While PWD is very good at focussing in depth it suffers difficulty in resolving blood velocities which are greater than one half the PRF. This phenomenon called aliasing, shows the frequencies in a false range. A familiar example of this is seen when making a movie of a turning wheel with spokes. The wheel appears to move slowly and backwards when the movie frame repetition rate is less than the 'spoke rate'. Fig. 22 illustrates the limitations of pulsed Doppler in following the maximum velocities which occur in stenosis of the carotid artery (Fig. 22). Aliasing occurs in any sampling process when the PRF is not high enough to follow the velocities of blood within the sample volumes. Thus, when the Doppler shift frequency exceeds one half the PRF the sampling process fails to represent the velocities in their proper frequency range, hence, the term aliasing.

Since the continuous-wave (CW) Doppler sound beam can pass through a broad region of blood velocities in the heart or a blood vessel without focussing in depth it provides a representation of many hemodynamic phenomena occurring along the beam sample volume. When the CW transducer is placed against the chest wall and directed at the heart, a rather confusing set of repetitive sounds are heard and displayed on the frequency spectrum display. Without filtering the spectrum is dominated by enormous low frequency energies from heart wall reflection which override the more subtle high frequencies present. These un-

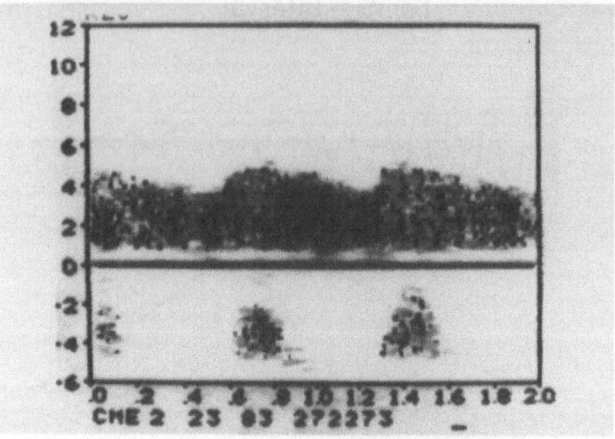

Figure 22. Effect of aliasing on the pulsed Doppler frequency spectrum in the presence of high velocities produced by carotid artery stenosis. Upward directed velocity spectrum is amputated at its peak which is displaced below the zero line.

wanted low frequency energies are conveniently removed by means of a high-pass filter which eliminates most of the frequency energies below 1 kHZ (Figs. 23A and 23B). These high energies are produced by reflections from the moving cardiac walls and valve structures while we are actually more interested in the more subtle frequencies representing the blood flow streams within the cardiac chambers. Another application of filter processing of the spectrum is that of using a high-pass filter or a 'high boost' to accentuate the high frequency, low amplitude components of the spectrum. The high pass and high boost filtering is very useful in stenosis of the arteries. As explained in the chapter on hemodynamics of arterial stenosis, these filter techniques bring out the maximum frequency (f_{max}) or pulse envelope frequency on the frequency spectral display.

Multigate pulsed Doppler

In concept, a multigate pulsed Doppler uses a regular pulse transmission train with a number of simultaneous listening gates. The received signals are range-gated at various time delays into a number of parallel channels for parallel processing. Applications of multigate pulsed Doppler in visualizing velocity profiles are discussed in Chapter 3 on Doppler Instrumentation.

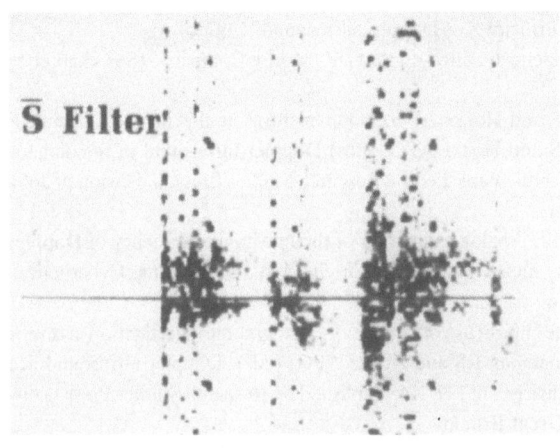

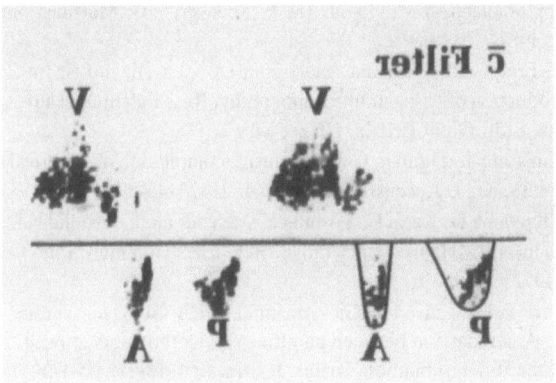

Figure 23A. Continuous wave Doppler generated frequencies from a probe held over the normal mitral valve.

Figure 23B. Application of a high-pass filter eliminates the high energy low frequencies present in '11A' and with further amplification the more meaningful velocity signals emerge. 'P' represents the passive inflow velocities upon opening of the mitral valve. '11A' represents the Doppler frequencies generated by atrial contraction. Both P & A represent velocities moving towards the transducer. 'V' equals the velocities moving away from the transducer in the ventricular outflow track.

References

1. Wells PNT: The possibility of harmful biological effects in ultrasonic diagnosis. In: Reneman RS, (ed), Cardiovascular applications of ultrasound. 1: 1–17, North-Holland Publishing Company, The Netherlands, 1974.
2. Reid JM. Sound and ultrasound. In: Spencer MP and Reid JM: (eds), Cerebrovascular evaluation with Doppler ultrasound. 2: 23–40, Martinus Nijhoff Publishers, The Netherlands. 1983.
3. Wells PNT. Biomedical ultrasonics. London/New York: Academic Press, 1977.
4. Reneman RS (ed): Cardiovascular applications of ultrasound. Amsterdam, London/New York: North Holland/American Elsevier Publishing, 1974.

5. Baum G. Fundamentals of medical ultrasonography. New York. G.P. Putnam & Sons. (See chapter 27, 'Principles of Doppler ultrasound'), 1975.

6. King DL. Diagnostic ultrasound. C.V. Mosby Company. (See chapter by Donald W. Baker). 1974.

7. Reneman RS and Hoeks APG. Doppler ultrasound-principle, advantages and limitations. In: Reneman RS and Hoeks APG, (eds),Doppler ultrasound in the diagnosis of cerebrovascular disease. 4: 77–101. Published by Research Studies Press, a division of John Wiley & Sons, Ltd., Great Britain.

8. Angelsen BAJ. Analog estimation of the maximum frequency of Doppler spectra in ultrasonic blood velocity measurements. Report 76-21-W. Div. of Eng. Cybernetics, N.T.H., Trondheim, Norway, 1976.

9. Mol JMF. The clinical use of Doppler hematographic investigation in cerebral circulation disturbances. In: Reneman RS and Hoeks APG; (eds), Doppler ultrasound in the diagnosis of cerebrovascular disease. 6: 129–156. Published by Research Studies Press, a division of John Wiley & Sons, Ltd., Great Britain.

10. Klepper JR. The physics of Doppler ultrasound and its measurement instrumentation. In: Cardiac Doppler diagnosis. 3: 19–31. (M.P. Spencer, ed). Martinus Nijhoff Publishers, The Netherlands. 1983.

11. Spencer MP. Frequency Spectrum Analysis in Doppler Diagnosis. In: Zwiebel WJ, (ed), 2nd Edition, Introduction of vascular ultrasonography. Research Studies Press Limited, a division of Wiley & Sons, Ltd., Great Britain. (In press).

12. Goss SA, Johnston RL, Dunn F. Comprehensive compilation of empirical ultrasonic parameters of mammalian tissue. J. Accoust. Soc. Am. 64: 2. 423–457.

13. Kikuchi Y, Okuyama D, Kasai C, Yoshida Y. Measurement of sound velocity and absorption of human blood in 1–10 MHz frequency range. Rec. Elec. Commun, Eng. Convers. Tohoku Univ. *41*: 152–159. 1972.

14. Bakke T, Gytre T, Haagensen A, Giezendanner L. Ultrasonic measurement of sound velocity in whole blood. A comparison between an ultrasonic method and convention packed-cell-volume test for hematocrit determination. Scand. J. Clin. Lab. Invest. *35* 473–478. 1975.

Doppler instrumentation

R.S. Reneman, A.P.G. Hoeks

The purpose of this chapter is to describe basic aspects of Doppler ultrasound instrumentation. Attention will be paid to such items as the Doppler principle, the transmission of ultrasound, with special emphasis on the differences between continuous wave and pulsed Doppler systems, and the methods used to process the Doppler signal. The information that can be obtained with the various systems will be discussed in some detail. This chapter may supply the user of this book with some basic information to facilitate the reading of the more clinically oriented chapters. For a more basic understanding of the Doppler effect, please refer to the Chapter on Ultrasound Physics.

Principle

In practical Doppler flowmeters a beam of ultrasonic waves (at the MHz level) is transmitted from a vibrating crystal diagonally through the vessel wall into the bloodstream. Some of the ultrasonic power is backscattered by the various structures in the body and received by another or the same crystal. The transducer crystals are mounted in a probe. Since ultrasound at the MHz level cannot be transmitted through air, acoustic gel is applied between the crystals and the skin to improve acoustic coupling (Fig. 1).

Ultrasound backscattered from particles in the flowing blood, mainly the red cells, is shifted in frequency by an amount proportional to the velocity of these particles. This frequency shift (the Doppler shift = f_d), which is retrieved by mixing the transmitted and received signals, is in the audio range and equals:

$$f_d = 2 f_e \, v \, \cos\alpha/c$$

in which f_e = emission frequency, v = velocity of the particles, α = the angle between the transmitted sound beam and the direction of the velocity of the particles; i.e. angle of interrogation (Fig. 1) and c = the velocity of sound in the medium (1560 m/sec in blood).

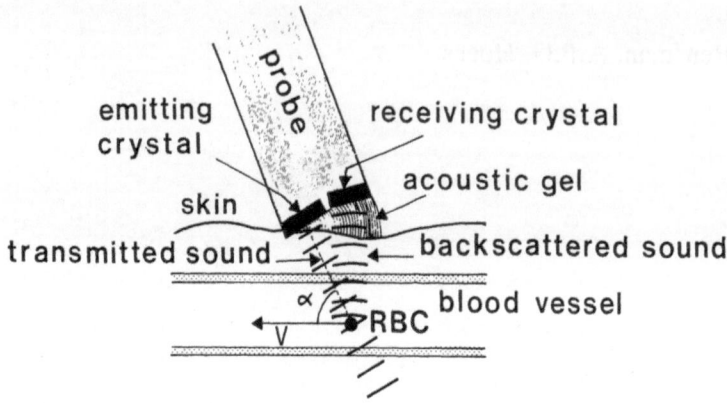

Figure 1. The principle of continuous wave Doppler flowmetry. The arrow indicates the flow velocity (v) direction. RBC = red blood cell and = the angle between the transmitted sound beam and the direction of flow, i.e. the angle of interrogation. From Reneman *et al.*, 1979; with permission of Angiology.

The Doppler signal does not contain one single frequency but a spectrum of frequencies (the Doppler spectrum). The frequency distribution depends on such factors as unequal distribution of the red blood cell velocity over the cross-sectional area of the vessel, variations in the blood cell interspace and divergence and non-uniformity of the sound beams, resulting in variations in the angle of interrogation when the red blood cells are passing the ultrasonic beam [1].

The amount of power received at the crystals is determined by the amount of backscattering from the red blood cell plasma interface and the quantity of sound absorption by the tissues. Both the amount of backscattering and the quantity of absorption increase at higher emission frequencies [2]. The higher the emission frequency the lower the penetration depth, but the better the ratio of power backscattered by particles in the blood and the power reflected by targets like vessel walls and tissue interphases. When the effects of reflection and absorption are combined, the backscattering from blood at a given distance from the transducer is strongest at a particular frequency [3]. For investigations on deeper vessels like the descending aorta and the iliac arteries, an emission frequency of 2–4 MHz has been found to be the most appropriate, while for the investigation of more superficial vessels, like the carotid arteries, the best results are obtained with frequencies in the range between 5 and 8 MHz. The higher the number of red blood cells moving in the ultrasonic beam, the higher the received Doppler power. The received signal contains power backscattered from the red blood cells as well as from the vessel wall. The signals induced by lateral wall motion are low in frequency, but high in amplitude. Their amplitude is approximately thirty times higher than that of the signals induced by moving red blood cells because the vessel wall-blood interface is a much better reflector than the red cell-blood interface.

Analogue signal processing

Originally in Doppler flowmeters the received signal was processed to an analog tracing, representing the average velocity as an instantaneous function of time. In this approach, however, valuable information, present in the Doppler signal, is ignored [4]. More recently audio spectrum analysis is used to analyze the received Doppler information. This processing technique, which yields detailed information about the Doppler signal will be discussed in detail in Chapter 5. In this section some aspects of analog signal processing, which might be of interest to clinicians, are delineated.

A simple method to retrieve the Doppler signal is mixing of the transmitted and received signals. This demodulation technique has the disadvantage that no information is obtained about the direction of blood flow (non-directional system). In directional systems a more complicated demodulation technique is used [5, 6]. In this technique the received signal is demodulated with two signals at the transmitter frequency shifted 90° in phase with respect to each other, resulting in two Doppler signals which are 90° out of phase. The sign of the phase shift between both signals indicates the sign of the frequency shift, i.e. the direction of blood flow. This demodulation technique gives a bidirectional velocity output, but interference between forward and backward flow cannot be prevented. Separation of positive and negative Doppler shifts, and hence between forward and backward flow, can be achieved with single side-band demodulation. Hence the presence of backward flow can be assessed when the net flow direction is antegrade and contaminating venous flow signals can be recognized when measuring arterial blood flow velocity. Adding of these flow signals, however, is only allowed when at least one of the outputs is zero. To diminish the influence of vessel wall motion signals and noise beyond the Doppler frequency band, the output of the demodulator is passed through a bandpass filter.

Determination of the mean frequency of the Doppler spectrum and conversion of the signal into an analog signal is usually performed with a zero-crossing meter. The output is an analog voltage proportional to the number of zero-crossings per unit of time. To diminish the counting of zero-crossings not related to blood flow velocity the comparator voltage of the Schmitt-trigger is set at such a level that the zero-crossing meter will not be activated by low level signals (e.g. noise). The analog tracing obtained with this technique approximates the average velocity as an instantaneous function of time (Fig. 2). A zero flow reference can easily be obtained by disconnecting the input to the signal processing system.

Difficulties encountered in this signal processing technique were examined [7, 8] and discussed previously [9]. The zero-crossing meter does not exactly measure the mean frequency of the Doppler spectrum, corresponding to the average velocity, but a value higher than the mean Doppler frequency [1, 10]. This systematic error depends on the shape and the width of the Doppler spectrum; the broader the spectrum with respect to its average frequency, the larger the

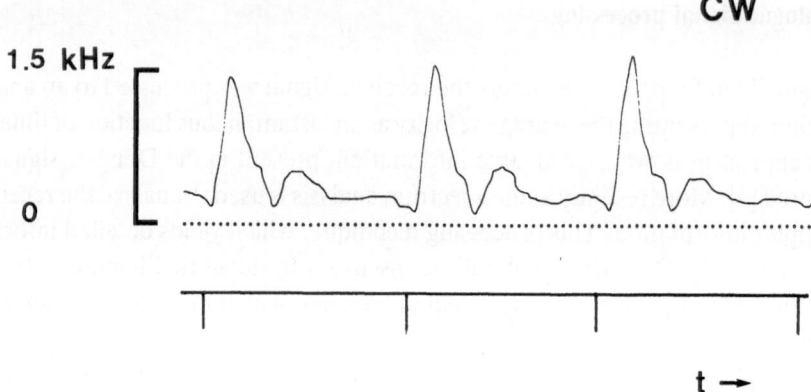

Figure 2. The instantaneous carotid artery flow velocity tracing as recorded with a 4 MHz continuous wave Doppler instrument, using a zero-crossing technique. This analog Doppler tracing represents the average velocity as an instantaneous function of time. The negative deflections coincide with the R-wave of the EEG.

error. The zero-crossing meter appears to be accurate only for a single frequency or a relatively narrow frequency spectrum.

An additional disadvantage of zero-crossing meters is that the output error is only negligible if the level of the audio signal exceeds the noise level by at least 10 times [8]. Proper adjustment of the threshold of the zero-crossing detector is required to prevent shifting of the instantaneous velocity tracing from the zero-line. This is essential because in cerebral vascular disease valuable information can be derived from the systolic and diastolic amplitudes of the analog velocity tracings of the common carotid artery [11]. Another disadvantage is that the output of the zero-crossing meter becomes unreliable if high amplitude low frequency components, induced by vessel wall motion, are present in the Doppler signal [8]. To reduce the noise contribution and vessel wall motion artefacts, a bandpass filter is used which limits the frequency range of the audio signal albeit at the cost of low and high velocity information. The upper frequency limitation can be a problem, especially in stenotic regions.

An alternative method has been described to determine the mean velocity from the Doppler spectrum [12, 13, 14]. This method looks promising because it properly takes into account the spectral distribution of frequencies.

In spite of this possible improvement in the processing of analog tracings, the use of these tracings has limitations. Although shape analysis and the systolic and diastolic amplitudes of the analog velocity tracings do give important information about the site and severity of arterial stenosis [15], valuable information, present in the Doppler signal, is eliminated in this technique. Therefore, the use of audio spectrum analysis is preferred in continuous wave and single-channel pulsed Doppler systems. Audio spectrum analysis yields insight into the flow pattern and, hence, into the disturbances in this pattern as induced by atherosclerotic lesions (Chapter 20). This method also detects arterial wall vibration as generated by high velocity turbulence just distal to a stenosis [16]. In multi-channel pulsed Doppler instruments zero-crossing meters can be used because of the narrow frequency spectrum in these systems. See section on 'CW versus pulsed Doppler instruments'.

Emission of ultrasound

In Doppler instruments ultrasound can be emitted continuously (CW Doppler) or intermittently (pulsed Doppler).

CW Doppler systems

In CW Doppler instruments the ultrasonic beam is usually transmitted from one crystal and the backscattered ultrasound received by another one (Fig. 1). These systems are easy to build and to operate, but vessel wall motion artefacts are often difficult to eliminate, at least without simultaneously eliminating the signals from blood flowing at low velocities. The high amplitude low frequency signals due to lateral wall motion strongly affect the shape of the frequency spectrum and, therefore, the accuracy of the mean velocity determination with the zero-crossing meter. Vessel wall motion signals can even mask the presence of high velocity information, necessitating additional attenuation at the lower end of the band-pass filter. An increase in roll-off rather than increasing the cut-off frequency is usually sufficient and preferable. This masking phenomenon is seen in analog signal processing with zero-crossing meters [8] as well as in audio spectrum analysis [16]. As discussed in section 3.2, the zero-crossing meter is only accurate for a single frequency or a narrow frequency spectrum. This limits the applicability of zero-crossing meters in combination with CW Doppler flowmeters, where a wide spectrum is fed into the meter. This wide spectrum results among other things from the variations in velocity of the red blood cells over the cross-sectional area of the blood vessel.

Pulsed Doppler systems

In pulsed Doppler flowmeters usually one single crystal, operating alternately as transmitter and receiver, is used. The crystal receives the backscattered signals from the red blood cells and the vessel wall during the interval between pulses. In pulsed Doppler systems, single-channel and multi-channel instruments can be distinguished.

34

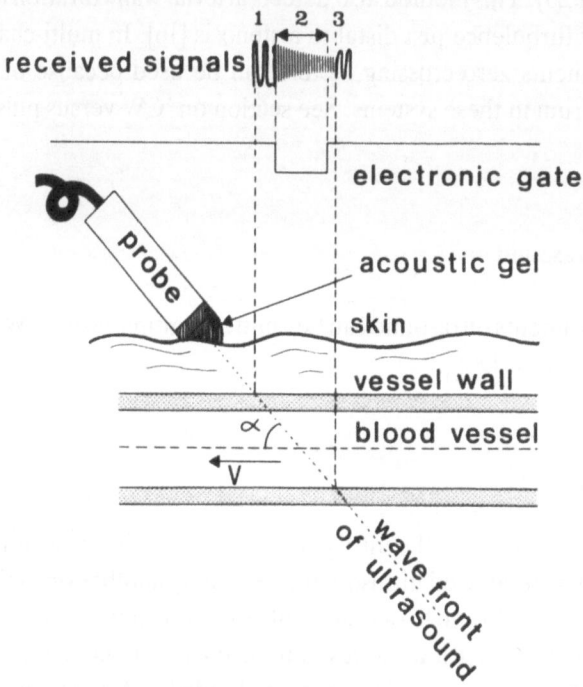

received signals

electronic gate

acoustic gel

skin

vessel wall

blood vessel

Figure 3. The principle of single-channel pulsed Doppler flowmetry. The arrow indicates the flow direction. 1 and 3 = ultrasonic power reflected from the anterior and posterior wall of the vessel, respectively. 2 = ultrasonic power backscattered from the red blood cells. The electronic gate is so adjusted that mainly the signal which contains the flow velocity information is processed. From Reneman *et al.*, 1979; with permission of Angiology.

Single-channel instruments

In single-channel pulsed Doppler systems an electronic gate allows selection of scatterings either from the vessel wall or the red blood cells at a given distance from the transducer (Fig. 3). This makes it possible to determine the mean velocity as an instantaneous function of time in a small sample volume at various sites in an artery, thus avoiding contamination of the desired signal by unwanted signals, like those from vessel wall and veins.

In principle, with single-channel pulsed Doppler systems, the velocity profile – that is the velocity distribution over the cross-sectional area of the vessel – can be determined. In these systems, however, during one cardiac cycle the velocity as an instantaneous function of time can only be determined at one site in the vessel. Therefore, synthesis of the velocity profiles during a cardiac cycle requires that the instantaneous velocity signals at various sites in an artery are assessed during consecutive heart beats. This may limit the applicability of these systems in the diagnosis of peripheral artery diseases because in the vicinity of stenotic lesions

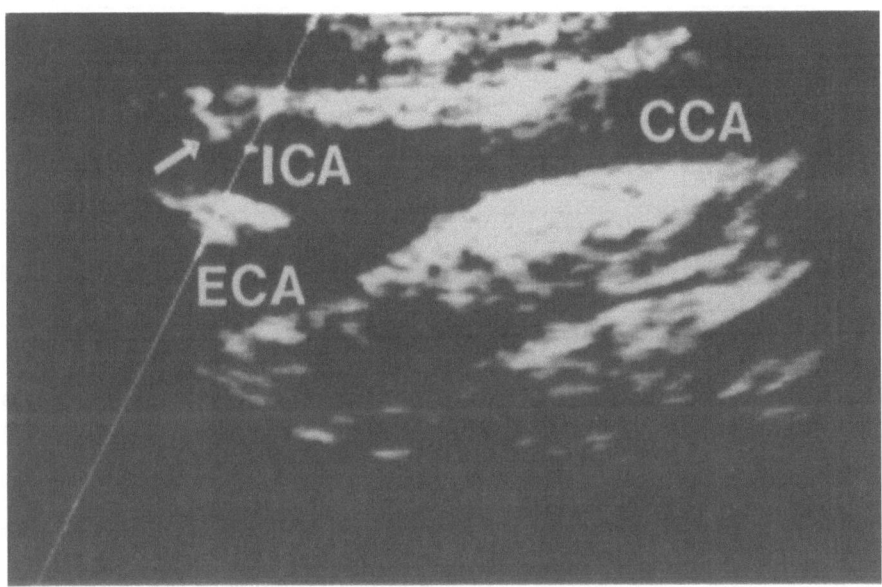

Figure 4. B-mode image of a carotid artery bifurcation as recorded with a mechanical sector scanner operating at 5 MHz. The line indicates the direction of the ultrasound beam and the marker the site of sampling. The arrow points to a vascular lesion in the internal carotid artery (ICA). CCA and ECA = common and external carotid artery, respectively.

the velocity profile was found to change locally during one cardiac cycle [17]. Besides, the positioning and maintenance of the sample volume at the site of interest requires some skill. The use of pulsed echo systems (e.g. B-mode imaging of the vessel wall) in combination with single-channel pulsed Doppler systems [18, 19] will facilitate this task (Fig. 4). Additional advantages of this approach are that information can be obtained about the angle between the sound beam and the direction of blood flow, and changes, if any, in the vessel wall may be detected, provided that the resolution of the B-mode system is adequate [20]. A drawback of using simultaneously pulsed Doppler and B-mode imaging techniques is that the maximum detectable velocity, which is already limited in pulsed Doppler systems (see below) is further reduced. In most of the commercially available systems this problem is overcome by freeze framing the image when the Doppler signal is recorded.

Multi-channel instruments

More recently multi-channel pulsed Doppler systems have been developed that have the ability to detect simultaneously and instantaneously velocities over the full range of interest [21, 22, 23, 24]. With these systems the mean velocity as an instantaneous function of time can be recorded on-line, simultaneously at various

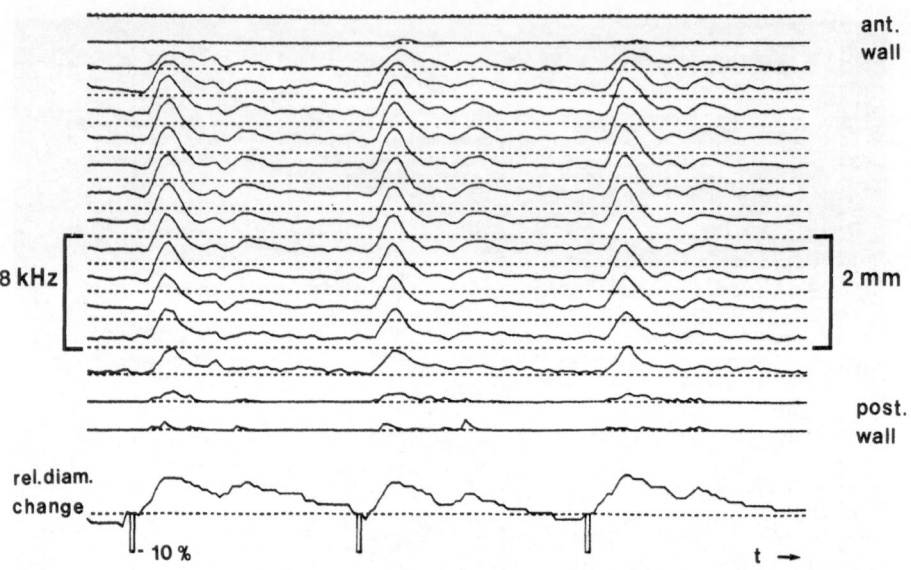

Figure 5. The mean velocity as an instanteneous function of time in the common carotid artery at various sites along the ultrasound beam as recorded wih a multi-channel pulsed Doppler system in a healthy volunteer (age: 26 years). The relative diameter changes of the artery during the cardiac cycle are shown as well. The negative deflection coincides with the R-wave of the ECG. Three cardiac cycles are presented.

sites along the ultrasound beam (Fig. 5), and hence the velocity profiles at discrete time intervals during the cardiac cycle (Figs. 6, 23, 24, 25, 26, 27, 28). To obtain reliable velocity profiles, the sample resolution has to be high and the sample distance along the ultrasonic beam must be small. A limited number of independent sample points along the cross-section of the vessel provides more parabolic velocity profiles and significantly overestimates vessel diameter [21]. Small sample volumes can only be obtained if the effective duration of the measurement is small and the beamwidth is narrow. The effective duration is set by the duration of emission combined with the bandwidth of the receiver section and the gate-width [29]. Increasing the bandwidth and shortening the duration of emission (high emission frequency) and the gate-width will reduce the sample volume, but will decrease the signal-to-noise ratio. To be adequately informed of the features of a pulsed Doppler system it is important to measure the size of the sample volume [30] rather than following the specifications provided by the manufacturer.

With multi-channel pulsed Doppler systems one can also determine the relative changes in artery diameter ($\triangle d/d * 100\%$) during the cardiac cycle [26, 27, 31] (Figs. 5 and 6). This assessment is based upon the detection of low frequency Doppler signals, originating from the sample volumes coinciding with the anterior and posterior walls [31]. Therefore, the vessel under investigation is interrogated under an angle of 60°. To ensure that the initial relative change at the

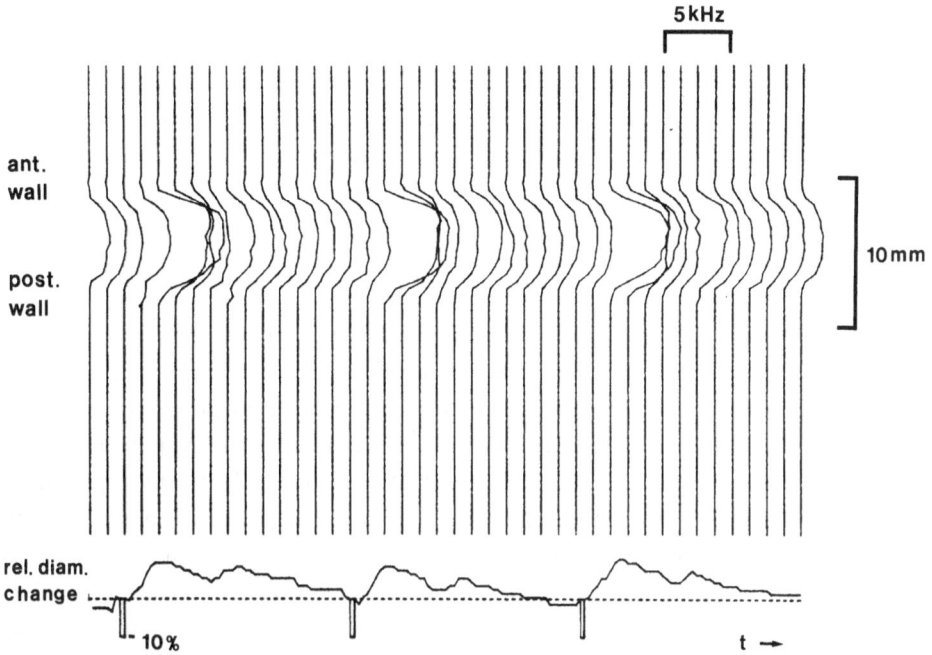

Figure 6. The axial velocity profiles at discrete time intervals during the cardiac cycle and the relative diameter changes during this cycle as simultaneously recorded in the common carotid artery of a healthy volunteer (age: 26 years) with a multi-channel pulsed Doppler instrument. Three heart beats are presented. Only a limited number of velocity profiles during one cardiac cycle, generally 10–20 out of 256, is presented for the sake of clarity. After Reneman, *et al.*[28]; with permission of the American Heart Association.

beginning of the cardiac cycle is constant, it is reset to zero by a trigger derived from the R-wave of the ECG. This trigger can also be used to mark the start of the cardiac cycle when velocities are recorded. The relative diameter changes are independent of the angle of interrogation and can be determined with an absolute accuracy of 0.5% [31]. The multi-channel system also allows the assessment of the absolute artery diameter from the A-mode of vessel wall displacement which is displayed continuously on a CRT. This A-mode differs from the A-mode as known in echo systems because of the rejection of stationary signals (cut-off frequency 5 Hz). The absolute artery diameters as obtained in this way are dependent on the angle of interrogation.

In multi-channel pulsed Doppler systems the vessel of interest can be localized easily without the use of a B-mode imager. For proper localization of the site of sampling, for example, in relation to the carotid artery bifurcation [28] or the diseased area, the combination of a multi-channel system and a B-mode or 2D-echo imager is preferred. The multi-channel systems presently in use in our laboratories (Pie Data, Maastricht, the Netherlands) can easily be connected to most of the commercially available ultrasonic devices.

CW versus pulsed Doppler instruments

CW Doppler instruments are easy to operate and they are inexpensive. The maximum frequency that can be detected unambiguously with these systems is theoretically unlimited. This is especially important when velocities are recorded within the stenosis to estimate the degree of artery narrowing. Velocity recording within a stenosis is rather easy because of the relatively wide ultrasound beam in CW systems.

In theory the average velocity over the cross-sectional area of an artery can be determined with CW Doppler, at least when the whole cross-sectional area of the blood vessel lies within the ultrasonic beam [15]. Quantitative assessment of this velocity, however, is still difficult, mainly because the angle of interrogation cannot be determined accurately and precise assessment of the average frequency of the Doppler spectrum is difficult to achieve (section 3.2). Besides, problems are encountered in processing the CW Doppler signal due to sampling over the full range. Vessel wall motion artefacts can mask the presence of high-velocity information, both when a zero-crossing meter and audio spectrum analysis is used. This is a special problem when high velocity turbulence distal to a stenosis leads to vessel wall vibrations [16].

A major advantage of pulsed Doppler devices is that small volume samples are taken along the vessel diameter, so that a narrow frequency spectrum is fed into the zero-crossing meter. Hence the error made in determining the mean frequency of the Doppler spectrum with this meter is small in pulsed systems. Obtaining information from small sample volumes at various sites along the ultrasound beam largely prevents contamination of the velocity signal by unwanted signals like those from the vessel wall and veins. Information about the angle between the ultrasound beam and the direction of blood flow can be obtained with pulsed systems when they are combined with B-mode imaging. Pulsed Doppler systems possess the possibility of determining transcutaneously the artery diameter. With multi-channel pulsed Doppler systems rather detailed information can be obtained on-line about the velocity distribution along the ultrasound beam during the cardiac cycle. Moreover, these systems allow the on-line assessment of the relative diameter changes of arteries ($\triangle d/d \star 100\%$) during the cardiac cycle. The accuracy of transcutaneous determination of the absolute artery diameter is still limited, but the relative changes in diameter can be determined rather precisely [31].

Although pulsed Doppler systems do have some obvious advantages, it should be noted that in these devices problems are encountered which are not met in CW systems. The circuitry of pulsed devices is more complex and the Doppler bandwidth of the system is limited. The maximum Doppler velocity that can be detected unambiguously depends on the distance between probe and vessel, and the transmitter frequency [9, 32]. This distance sets an upper bound to the pulse repetition frequency, which theoretically should exceed the maximum Doppler frequency at least twice. However, recently a frequency estimator for sampled Doppler signals has been developed that tracks frequencies close to and beyond the Nyquist frequency (half the pulse repetition frequency), significantly increasing the maximum Doppler frequency that can be detected unambiguously [24]. The limited bandwidth of pulsed Doppler devices is especially a problem when maximum velocities have to be recorded within tight arterial stenoses. An additional problem encountered under these circumstances is the positioning and maintenance of the sample volume in tight stenoses, especially when the sample volume is small, a requirement for accurate assessment of the velocity profile (section 4.2).

Probe construction is more complicated in pulsed than in CW systems. To obtain a sharp pulse of short duration, necessary for adequate axial resolution, matching of the characteristic impedance of the crystals to the backing and loading media is more critical than in CW probes.

Atherosclerotic lesions associated with substantial narrowing of the carotid arteries can be detected rather accurately, with both CW [33, 34, 35] and pulsed Doppler instruments [34, 37, 38, 39]. These techniques can also distinguish high grade stenosis ($>90\%$ diameter reduction) from total occlusion. This indicates that in the detection of these lesions there is no specific need for pulsed Doppler systems. However, at the present state of the art no definite conclusions can be made about which of these systems is most accurate in quantifying this type of lesions. In the diagnosis of lesions without substantial narrowing of the carotid arteries pulsed Doppler systems are likely to be more suitable than CW Doppler devices.

Acknowledgements

The authors are indebted to Mariet de Groot and Jos Heemskerk for typing the manuscript and to Paul Hick for making the illustrations. The investigations were supported by the Dutch Heart Foundation and FUNGO, which is subsidized by the Netherlands Organization for the Advancement of Pure Research.

References

1. Peronneau PA, Hinglais J, Pellet M, and Leger F: Velocimetre sanguin par effect Doppler a emission ultra-sonore pulsee. L'Onde electrique 50: 369–384, 1970.
2. Wells PNT: Physical principles of ultrasonic diagnosis. Academic Press, London, 1969.
3. Reid JM and Baker DW: Physics and electronics of the ultrasonic Doppler method. In: Bock J and Ossoinig K. (eds) Ultrasonographia medica, pp. 109–120. Verlag der Wiener Medizinischen Akademie, Wien, 1971.
4. Gosling RG: General discussion: the usefulness of zero-crossing meters. In: Reneman RS (ed) Cardiovascular applications of ultrasound, pp. 455–456. North-Holland/American Elsevier, Amsterdam-Londen-New York, 1974.

5. McLeod FD: A directional Doppler flowmeter. Digest of seventh International Conference on Medical and Biological Engineering, 213, 1967.

6. Strandness DE, Kennedy JW, Judge TP, and McLeod FD: Transcutaneous directional flow detection: A preliminary report. Am Heart J 78: 65–74, 1969.

7. Reneman RS, Clarke HF, Simmons N, and Spencer MP: In vivo comparison of electromagnetic and Doppler flowmeters; with special attention to the processing of the analogue Doppler flow signal. Cardiovasc Res 7: 557–566, 1973.

8. Reneman RS, and Spencer MP: Difficulties in processing of an analogue Doppler flow signal; with special reference to zero-crossing meters and quantification. In: Reneman RS (ed) Cardiovascular applications of ultrasound (Reneman RS, ed.), pp. 32–42. North-Holland/American Elsevier, Amsterdam-London-New York, 1974.

9. Reneman RS, and Hoeks A: Continuous wave and pulsed Doppler flowmeters – A general introduction. In: Bom N (ed.) Echocardiology with Doppler applications and real time imaging, pp. 189–205. Martinus Nijhoff, The Hague, 1977.

10. Rice SO: In selected papers and noise and stochastic processes (Wax W, ed.), pp. 133–294. Dover Publications, New York, 1954.

11. Mol JMF: The clinical use of Doppler hematographic investigation in cerebral circulation disturbances. In: Reneman RS and Hoeks APG (eds.), Doppler ultrasound in the diagnosis of cerebrovascular disease, pp. 129–156. Research Studies Press – A division of John Wiley, Chichester-New York-Toronto, 1983.

12. Arts MGJ, and Roevros JMJG: On the instantaneous measurement of blood-flow by ultrasonic means. Med Biol Engng 10: 23–34, 1972.

13. Reid JM, Davis DL, Ricketts HJ, and Spencer MP: A new Doppler flowmeter system and its operations with catheter mounted transducers. In: Reneman RS (ed) Cardiovascular applications of ultrasound, pp. 183–192. North-Holland/American Elsevier, Amsterdam-London-New York, 1974.

14. Angelsen BAJ: Transcutaneous measurement of aortic blood velocity by ultrasound; a theoretical and experimental approach. PhD-thesis no. 75–78W, NTH, Trondheim, Norway, 1975.

15. Reneman RS, Hoeks A, and Spencer MP: Doppler ultrasound in the evaluation of the peripheral arterial circulation. Angiology 30: 526–538, 1979.

16. Reneman RS, and Spencer MP: Local Doppler audio spectra in normal and stenosed carotid arteries in man. Ultrasound Med Biol 5: 1–11, 1979.

17. Wille SO: Numerical models of arterial blood flow. Thesis, Institute of Informatics, University of Oslo, Norway, 1979.

18. Barber FE, Baker DW, Strandness DE, and Mahler GD: Duplex scanner II. Ultrason Symp Proc IEEE Cat. = 74 CHO 8961 Trans Sonics Ultrasonics, 1974.

19. Pourcelot L: Echo-Doppler Systems – Applications for the detection of cardiovascular disorders. In: Bom N (ed.) Echocardiology with Doppler applications and real time imaging, pp. 245–256. Martinus Nijhoff, The Hague, 1977.

20. Hennerici M, Reifschneider G, Trockel U, and Aulich A: Detection of early atherosclerotic lesions by Duplex scanning of the carotid artery J Clin Ultrasound 12: 455–464, 1984.

21. Anliker M: Diagnostic analysis of arterial flow pulses in man. In Cardiovascular system dynamics (Baan J, Noordergraaf A, and Raines J, eds.), pp. 113–123, MIT Press, Cambridge, 1978.

22. Brandestini M: Topoflow – A digital full range Doppler velocity meter. IEEE Trans. Sonics Ultrasonics SU-25: 287–293, 1978.

23. Hoeks APG, Reneman RS, and Peronneau PA: A multi-gate pulsed Doppler system with serial data processing. IEEE Trans Sonics Ultrasonics SU-28: 242–247, 1981.

24. Hoeks APG, Peeters HPM, Ruissen CJ, and Reneman RS: A novel frequency estimator for sampled Doppler signals. IEEE Trans Biomed Eng BME-31: 212–220, 1984.

25. Keller HM, Meier WE, Anliker M, and Kumpe DA: Noninvasive measurement of velocity profiles and blood flow in the common carotid artery by pulsed Doppler ultrasound. Stroke 7: 370–377, 1976.

26. Reneman RS: What measurements are necessary for a comprehensive evaluation of the peripheral arterial circulation. Cardiovasc Dis 8: 435–454, 1981.

27. Reneman RS, Van Merode T, Hick P, and Hoeks APG: Noninvasive detection of atherosclerotic lesions in cervical carotid arteries at an early stage of the disease. J Cereb Blood Flow Metabol 2, Suppl. 1: 32–34, 1982.

28. Reneman RS, Van Merode T, Hick P, and Hoeks APG: Flow velocity patterns in and distensibility of the carotid artery bulb in volunteers of varying age. Circulation 71: 500–509, 1985.

29. Peronneau PA, Bournat JP, Bugnon A, Barbet A, and Xhaard M: Theoretical and practical aspects of pulsed Doppler flowmetry: real-time application to the measure of instantaneous velocity profiles in vitro and in vivo. In: Reneman RS (ed.) Cardiovascular applications of ultrasound, pp. 66–84. North-Holland/American Elsevier, Amsterdam-London-New York, 1974.

30. Hoeks APG, Ruissen CJ, Hick P, and Reneman RS: Methods to evaluate the sample volume of pulsed Doppler systems. Ultrasound Med Biol 10: 427–434, 1984.

31. Hoeks APG, Ruissen CJ, Hick P, and Reneman RS: Transcutaneous detection of relative changes in artery diameter. Ultrasound Med Biol 11: 51–59, 1985.

32. Hoeks APG, Reneman RS, Ruissen CJ, and Smeets FAM: Possibilities and limitations of pulsed Doppler systems. In: Lancee ChT (ed.) Echocardiology, pp. 413–419. Martinus Nijhoff. The Hague-Boston-London, 1979.

33. Barnes RW, Rittgers SE, and Putney WW: Real-time Doppler spectrum analysis: predictive value in defining operable carotid artery disease. Arch Surg 117: 52–57, 1982.

34. Padayachee TS, Lewis RS, and Gosling RG: Detection of carotid bifurcation disease: comparison of ultrasound tests with angiography. Br J Surg 69: 218–222, 1982.

35. Van Baalen JM, Jakimowicz JJ, and Reneman RS: Noninvasive evaluation of carotid artery stenosis – Comparison of direct and indirect techniques. Vasc Surg 18: 88–95, 1984.

36. Blackshear WM, Phillips DJ, Thiele BL, Hirsch JH, Chikos PM, Marinelli MR, Ward CJ, and Strandness DE: Detection of carotid occlusive disease by ultrasonic imaging and pulsed Doppler spectrum analysis. Surgery 86: 698–706, 1979.

37. Fell G, Phillips DJ, Chikos PM, Harley JD, Thiele BL and Strandness DE: Ultrasonic Duplex scanning for disease of the carotid artery. Circulation 64: 1191–1195, 1981.

38. Breslau PJ: Ultrasonic duplex scanning in the evaluation of carotid artery disease. Thesis, University of Limburg, Maastricht, The Netherlands, 1982.

39. Langlois Y, Roederer GO, Chan A, Phillips DJ, Beach KW, Martin D, Chikos PM and Strandness DE: Evaluating carotid artery disease – The concordance between pulsed Doppler/spectrum analysis and angiography. Ultrasound Med Biol 9: 51–63, 1983.

Normal anatomy, anatomical anomalies and collateral pathways of the blood supply to the brain

R. Ackerstaff

The blood supply to the brain and the cranial part of the spinal cord is derived from the great vessels which arise from the aortic arch in the superior mediastinum: the brachiocephalic trunk, and the left common carotid and subclavian arteries. Most interest about the detection and treatment of cerebral atherosclerosis concerns the internal carotid arteries because about 80% of the total blood flow through the brain tissue is transported by these vessels. Moreover, this part of the cerebrovascular tree is easily accessible to diagnostic techniques and surgical procedures. However, since the vertebral arteries are often as large as, and sometimes larger than, the internal carotid arteries at the point where they penetrate the dura and since they supply the vital centers of the brain stem, a careful and reliable investigation of the innominate subclavian-vertebral arterial system in patients with cerebral arterial disease is also important.

Any discussion on disease of the carotid and the vertebrobasilar arterial systems should begin with the origin of these vascular systems, because obstructive disease, ulcerative plaques or anatomical anomalies anywhere in the cerebrovascular tree may produce stroke or symptoms of insufficiency. For a good understanding of the possibilities and limitations of the many Doppler techniques available at present, knowledge of the normal anatomy and anatomical variations of the cerebrovascular tree is essential.

This chapter contains a review of the anatomy of the arch vessels, the internal and external carotid as well as the vertebral and basilar arteries. Besides the normal anatomy, anatomical anomalies are briefly described. In order to estimate symptoms of cerebrovascular insufficiency, a survey of the different parts of the central nervous system which are supplied by branches of the cerebral arteries is also given in this chapter. The reader is referred to anatomical tests for further guidance [1, 2].

The vital role of collateral circulation and its interplay in cerebrovascular disease has now become an important diagnostic consideration. When evaluating symptoms of cerebrovascular insufficiency, clinicians and technicians must be aware of the potential collateral circulation and its influence on diagnostic tests.

The potential collateral pathways of both the carotid and vertebral arteries are discussed at the end of this chapter.

Branches of the aortic arch

The arch of the aorta begins behind the manubrium sterni at the level of the upper border of the second right sternocostal articulation, and at first runs upwards and backwards to the left of the trachea. It is then directed backwards on the left side of the trachea. Finely, it passes downwards on the left side of the body of the fourth thoracic vertebra, at the lower border of which it is continuous with the descending aorta. Its termination corresponds to the sternal extremity of the second, left costal cartilage. Thus, it has two curvatures: one with its convexity upwards, the other with its convexity forward and to the left. Its upper border is usually about the level of the middle of the manubrium sterni, but it may be considerably higher or lower than this.

Anatomical variations of the aortic arch may result in an abnormal origin and location of its branches. They are briefly summarized here and some of them are shown in Fig. 1. Sometimes the aorta arches over the root of the right lung instead of that of the left lung. This right aortic arch passes downwards on the right side of the vertebral column. In this condition, which is normal in birds, there is usually a transposition of the thoracic and abdominal viscera. Less frequently, after arching over the root of the right lung, the aorta passes behind the oesophagus to gain its position on the left side of the vertebral column. This anatomical pecularity is not associated with transposition of the viscera. In this case the left subclavian artery arises as the last branch from that arch, and crosses behind the oesophages en route to the left upper extremity.

The aorta occasionally divides, as in some quadricepts, into an ascending and descending trunk. The former is directed vertically upwards, and subdivides into three branches to supply the head and the upper limbs. Sometimes the aorta subdivides near its origin into two branches, which soon reunite. In this condition, which is normal in reptiles and is due to persistence of a part of the right dorsal aorta, the oesophagus and the trachea usually pass through the interval between the two branches.

Three branches arise from the upper aspect of the aortic arch: the brachio-cephalic trunk, the left common carotid and the left subclavian arteries. At their origins the distance between these vessels varies. The most frequent variation in this respect is the approximation of the left common carotid artery to the brachiocephalic trunk. The braches may arise from the commencement of the arch or upper part of the ascending aorta.

The number of primary branches may be reduced to one. More commonly there are two (Fig. 1a): in 7% of the cases the left common carotid artery arises from the brachiocephalic trunk [15, 3]. More rarely the common carotid and

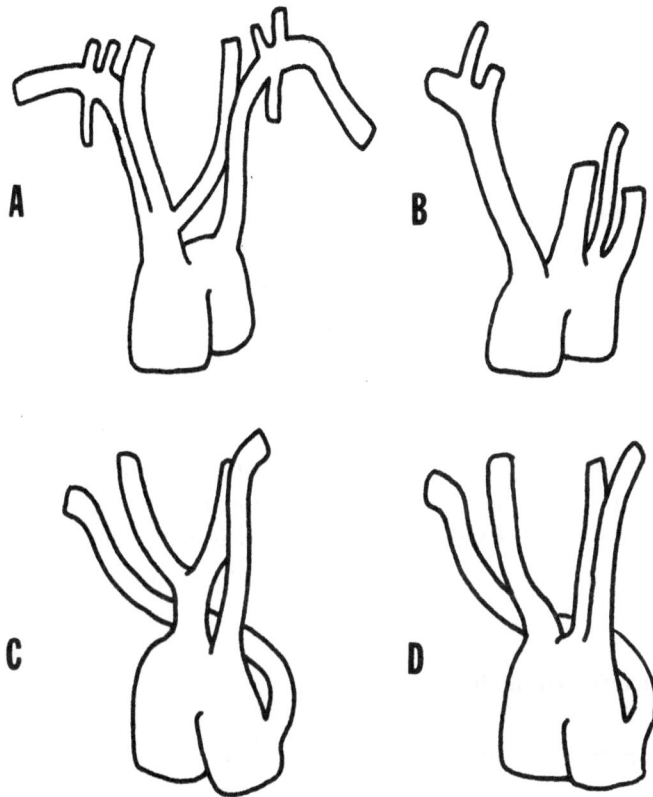

subclavian arteries of the left side arise from a left brachiocephalic trunk. But the number of branches may increase to four, because the right common carotid and the subclavian arteries may arise directly from the aorta. In most of these cases the right subclavian artery arises from the left end of the arch and passes to the right behind the aorta [4]. This anomaly was found in 0.25% of the 400 autotopsy specimens in their series (Fig. 1d). A more common variation, in which there are four primary branches, is the left vertebral artery arising from the arch of the aorta between the left common carotid and subclavian arteries (Fig. 1b). The figures of this anomaly vary between 2.46% and 6% [4, 5]. Very rarely the external and internal carotid arteries arise separately from the aortic arch, the common carotid being absent on one or both sides. In a few cases both vertebral arteries originate directly from the arch of the aorta.

When the aorta arches to the right side, the arrangement of the three branches of the arch is reversed. There is a left brachiocephalic trunk, and the right common carotid and right subclavian arteries arise separately. In other cases, where the aorta takes its usual course, the two common carotid arteries may be joined in a single trunk and the subclavian arteries arise separately from the arch. In this condition the right subclavian artery generally arises from the left end of the arch (Fig. 1c).

Other arteries may branch from the arch of the aorta. Most common are one or two bronchial arteries and the thyroidea ima artery. The latter is a small and inconstant artery that ascends in front of the trachea to the isthmus of the thyroid gland. It occasionally arises from the aorta, the brachiocephalic trunk, or the right common carotid, subclavian or internal thoracic arteries.

The brachiocephalic trunk or innominate artery is the first and largest branch of the arch of the aorta. It is 4 to 5 cm in length and arises from the convexity of the arch, posterior to the center of the manubrium sterni. It passes obliquely upwards, backwards and to the right, lying at first in front of the trachea and then on its right side. At the level of the upper border of the right sternal clavicular joint it divides into the right common carotid and subclavian arteries. The root of the innominate artery is crossed anteriorly by the left brachiocephalic and right inferior thyroid veins. On its right side are the right brachiocephalic vein and the upper part of the vena cava superior. The innominate artery is usually devoid of branches other than its terminal ones, but occasionally the thyroidea ima may arise from it, or it gives off a thymic or bronchial branch.

Anterior arterial circulation

Cervical arterial anatomy

The principle arteries of the head and the neck are the two common carotid arteries. Each artery ascends in the neck as far as the upper border of the thyroid cartilage, where it divides into the external and internal carotid arteries. The common carotid arteries differ in length and in their mode of origin. Usually the right common carotid artery begins at the bifurcation of the innominate artery behind the right sternoclavicular joint and is confined to the neck. However, in twelve percent of subjects the artery arises above the level of this joint. The left common carotid artery springs from the highest part of the arch of the aorta immediately behind and to the left of the innominate artery. Its thoracic part ascends from the aortic arch to the level of the left sternoclavicular joint, where it is continuous with its cervical portion.

At its point of division, the common carotid artery shows a dilatation, termed the carotid sinus, which usually involves, and may be restricted to, the proximal part of the internal carotid artery. The structure of the walls of the sinus enables it to react readily to changes in the arterial blood pressure and to bring about appropriate reflex modifications. Its function as a baroreceptor mechanism enables it to exercise control over intracranial pressure. The carotid body, which lies behind the point of division of the common carotid artery, acts as a chemoreceptor. The common carotid artery is contained in the carotid sheath which also encloses the internal jugular vein. This vein lies laterally to the artery.

The left common carotid artery varies in its origin more frequently than the right. In the majority of abnormal cases it arises together with the innominate artery. If that artery is absent the two common carotid arteries arise usually by a single trunk. It is rarely joined with the left subclavian artery except in the event of transposition of the aortic arch. The common carotid artery very rarely ascends in the neck without undergoing division, either the internal or the external carotid artery is absent. In a few cases the common carotid artery itself was absent and the internal and external carotid arteries arose directly from the aortic arch. In some cases, this peculiarity may occur on one side and on both sides in others. The common carotid arteries usually have no branches. However, they may give rise to the vertebral, the superior thyroid or its laryngeal branch, the ascending pharyngeal, the inferior thyroid or the occipital arteries.

The bifurcation of the common carotid artery can vary considerably in level. It may occur higher than usual, at or about the level of the hyoid bone. More rarely it is located below the usual level, opposite the middle of the larynx, or at the lower border of the cricoid cartilage. Although the level of the carotid bifurcation tends to be symmetrical, it is important in Doppler examinations to realize that in some subjects it is located very asymmetrical. At the level of the bifurcation, the external carotid artery usually is located in an anteromedial and the internal carotid artery in a posterolateral position.

In about 50% of the cases [6] the external carotid artery begins opposite at the level of the disc between the fourth and fifth cervical vertebrae. It takes a slightly curved course, passes upwards and forwards and then inclines backwards to a point behind the neck of the mandible, where, in the substance of the parotid gland, it divides into its terminal branches: the maxillary and superficial temporal arteries. It diminishes rapidly in size, owing to the number and large size of its branches. The branches of the external carotid artery are: the superior thyroid, the ascending pharyngeal, the lingual, the facial, the occipital, the posterior auricular, the superficial temporal and the maxillary arteries. Most of these branches are very important as potential collateral pathways and will be discussed in more detail in the last section of this chapter.

The internal carotid artery supplies the greater part of the cerebral hemisphere, the eye and its accessory organs and sends branches to the forehead and nose. Its length naturally varies with the length of the neck and with the level of the carotid bifurcation. It very rarely rises directly from the aortic arch, and then has been found medial to the external carotid artery as far as the larynx, where it crosses behind the latter vessel to reach its usual position. For convenience sake the internal carotid artery may be divided into four segments.

The first (cervical) segment begins at the bifurcation of the common carotid artery and ascends vertically in the neck to the base of the skull. Usually it is located posterior and slightly medial to the external carotid artery and anterior to the internal jugular vein. It lies relatively deeply to the sterno-cleidomastoid muscle and the parotid gland. The course of the cervical segment, instead of being straight, may be very tortuous. When this occurs the vessel approaches nearer to the pharynx than usual. The cervical segment of the internal carotid artery has no branches.

Intracranial arterial anatomy

At the base of the skull, the cervical segment enters the carotid canal of the temporal bone, where it becomes the petrous segment. At first this segment ascends a short distance, and then curves forwards and medially to assume a horizontal course, anterior to the tympanic cavity and cochlea. As it leaves the canal to enter the cranial cavity it runs upwards and medially to enter the posterior portion of the foramen lacerum. Finally, it ascends to a juxtasellar location, piercing the dural layers of the cavernous sinus to become the cavernous segment. The petrous segment of the internal carotid artery is surrounded by a plexus of small veins.

When the internal carotid artery is in the cavernous sinus it is covered by the vascular membranes lining the sinus and follows a sinuous course. It passes anteriorly and then superomedially to exit the sinus just medial to the anterior cliniod process. The artery once again pierces the dura at this point. The petrous and cavernous segments of the internal carotid artery give rise to several small and sometimes inconstant branches. Although some of these branches can be demonstrated by arteriography in patients with severe cerebral atherosclerosis, mostly they are too thin to function as hemodynamically significant collaterals.

The supraclinoid or cerebral segment ascends slightly backwards below the optic nerve, and then passes between the optic and oculomotor nerves to the anterior perforated substance, where it divides into its terminal branches. Normally, the ophthalmic artery is a branch from the internal carotid artery as it emerges form the cavernous sinus. It forms the most important collateral pathway between the internal and external carotid arteries. Some authors [7] have described an unusual origin of the ophthalmic artery from the middle meningeal, the anterior cerebral, the middle cerebral or posterior communicating arteries.

The anterior cerebral artery is the smaller of the two terminal branches of the internal carotid artery. It starts at the medial end of the lateral cerebral sulcus and passes horizontally and anteriomedially above the optic nerve, to enter the interhemispheric fissure at the midline. Here it comes into close proximity with the opposite artery and is joined to it by a short (about 4 mm) and sometimes duplicated transverse trunk, called the anterior communicating artery. From this point, the two anterior cerebral arteries run side by side in the longitudinal cerebral fissure, curving around the genu of the corpus callosum, and running backwards along the upper surface of this structure to its posterior extremity. Here they end by anastomosing with branches of the posterior cerebral arteries. In their course they give off many central and cortical branches. It is to be noted that the frontal branches supply the leg area of the cortex. The origin of the anterior cerebral artery, on one side may be hypoplastic, in which case the contralateral anterior cerebral artery supplies the distal branches via the anterior communicating artery.

The middle cerebral artery is the larger terminal branch of the internal carotid artery. It arises just lateral to the optic chiasm and at first runs laterally in the lateral cerebral sulcus and then backwards and upwards on the surface of the insula, where it gives rise to branches distributed to the insula. Finally, it runs to the lateral surface of the cerebral hemisphere where it divides into many cortical arteries. The branches to the cerebral convexity vary, but ascending frontal, precentral, central, anterior and posterior parietal, and angular, anterior and posterior temporal branches are fairly common. The terminal branches of the middle cerebral artery anastomose at the cerebral convexity with terminal branches of the anterior and posterior cerebral arteries. It is to be noted that the cortical branches of the middle cerebral artery supply the greater part of the motor and auditory areas. The medial and lateral lenticulostriate arteries are small branches from the commencement of the middle cerebral artery which enter the brain through the anterior perforated substance. They supply the lentiform and caudate nuclei, the superior half of the internal capsule, the adjacent corona radiata, and the putamen.

The anterior choriodal artery is a small but constant branch of the internal carotid artery. It arises near the posterior communicating artery, passes back-wards above the medial part of the uncus, and crosses inferior to the optic tract to reach the crus cerebri. Finally, it turns laterally, recrossing the optic tract, enters the inferior horn of the lateral ventricle and ends in the choroidal plexus. It supplies the crus cerebri, the lateral geniculate body, the globus pallidus, the optic tract and radiation, the posterior limb of the internal capsule, the hippocam-pus, and the fimbria.

The posterior communicating artery runs backwards from the internal carotid artery, above the oculomotor nerve, and anastomoses with the posterior cerebral artery, a branch from the basilar artery. Although usually a small vessel, it gives rise to several small central branches which pierce the posterior perforated substance and supply the medial surface of the thalamus and the walls of the third ventricle.

Posterior arterial circulation

The first part of the subclavian arteries differ from one another in their origin, length, course and relations. The right subclavian artery originates behind the right sternoclavicular joint. It passes upwards and laterally to the medial margin of the anterior scalenus muscle. It ascends about two centimeters above the clavicle, but the height it reaches varies considerably. At its start it is behind the origin of the right common carotid artery. More laterally it is crossed by the internal jugular and vertebral veins. The left subclavian artery is the third branch of the arch of the aorta. It arises behind the left common carotid artery, usually at the level of the disc between the third and fourth thoracic vertebra. It ascends to the root of the neck and arches laterally as far as the medial border of the left anterior scalenus muscle. Within the thorax it is related anteriorly to the left common carotid artery and the commencement of the left brachiocephalic vein.

The subclavian arteries can be represented by a broad line, convex upwards, drawn from the sternoclavicular joint to the middle of the clavicle. As a result of its origin from the arch of the aorta the left subclavian artery is more posterior in its first part than the right one, and, as a rule, it does not reach quite as high a level in the neck.

On both sides the vertebral artery is the first branch of the subclavian artery, arising from the upper and posterior wall of the first part of this vessel. Especially the origin of the left vertebral artery from the left subclavian artery may vary considerably in height. Sometimes the thyrocervical trunk is the first branch, the vertebral artery arises from the subclavian artery lateral to or as a common trunk with the thyrocervical trunk. There may be an anomalous origin of the vertebral artery from the aorta, innominate or common carotid arteries.

The vertebral artery is generally divided into four segments. The first (prevertebral) segment ascends upwards and backwards between the longest colli and scalenus anterior muscles to enter the transverse foramina of the cervical spine at the level of the sixth servical vertebra. This segment of the artery is usually 4 to 5 centimeters in length. Anteriorly it is related to the common carotid artery and the vertebral vein and is crossed by the inferior thyroid artery. Posteriorly, it is related to the transverse process of the seventh cervical vertebra. In many cases the vertebral artery shows a postero-inferior flat curve just distal to its origin from the subclavian artery. Occasionally the vertebral artery may enter the fifth, fourth or seventh cervical vertebrae. Branches which arise from the prevertebral segment of the vertebral artery are rare. The inferior thyroid artery was found to be a branch of the vertebral artery in 0.64% of cases [4]. In 0.81% of the cases the costo-cervical trunk arose as a branch from this part of the vertebral artery.

The second (cervical) segment has a straight course encased in the bony canal formed by the transverse foramina of the upper six cervical vertebrae. It pursues an almost vertical course as far as the transverse process of the axis, through which it runs upwards and laterally to the transverse foramen of the atlas. It is associated with a plexus of veins which unite to form the vertebral vein in the lower part of the neck. The artery passes anteriorly to the vertebral rami of the cervical nerves (C6–C2) and lies in apposition with each successive nerve. The nerve sheath is often grooved as the vessel passes upwards. On its medial aspect the vertebral artery bears an intimate relationship to the neurocentral joint. This is the junction of the centrum and lateral masses in development of the vertebrae, and is also known as Luschka's joint or the uncovertebral joint. There is disagreement on whether this is a true joint or not [6]. The anatomical relationship of the vertebral artery to the uncovertebral joint is assumed to be important when the cervical vertebrae are effected by degenerative osteo-arthritic change.

The third (atlantic) segment issues from the transverse foramen of the atlas on the medial side of the rectus capitis lateralis. It curves horizontally backwards and medially around the articular process of the atlas, lying in a groove on the upper surface of the posterior arch of the atlas. The artery enters the vertebral canal by passing below the lower, arched border of the posterior atlanto-occipital membrane. This part of the artery is contained in the suboccipital triangle and is covered by the semispinalis capitis.

The fourth (intradural) segment pierces the dura and arachnoid mater, ascends in front of the roots of the hypoglossal nerve and inclines medially to the front of the medulla oblongata where, at the lower border of the pons, it unites with the opposite artery to form the basilar artery.

The branches of the vertebral artery may be divided into two sets: cervical branches which arise in the neck, and cranial branches which arise from the intradural segment of the artery. These branches are briefly mentioned here from a proximal to a distal position.

The spinal branches arise from the cervical segment of the vertebral artery and enter the vertebral canal through the intervertebral foramina. They give rise to anterior and posterior radicular arteries which approach the spinal cord along the ventral and dorsal nerve roots. According to Lazorthes [9] only two or three spinal branches of the vertebral artery actually vascularize the middle segments (C4–C6) of the cervical part of the spinal cord, the so-called radiculomedullary arteries. The other spinal branches terminate in the nerve roots (the radicular arteries sensu strictiori) or do not extend beyond the pial leptomeningeal arterial plexus (the radiculopial arteries).

The muscular branches arise from the cervical and atlantic segments of the vertebral artery as it curves round the lateral mass of the atlas. They supply the deep muscles of this region and anastomose with the occipital artery, and with the ascending and deep cervical arteries (Fig. 3).

At the upper end of the second and third segments a small anterior and a larger posterior meningeal branch originate respectively. The former supplies the dura of the anterior margin of the foramen magnum, and the latter supplies the posterior rim of the foramen magnum, the falx cerebelli and the posteromedial portion of the dura of the posterior fossa. The posterior meningeal branch may extend superiorly to supply the posterior portion of the falx cerebri. The arteries supplying the meninges freely anastomose among themselves and with their counterparts from the opposite side of the skull.

The posterior inferior cerebellar artery is the largest branch of the vertebral artery, but is frequently absent. Usually it springs from the intradural segment of the vertebral artery. Occasionally it arises from the basilar artery. It finally divides into a medial and a lateral branch. The medial branch runs backwards between the cerebellar hemisphere and the inferior vermis, supplying branches to both; the lateral branch supplying the undersurface of the hemisphere, as far as its lateral border, and anastomoses with the anterior inferior cerebellar and superior cerebellar branches of the basilar artery. The trunk of the posterior inferior cerebellar artery supplied the medulla oblongata and the choroid plexus of the fourth ventricle. It also sends a branch upwards lateral to the tonsil to supply the dentate nucleus of the cerebellum. The area supplied in the medulla oblongata lies dorsal to the olivary nucleus and lateral to the nucleus and emerging fila of the hypoglossal nerve.

The posterior spinal artery may arise from the vertebral artery at the side of the medulla oblongata, but most frequently originates from the posterior inferior cerebellar artery. It passes backwards and then descends as two branches, one in front and the other behind the dorsal roots of the spinal nerves.

The anterior spinal artery is a small branch, which arises near the termination of the vertebral artery. It descends in front of the medulla oblongata and unites with its counterpart of the opposite side. The single trunk thus formed descends on the front of the spinal cord. The anterior spinal artery supplies the medial part of the medulla oblongata and the main part of the superior cervical segments (C1–C4).

The medullary arteries are several minute vessels which originate from the vertebral artery and its branches and are distributed to the medulla oblongata.

The basilar artery is formed by the junction of the two vertebral arteries at the level of the pontomedullary sulcus between the two abducens nerves. It extends from the lower to the upper border of the pons, where it divides into two posterior cerebral arteries.

The pontine arteries are numerous, small, penetrating branches of the basilar artery, and can be divided into medial and lateral groups. The lateral group not only supplies the pons, but also the ventrolateral aspect of the cerebellar cortex. Towards its upper end, the basilar artery gives off several penetrating branches that supply the inferior portion of the midbrain.

The anterior inferior cerebellar artery arises from the lower part of the basilar artery. At first it passes ventrally, then horizontally across the inferior portion of the pons, and finally through the cerebellar pontine angle cistern, along with the facial and vestibulocochlea nerves to reach the internal auditory meatus. It then loops on the antero-inferior surface of the cerebellum, supplying the middle cerebellar peduncle and adjacent areas of the cerebellar hemisphere. In its pontine course it gives rise to many pontine perforating branches. The internal auditory artery may arise directly from the basilar artery but is more often derived from the anterior inferior cerebellar artery. It enters the internal auditory canal, contributing to the blood supply of the dura mater of the canal and sending branches to the cochlea, the labyrinth and the horizontal portion of the facial nerve.

The superior cerebellar artery arises from the basilar artery, just proximal to its termination. It passes laterally just caudal to the oculomotor nerve to circle the cerebral peduncle or upper pons just below the trochlear nerve. It sends multiple branches to the midbrain, adjacent pons and the superior cerebellar peduncle. On the upper surface of the cerebellum it divides into branches which ramify in the pia mater, supplying this aspect of the cerebellum. In addition branches are given off to the pineal body, the superior medullary velum, and the tela choroidea of the third ventricle.

The posterior cerebral artery arises from the terminal bifurcation of the basilar artery. While this artery predominantly supplies the supratentorial structures of the brain, it also contributes to the blood supply of the upper part of the midbrain. The proximal segment of the posterior cerebral artery from its origin to its junction with each posterior communicating artery constitutes a distinctive arterial segment, called the mesencephalic artery. From this segment of the posterior cerebral artery arise complex penetrating vessels destined chiefly for the thalamus, subthalamus, rostral midbrain-subthalamic junction, and adjacent structures. It should be noted that the posterior cerebral artery also supplies the visual area of the cerebral cortex.

Collateral pathways

Once it was believed that arteries in the brain were end arteries. Now it is known that capillary and precapillary anastomoses are common. To further appreciate these collateral pathways, it should be noted that there are two types of arteries supplying the brain. The more important in terms of neuronal function and nutrient supply are the penetrating arteries. However, it is the diffuse superficial arteries spreading over the entire surface of the central nervous system through which collateral circulation takes place. The circle of Willis and the major arterial trunks are included in this superficial system.

The circulus arteriosus of Willis [10], which is really more polygonal then circular, is situated in the cisterna interpeduncularis at the base of the brain. It connects the two internal carotid and the basilar arteries. Anteriorly, this circle is formed by the horizontal segment of the anterior cerebral arteries and the anterior communicating artery. Posteriorly, it is formed by the posterior communicating arteries and the proximal segment of the posterior cerebral arteries. In general the circle of Willis is considered to be the most important source of collateral blood flow in patients with cerebrovascular obstructive disease. However, its elaborate embryological evolution and the shifting patterns which precede its definitive form predispose it to abnormal development which may influence its capacity as a collateral. When reviewing the literature an abnormal circle of Willis is found in 50–80% of the reported cases [11, 12, 13]. Probably the exact number depends on the neurological status of the patients involved. The most frequent anomaly is a stringlike calibre of one of the component vessels. Variations are more frequent in the posterior than in the anterior part of the circle. For example, an anomalous origin of the posterior cerebral artery from the internal carotid artery has been frequently encountered. In many of these conditions the anterior or posterior circulation may be isolated and therefore susceptible to a pressure reducing lesion.

Second only to the circle of Willis in importance is the complex of intracranial-extracranial anastomoses. When evaluating Doppler techniques of the carotid and vertebrobasilar arterial systems one should be conversant with the anatomy of these potential collaterals. For the carotid system this network connects the internal and external carotid arteries via the ophthalmic and orbital arteries. Usually, the opthalmic artery originates from the distal part of the carotid syphon. It enters the orbital cavity through the optic canal together with the optic nerve. At first it runs for a short distance anterolaterally in the orbital cavity. It next crosses obliquely above the optic nerve to reach the medial wall of the orbit. Then it runs forwards, where, at the medial end of the upper eyelid, it divides into two branches, named the supratrochlear and dorsal nasal arteries. The supraorbital artery leaves the ophthalmic artery more proximally. It runs forwards and leaves the orbital cavity through the supra-orbital foramen or notch. These branches of the ophthalmic artery turn upwards and pass into the subcutaneous tissue of the forehead, where they anastomose with the frontal branches of the superficial temporal artery. Other communications between the ophthalmic artery and branches of the external carotid artery occur through the ethmoidal and lacrimal arteries. The maxillary branch of the external carotid artery needs to be particularly considered because of its contribution to the collateral blood supply of the carotid syphon. Several authors [14, 15, 16, 17] made the suggestion that these orbital anastomoses offer little in the way of effective collateral circulation to the brain, that they probably only play a passive role, and that they may mainly be indicative of the inadequacy of the collateral circulation via the circle of Willis.

For the vertebrobasilar arterial system the intracranial-extracranial network connects the occipital branch of the external carotid artery, the deep cervical artery and the ascending cervical artery with branches of the vertebral artery. The thyrocervical trunk is a short and wide vessel which arises from the upper and front part of the first segment of the subclavian artery, usually a half to two centimeters lateral to the origin of the vertebral artery. It divides almost immediately into three branches: the inferior thyroid, the suprascapular, and superficial cervical arteries. Of these the former runs upwards in front of the medial border of the scalenus anterior. It then turns medially in front of the vertebral vessels and behind the carotid sheath. It finally descends on the longus colli muscles to the lower border of the lobe of the thyroid gland. The ascending cervical artery is a small branch which arises from the inferior thyroid artery as that vessel turns behind the carotid sheath. It ascends on the anterior tubercles of the transverse processes of the cervical vertebrae in the interval between the scalenus anterior and the longus capitis muscles. Besides small branches to the muscles of the neck it sends off one or two spinal branches into the vertebral canal through the intervertebral foramina. It anastomoses with muscular branches of the vertebral artery and with the occipital and deep cervical arteries.

The costocervical trunk arises from the back of the second part of the subclavian artery on the right, but from the terminal portion of the first part of that vessel on the left. It arches backwards above the cervical pleura to the neck of the first rib and divides into the superior intercostal and deep cervical arteries. Occasionally the latter is a separate branch from the subclavian artery. Passing backwards between the transverse process of the seventh cervical vertebra and the neck of the first rib it gives off a spinal branch which enters the vertebral canal through the foramen between the seventh cervical and first thoracic vertebrae. It ascends in the back of the neck, between the semispinalis capitis and cervicis muscles as high as the second cervical vertebra. It supplies the adjacent muscles, and anastomoses with the deep division of the occipital artery and the muscular branches of the vertebral artery.

The occipital artery arises from the back of the external carotid artery, opposite to the facial artery. It passes backwards, crossing in its course the internal carotid artery and the internal jugular vein. Reaching the interval between the transverse process of the atlas and the mastoid process of the temporal bone, it comes into contact with the lateral border of the rectus capitis lateralis. It then runs in the occipital groove on the temporal bone, and finally turns upwards and pierces the cranial attachment of the trapezius and sternocleidomastoid muscles. The descending branch arises from the occipital artery as the latter lies on the oblique capitis superior and divides into superficial and deep branches. The deep branch descends between the semispinalis capitis and cervicis muscles, and anastomoses with the deep cervical artery, and with the vertebral artery.

References

1. Netter F: The Ciba Collection of Medical Illustrations. Nervous System, Anatomy Physiology, Vol. 1, Part I, 1983.
2. Pernkoff E: Atlas of Topographical and Applied Human Anatomy. Head and Neck (Saunders WB, publishers). Philadelphia, 1963.
3. Wright ML: Dissection study and measuration of the human aortic arch. Journal of Anatomy, 104: 377–385, 1969.
4. Daseler EH, Anson BJ: Surgical anatomy of the subclavian artery and its branches. Surgery, Gynaecology and Obstetrics, 108: 149–174, 1959.
5. Bosniak MA: An analysis of some anatomic-roentgenologic aspects of the brachiocephalic vessels. American Journal of Roentgenology, 91: 1222–1231, 1964.
6. Jonkman EJ, Mosmans PC: Basic anatomy, physiology and pathology of human cerebral circulation. In: Reneman RS, Hoeks APG, John Wiley and Sons, Ltd (eds.), Doppler ultrasound in the diagnosis of cerebrovascular disease, 1–28, 1982.
7. Picard L, Vignaud J, Lombardi G, Roland J: Radiological anatomy of the origin of the ophthalmic artery. In: Modern Problems in Ophthalmology, Vol. 14, Karger, Basel 164–169, 1975.
8. Payne EE, Spillane JD: The cervical spine. An anatomico-pathological study of 70 specimens

(using a special technique) with particular reference to the problem and cervical spondylosis. Brain, 80: 571–596, 1957.

9. Lazorthes G: Pathology, classification and clinical aspects of vascular diseases of the spinal cord. In: Vinken PJ, Bruyn GW (ed.), Handbook of Clinical Neurology, Vol. 12, North-Holland Publishing Company, Amsterdam, 492–506, 1972.

10. Willis T: Opera omnia: cerebri anatome, cui accesit nervorum descriptio et usus, Flesher J, London, 1664.

11. Padget DH: The circule of Willis. Its embryology and anatomy. In: Intracranial arterial aneurysms, ed. Danoy WE, Cormstock Publishing Company, New York, 1947.

12. Alpers BJ, Berry RG: Circle of Willis in cerebrovascular disorders. The anatomical structure. Archives of Neurology, 8, 398–402, 1963.

13. Riggs HE, Rupp CH: Variations in form of circle of Willis. The relation of the variations to collateral circulation: anatomic analysis. Archives of Neurology, 8: 8–14, 1963.

14. Fetterman GH, Moran TJ: Anomalies of the circle of Willis in relation to cerebral softening. Archives of Pathology, 32, 251–257, 1941.

15. Pitts FW: Variations of collateral circulation in internal carotid occlusion. Comparison of clinical and x-ray findings. Neurology 12: 467–471, 1962.

16. Kameyama M, Okinaka S: Collateral circulation of the brain. With special reference to atherosclerosis of the major cervical and cerebral arteries. Neurology, 13: 279–286, 1982.

17. Fogelholm R, Vuolio M. The collateral circulation via the ophthalmic artery in internal carotid aratery thrombosis. Acta Neurologica Scandinavica, 45: 78–86, 1969.

Normal blood flow in the arteries

M.P. Spencer

The arterial system is a many-branched elastic conduit for distribution of blood from the heart to all body tissues. Its calibre ranges from 4 cm for the human aorta to 4 micrometers for the capillaries. Over this wide range, the dynamics of each vascular segment may be described by various combinations of three fundamental physical properties: Resistance, Inertance and Compliance, collectively referred to as 'Impedance'. The term 'flow' refers to volumetric flux and is defined in units of volume per unit time such as ml/min or m^3/sec. 'Velocity' is a term which is expressed in distance per unit time such as cm/sec or m/sec. Acceleration is expressed in distance/time^2 expressed such as cm/sec/sec or m/sec/sec. 'Perfusion' is a term applied to the amount of flow per unit of tissues e.g. ml/min/100 grams.

Discrete arterial elements

Resistance arises from viscous losses in the blood flowing through the vessel segment. Hemodynamic resistance is analogous to electrical resistance which we symbolize ⎓⎓⎓ . Just as electricity is impelled by a voltage difference, blood always flows in the direction of the pressure gradient or pressure difference (Fig. 1). Resistance is normally found in the small arterials and a peripheral resistance unit (PRU) [1] is defined as one mmHg/min. The large arteries such as the aorta and its larger branches normally have very low resistance because they are so wide that very little pressure drop occurs as the blood flows through them. Only when abnormally narrowed do they develop a significant resistance. Resistance decreases with the 4th power of the radius of the artery lumen and increases directly with its length. According to Poiseuille, a French physician

$$R = \eta \frac{8\,l}{\pi r^4}$$

where R = resistance) η = the viscosity of blood) l & r = length and radius of the vessel segment.

RESISTANCE

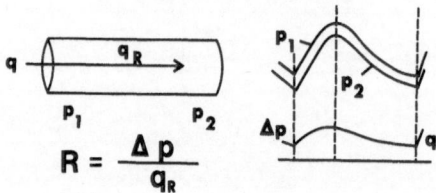

$$R = \frac{\Delta p}{q_R}$$

Figure 1. Relationship between pressure and flow through a vascular resistance vessel segment, q_R = volumetric flow p_1–p_2 represent two pressures along the vessel axis and $p = p_1$–p_2. During pulsating flow the pressure and flow waveforms rise and fall in phase with each other. This concept may be applied to the region of an arterial territory on the entire peripheral resistance.

The viscosity acts to produce a distribution of velocities across the diameter of the blood vessel. If flow is steady, the distribution assumes a parabolic shape (Fig. 2). This distribution of velocities in cross-section produces an even representation of velocities and a Doppler frequency spectrum of evenly distributed frequencies as shown in Fig. 2.

When the blood is accelerating due to the pumping action of the heart, the hemodynamics becomes more complex in the larger vessels and resistance alone no longer describes the pressure flow relationships. Two other important parameters, inertance and compliance called reactances come into play to greatly affect the pulsatile hemodynamics.

Inertance is most apparent in the heart aorta and larger arteries where resistance is small. Inertance arises primarily from the density (mass or weight) of the

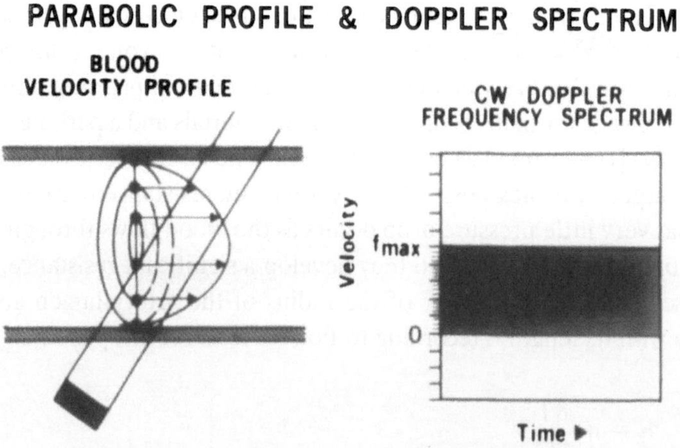

PARABOLIC PROFILE & DOPPLER SPECTRUM

**BLOOD
VELOCITY PROFILE**

**CW DOPPLER
FREQUENCY SPECTRUM**

Figure 2. Effect of fluid viscosity and laminar flow on the velocity profile. In a steady flow state a parabolic profile is developed with the slowest flow streams near the wall. Each flow stream nearer the vessel axis moves faster than the one outside. The right hand panel illustrates how the Doppler frequency spectrum represents a parabolic profile.

INERTANCE

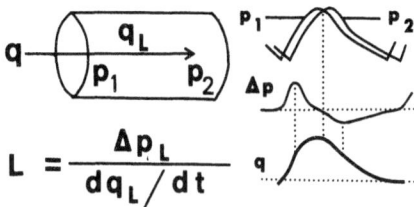

$$L = \frac{\Delta p_L}{dq_L/dt}$$

Figure 3. Relationship between pulsating pressure and flow in a large blood vessel segment where inertance is dominant and resistance is low. q and q_L represent blood flow while p_1 and p_2 represent upstream and downstream pressures respectively. $\triangle p$ represents the instantaneous pressure drop and dq_L/dt represent acceleration of the blood. Note that the peak of the $\triangle p$ curve occurs at the time of maximum acceleration of q and q reaches a peak when $\triangle p$ crosses zero.

blood and is analogous to electrical inductance symbolized as ⬛. Any *change* in electrical current through a coil of wire of an electrical inductance requires an initial peak of voltage difference in the direction of current flow to overcome the inductance of the coil. Similarly, any acceleration of the blood is attended by an acceleration transient in the blood pressure gradient along the segment of acceleration necessary to overcome the inertance of the blood mass (Fig. 3). A familiar example of the inertance property is apparent when pushing a person on an ice sled. One must push hard against the sled to accelerate it in order to get it going and pull back to stop it. During constant speed only enough push must be applied to overcome the small friction (resistance) between the runners and the ice.

Because inertance is defined in terms of volumetric acceleration the larger the lumen cross-section the smaller will be the inertance per unit length of vessel. Inertance increases directly with increase in length of the vessel. Because resistance is low in the larger vessels inertance produces large pulsations in blood flow.

The property of inertance in the aorta was first demonstrated [2] by direct measurement of the pressure difference along a 4 cm segment of the aorta through which volumetric flow was simultaneously measured. Fig. 4A illustrates the experimental arrangement for measurement of two pressures simultaneously along the aorta. By subtracting the downstream pressure (p_2) from the upstream pressure (p_1), the instantaneous pressure difference ($\triangle p$) across the segment was recorded. The instantaneous blood flow was recorded with the electromagnetic flowmeter applied to the aorta between the pressure recording needles. By inspection of Fig. 4B, one can see that during the systolic upslope of the flow pulse $\triangle p$ reaches a maximum positive value and during the following downstroke of flow $\triangle p$ reaches a maximum negative value. This phase lead of the pressure drop ahead of flow continues throughout subsequent oscillations in the heart cycle. This phase lead is a direct demonstration of the property of inertance in the large arteries. The periodic oscillation seen on the tracings of both flow and pressure drop is known as the arterial 'resonant wave'.

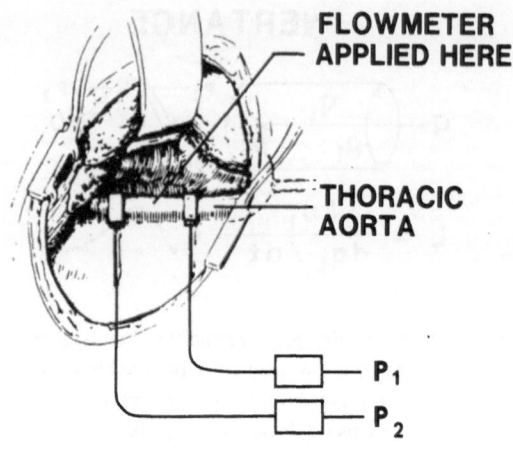

AORTIC FLOW AND DIFFERENTIAL PRESSURE

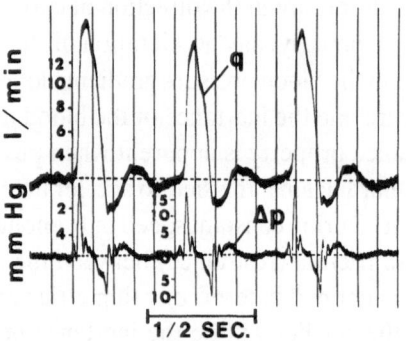

Figure 4A. Experimental arrangement for recording the instantaneous pressure drop along the descending thoracic aorta. p_1 was recorded upstream (nearer the heart) and p_2 downstream by means of hypodermic needles passed through the aorta wall and held stable by means of metal c-rings. Blood flow was recorded with the square wave electromagnetic flowmeter.

Figure 4B. Relationship between flow and $\triangle p$ in the dog's descending thoracic aorta recorded by the methods of Figure 4A. Each recorded flow acceleration is accompanied by a positive deflection seen on the $\triangle p$ tracing and each deceleration is accompanied by a negative deflection in $\triangle p$. Two backflow phases are seen on the flow tracing during diastole representing a resonant wave of blood oscillating back and forth in the aorta during diastole and with the same 90° phase shift compared to $\triangle p$.

The pulsation of flow streams in the arteries modifies the parabolic profile of a steady flow. During acceleration a more blunt profile is assumed which has a visible effect on the Doppler frequency spectrum. Fig. 5. During deceleration and during diastole the flow profile returns to a more parabolic shape.

Compliance is a property of the arterial wall arising from its distensibility and chiefly resides in the elastic fibers but also is contributed to by smooth muscle and

TEMPORAL ACCELERATION

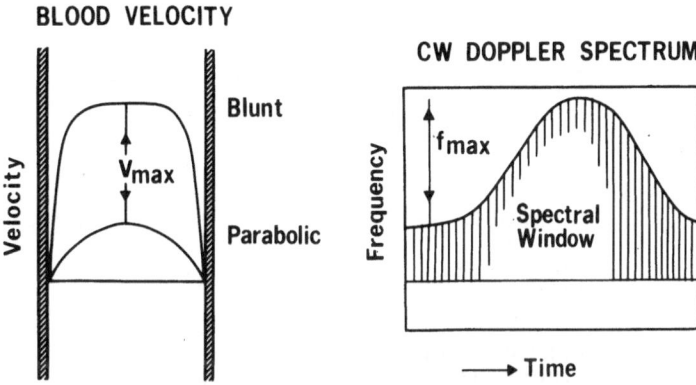

Figure 5. Effect of temporal acceleration on velocity profile and the Doppler frequency spectrum. Acceleration of blood produces a blunt blood velocity profile represented by a concentration of Doppler frequency spectral energies near f_{max}.

fibrous tissue. Vascular wall compliance is analogous to electrical capacitance which is symbolized as ⊣⊢. Just as an electrical capacitance represents the ability to accumulate a charge of electricity and discharge it back into the same circuit so compliance presents the ability of the arteries to expand and take up a volume of blood during systole then discharge it along the arteries during diastole. The action of compliance in a short arterial segment is diagrammed and defined in Fig. 6.

Combined arterial models

The property of compliance was represented in the early 'windkessel' concept of

COMPLIANCE

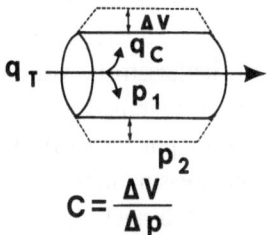

$$C = \frac{\Delta V}{\Delta p}$$

Figure 6. Diagrammatic and mathematical definition of compliance. q_T represents the flow into the segment which then is divided into an axial and radial component. q_c = radial component ΔV is the change in volume of blood in the vesel segment and Δp is the pressure difference between the inside of the vessel and the outside of the vessel. ΔV = the change in volume of the segment. The dotted lines represent the expansion and collapse of the vessel under the force imposed by Δp.

WINDKESSEL MODEL OF AORTA

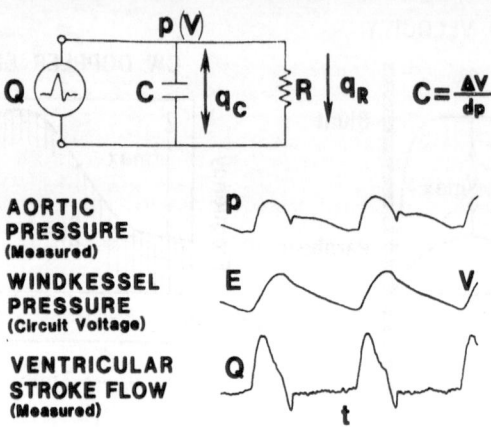

Figure 7. The 'Windkessel' concept is illustrated as a simple electrical analogy. The heart is represented as a flow generator with a stroke flow (Q). The fraction of Q in and out of the compliance (C) is designated q_C and that fraction flowing through the peripheral resistance (R) is designated q_R. Both Q and p were measured in the dog's aorta while the voltage (E) in the model was generated by inputting an electrical current shaped as Q into the circuit. The difference in shape between p and E are primarily due to the absence of an inertial component in the model.

the aorta which considered it to rapidly take up the cardiac stroke volume during systole and slowly discharge it during diastole through the peripheral resistance. Fig. 7 illustrates the 'windkessel' concept as a two component electrical analogy. The windkessel model of the arterial tree explains the overall rise and fall characteristic of the arterial pressure and demonstrates how flow runs off through the peripheral resistance during systole as well as diastole. The windkessel model does not explain how there is a higher systolic pressure in the legs than in the arm. A more complete and clinically useful model of the hemodynamics of the aorta and its major branches is illustrated in Fig. 8 [3]. Here the model of the arterial tree is expanded to two windkessels represented by two R-C circuits one for the aortic arch and its branches (R_1C_1) and one for the abdominal aorta and its branches (R_2C_2). They are connected by the single inertial element (L) representing the mass of blood in the aorta. The heart pumps directly into R_1C_1. The R_1C_1 windkessel absorbs the left ventricular stroke volume in systole while the inertiance of blood in the descending aorta impedes flow into R_2C_2. The acceleration pressure wave then moves the flow pulse (q_a) through (L) down the aorta, to enter the R_2C_2 windkessel. As the pressure in the lower windkessel then peaks the flow and pressure waves are reflected back up the aorta producing a resonate wave seen strongly in the descending aorta. Of course, this model still lumps the elements together while a distributed many element model would be more accurate but the model of Fig. 5 serves to understand many clinically important observations.

According to this model the arterial tree is a liquid-filled elastic tube which is

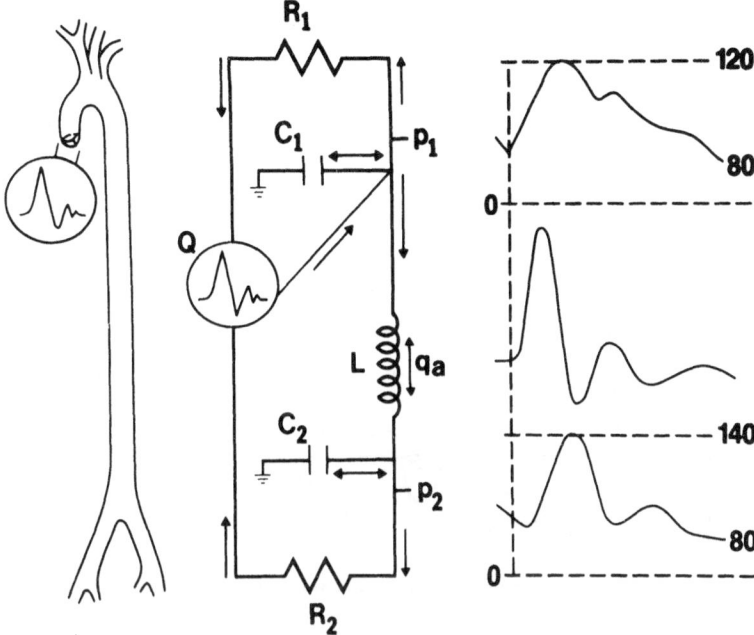

Figure 8. A model to explain the major pressure and flow relationships of the aorta and its major branches. See text for explanation of symbols. This model explains the resonant wave and how the systolic pressure in the arms is higher than in the legs. On the right are seen analog tracings of p_1 and flow (qa) through the inertance element.

caused to resonate each time the heart beats. The combination of the two capacitances with the blood produces resonant flow waves. The resonant wave and the 'standing' pressure wave of Hamilton [4] are necessary components of the interaction of inertiance and compliance. The dichrotic notch so prominent in the peripheral pressure and volume pulses is a representation of the standing wave. The peak systolic pressure in the legs is higher than in the arms because the compliance of the lower aorta and branches is smaller than that of the upper aorta, i.e., $C_2 < C_1$.

Flow pulses in the extremities

The amplitude of the resonant wave including backflow phases seen in peripheral arteries is affected by the peripheral resistance in the smaller arterioles, Fig. 9. Two conditions diminish the resonant wave amplitude: vasodilation of the downstream small arteries and obstruction of the proximal artery. Vasodilation raises the diastolic flow and dampens the resonant wave. This can be demonstrated on a normal subject by listening to the Doppler sound from the brachial artery while making a tight fist then releasing. While the fist is clenched the resonant wave in the arm persists as systolic forward and reverse flow only while the diastolic and

Carotid and Extremity Arteries

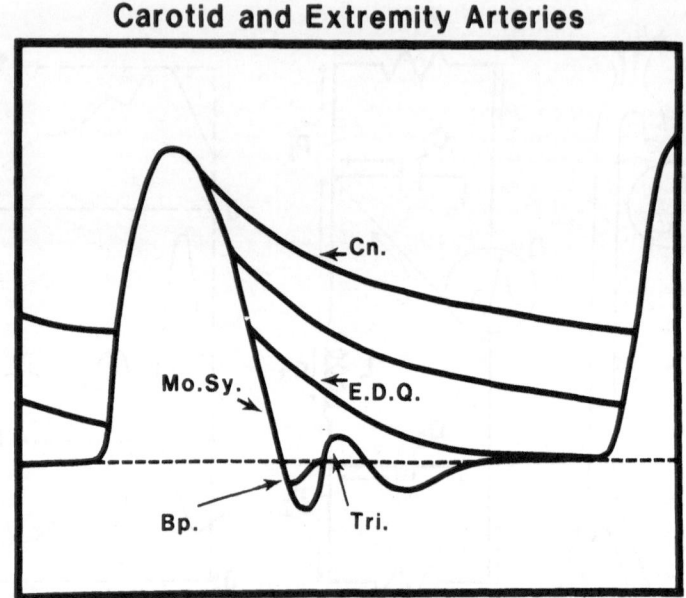

Figure 9. Diagram of blood flow velocity waveforms found in carotid and other peripheral arteries. Standard terminology is abbreviated. Cn = Continuous, EDQ = Early Diastolic Flow, Mo = Monophasic, Sy = Systolic, Bp = Biphasic and Tri = Triphasic.

mean flow are reduced by muscular compression of the downstream small arteries. Upon release of the clenched fist, reactive hyperemia in the distal bed produces vasodilation and increased flow velocity. During the reactive hyperemia response two features are particularly noticeable: 1) high diastolic flow, and 2) a decrease in the pulsatility of the resonant wave. Further discourse on flow pulses in the extremities and the effect of arterial obstructions is recommended for those interested [5, 6].

Characteristics of normal carotid artery blood flow

Fig. 10 illustrates the normal pulsatile wave form of human internal carotid blood flow signals measured with the electromagnetic flow meter simultaneously with P_1, P_2, and $\triangle p$. It is seen that the flow pulse waveform closely tracks the internal arterial pressure pulse, both of which are superimposed on a large static component. This characteristic indicates flow is primarily influenced by a low peripheral resistance. The brain vascular resistance is one of the lowest in the body. Both carotid and vertebral flow patterns are similar because they both feed the brain. The pattern of renal arterial flow will be found to be similar because the kidney also has a low vascular resistance.

Close inspection of the pressure difference in Fig. 10 discloses subtle features of

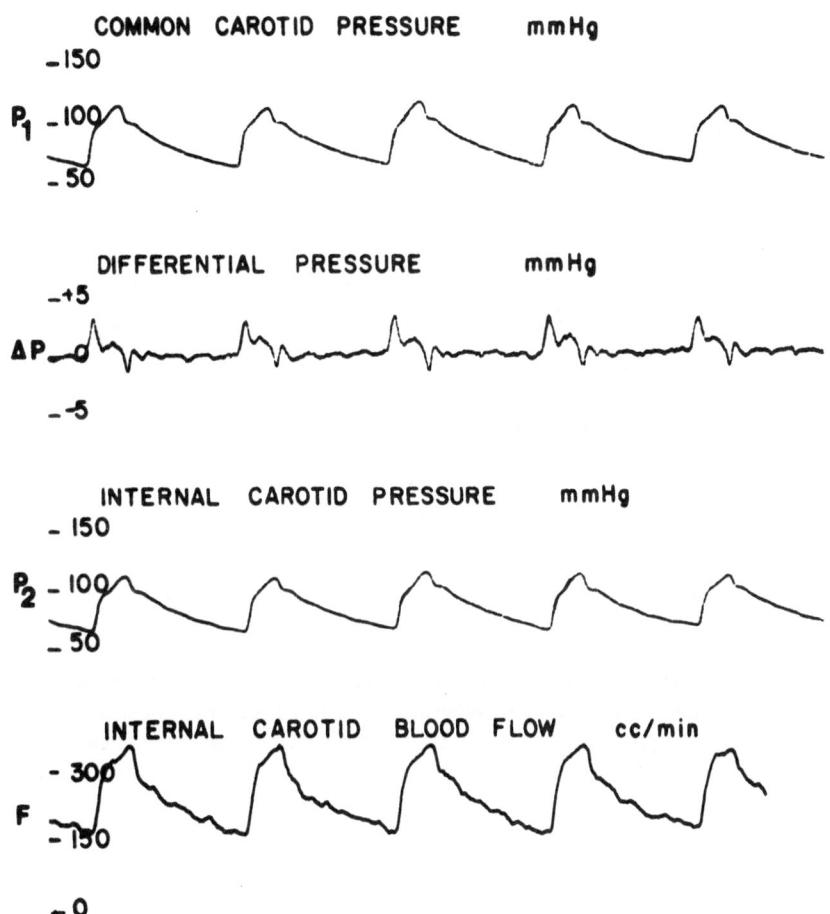

Figure 10. Relationship between pressure and flow in the normal human internal carotid artery measured during surgical anesthesia. The square-wave electromagnetic flowmeter was applied to the internal carotid to obtain the flow tracing (F). Two pressures were simultaneously recorded with high resolution strain gauges attached to needles puncturing the common carotid (p_1) and the internal carotid artery beyond the flowmeter (p_2). $\triangle p$ (differential pressure) is a tracing made by electrical substraction of p_1 and p_2. The similarity between p_1, p_2 and F is apparent indicating flow is primarily controlled by resistance. Subtle differences seen are explained in the text.

inertial flow superimposed on resistive flow. The first peak of $\triangle p$ in early systole and corresponds in time to the upstroke of the pressure flow tracings where a slight time lag produces an acceleration transient. Immediately following this transient, in mid-systole, a more rounded wave is seen on $\triangle p$ which corresponds to the time of maximum systolic flow. This mid-systolic pressure gradient is an expression of the small amount of resistance present in the short segment of artery between the pressure points. This is followed immediately by a decelaration transient. During diastole an almost imperceptible pressure gradient exists because the carotid artery is a low resistance artery.

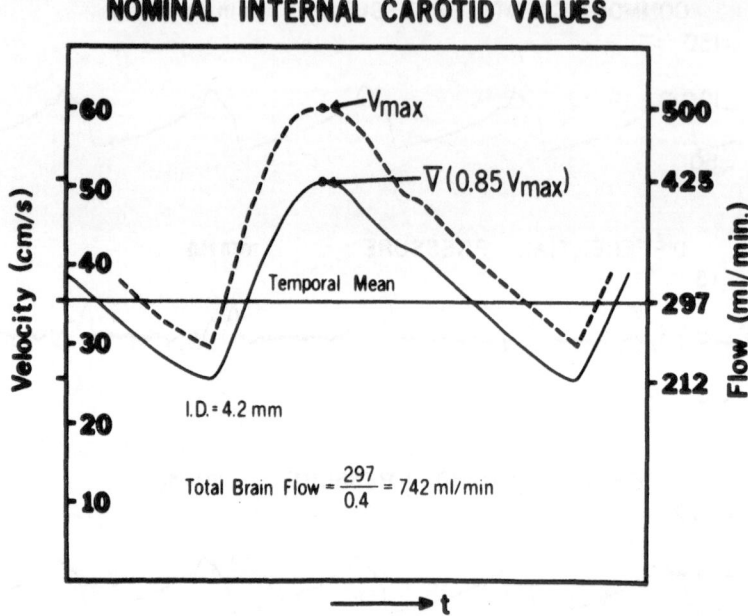

Figure 11. Representative blood velocity and corresponding flow values for the normal human internal carotid artery 4.2 mm in diameter. Total brain flow of 742 ml/m is assumed to be 40% supplied by one internal carotid. v represents instantaneous spatial velocity at the point of measurement. v_{max} is the maximum axial velocity seen on the Doppler frequency spectrum as f_{max}. $\bar{v}$ is the mean spatial velocity.

Fig. 11 presents some idealized characteristics of blood flow in the human internal carotid artery and some important definitions. The instantaneous mean velocity is approximately 85 percent of the maximum velocity. The lower pulse represents the spatial mean velocity extracted from the spatial mean frequency of the Doppler spectrum. The temporal mean flow (average over a complete heart cycle) is characteristic of an artery 4.2 mm in diameter supplying 40 percent of the brain's total blood flow.

A feature often seen on flow and velocity pulses of the internal carotid artery is a 'spike' on the early systolic phase and a 'dip' at the end of systole Fig. 12. This feature is particularly prominent in young persons less than 20 years of age where this spike and dip appear to represent more compliance of young arteries. It tends to disappear with age as the arteries become more stiff and is also less prominent in individuals who have a low peripheral resistance. Fig. 13 illustrates a CW Doppler spectrum with an early systolic spike and late systolic dip.

Doppler indices of peripheral resistance

Measurement of volumetric flow has proven difficult with Doppler because of problems in obtaining the angle between the soundbeam and the velocity direc-

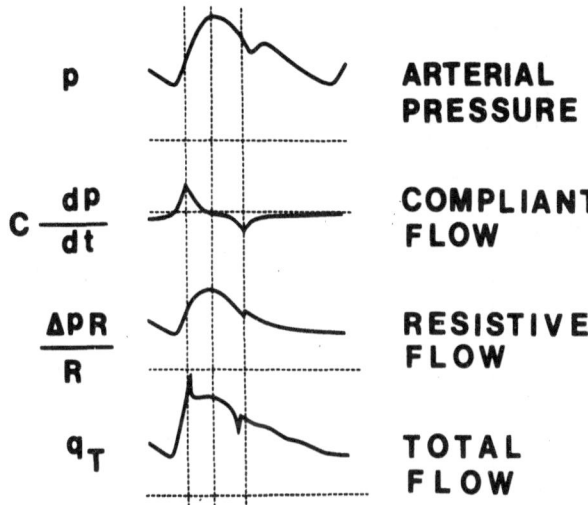

Figure 12. Combination of effects of compliant and resistive flow as often seen in the carotid arteries. Diagrammic representation of how a commonly seen flow waveform in the carotid arteries (q_T) is a summation of both wall compliance and peripheral resistance.

tion and also because the cross-sectional area is critical and difficult to measure. The flow waveform, however, is independent of the angle and has been used in estimating the peripheral resistance by the use of a pulsatility index (PI). Because internal carotid artery flow supplies the low resistance bed of the brain the magnitude of the diastolic component of the velocity pulse is particularly elevated

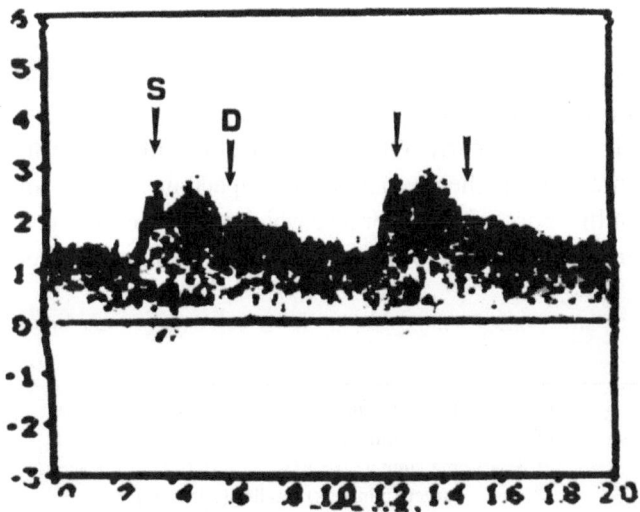

Figure 13. Doppler frequency spectrum of a normal signal from the internal carotid artery showing the 'Spike (S) and dip (D)' feature indicated by the arrows on the upper f_{max} edge. This results from the compliance of the artery distal to the site of measurement.

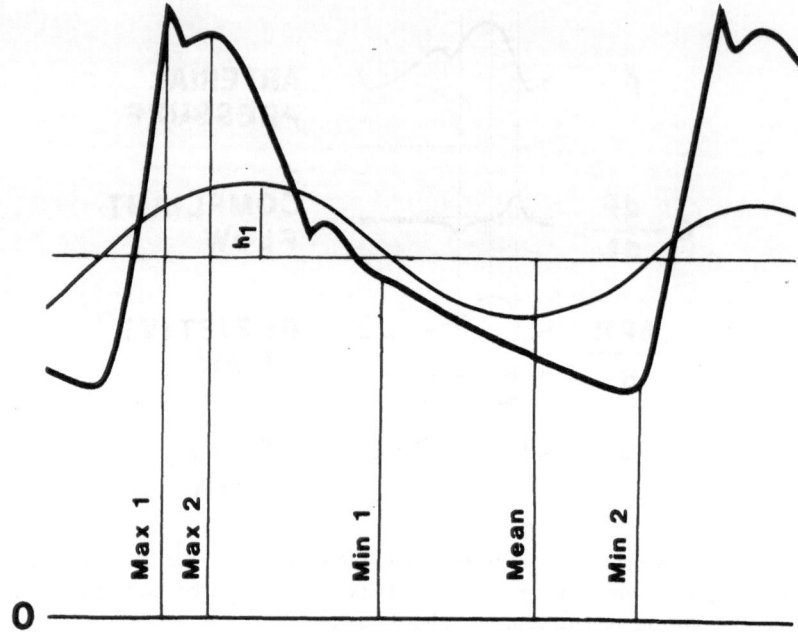

Figure 14. Diagram showing points of measurement for calculation of various pulsatility indices. Max 1 and 2 represent two choices for peak systolic measurement. Min 1 and 2 represent two choices for diastolic measurement. hl represents the amplitude of the first harmonic of the Fourier series computed from the waveform over the pulse cycle. 'Mean' represents the temporal mean valve averaged over the pulse cycle.

in comparison to the peripheral arteries. Table 1 lists several pulsatility indices in use. Fig. 14 diagrams the various points of measurement for calculation of pulsatility.

Gosling's index [7] was developed for lower extremity arteries but may be applied to the carotid arteries. The maximum peak occurring in systole may be the capacitative spike in early systole or may be the mid-systolic maximum which does not reflect the higher harmonics of capacitance. Mol's index [9] takes advantage of the more subtle difference which sometimes occurs between external and internal carotid waveforms occurring in early diastole. Archie's index [11]

Table 1.

Gosling [7]	1974	=	max2-min/mean
Pourcelot [8]	1974	=	max1-min/max
Mol [9]	1973	=	max/min 1
Archie [10]	1981	=	larger (min/max) smaller (min/max)
			comparing right and left carotids
Aaslid [11]	1986	=	1st harmonic/mean
Roederer [12]	1982	=	max – D1/max

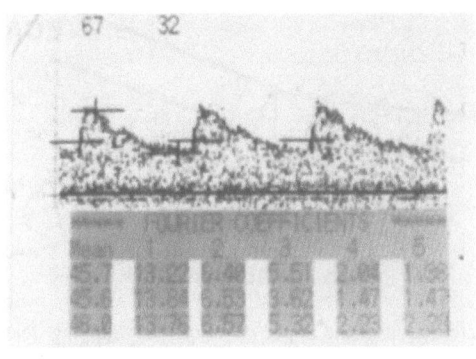

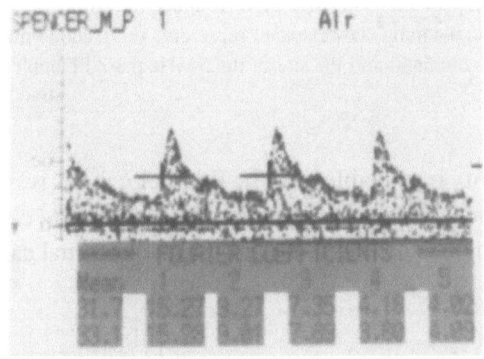

Figure 15. Velocity profiles present at the bifurcation of the normal common carotid artery (CCA). ECA and ICA designate the external and internal carotid arteries. A stagnant zone (shaded) may give rise to reversed flow eddies.

is useful in comparing one common carotid with the opposite when seeking the resistance of obstruction in one internal carotid artery vs the other.

The 'harmonic index' suggested by Gosling [7] and implemented by Aaslid *et al.*, [11] is the ratio of the amplitude of the 1st harmonic in the Fourier series to the mean value (h1/mean), Figure 15A and B. The second harmonic (h2) or higher harmonics may be used and may be more sensitive, however, accurate higher frequency recording of the signals applied to the Fourier analyzer must be assured.

Pourcelot [8] found the normal PI for the common carotid to range from 0.55 to 0.75 and in the case of thrombosis of the MCA was greater than 0.75. One must avoid the use of the early systolic spike in the use of mid-systolic maximum in applying this index. The pulsatility of velocities in the common carotid artery is always greater on the side of the occlusion of an internal carotid than on the nonobstructed side.

In summary, all of the pulsatility indices mentioned have validity and are useful. The user should validate the method he choses and establish numerical criteria for disease in his own laboratory. This author prefers the harmonic index

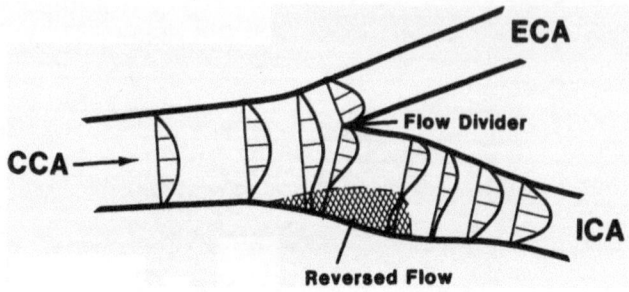

Figure 16. Spectral representation in the upper panel of the 'whipping' feature at peak maximum systole found using Doppler within the bulb of the normal internal carotid artery. Arrows indicate a transient peak on the top of the otherwise more rounded spectrum f_{max}. This feature does not represent atherosclerotic plaquing. Lower panel represents the B-mode image of the artery from which the spectrum was obtained and the site of the 5 MHz pulsed Doppler sample in the normal carotid sinus.

if computer capability is available, but the Pourcelot index is simpler to calculate. Even if no calculations are made, attention to the common carotid waveforms is helpful in separating occluded from non-occluded internal carotid arteries.

Special dynamics at the normal common carotid bifurcation

The bifurcation of the normal common carotid artery provides a situation where flow and pressure produce special effects which can be recognized in the Doppler frequency spectrum. An enlargement or bulb is present on the origin of the internal carotid artery which continues for 2–3 cm distal where the lumen then narrows to a constant diameter on to the base of the cranium. This enlargement called the carotid sinus or the 'bulb' may also include the end of the common carotid. The apparent purpose of the carotid sinus is to enhance the action of the 'stretch receptors' particularly concentrated at the carotid bifurcation. These 'pressure' receptors act through the sympathetic nervous system to control changes in arterial pressure insuring adequate pressure for brain perfusion when standing up from a recumbent position.

As the blood flow streams pass into the bifurcation and enter the bulb, their momentum carries the center of maximum velocities near the side of the flow divider that separates the origin of the internal from the origin of the external carotid artery. On the side of the bulb opposite to the flow divider a stagnant region develops where flow may even circulate in a reverse direction [13], Fig. 16. Maximum velocities and representative Doppler frequencies in the bulb are often lower than in the common carotid because of the dilatation there but accelerate again where the lumen narrows. Other phenomena of disturbed flow occur such as formation of helical flow streams tangential to the axis of the vessel. Turbulences may also develop in otherwise normal vessels at peak systole where the flow streams strike against the flow divider.

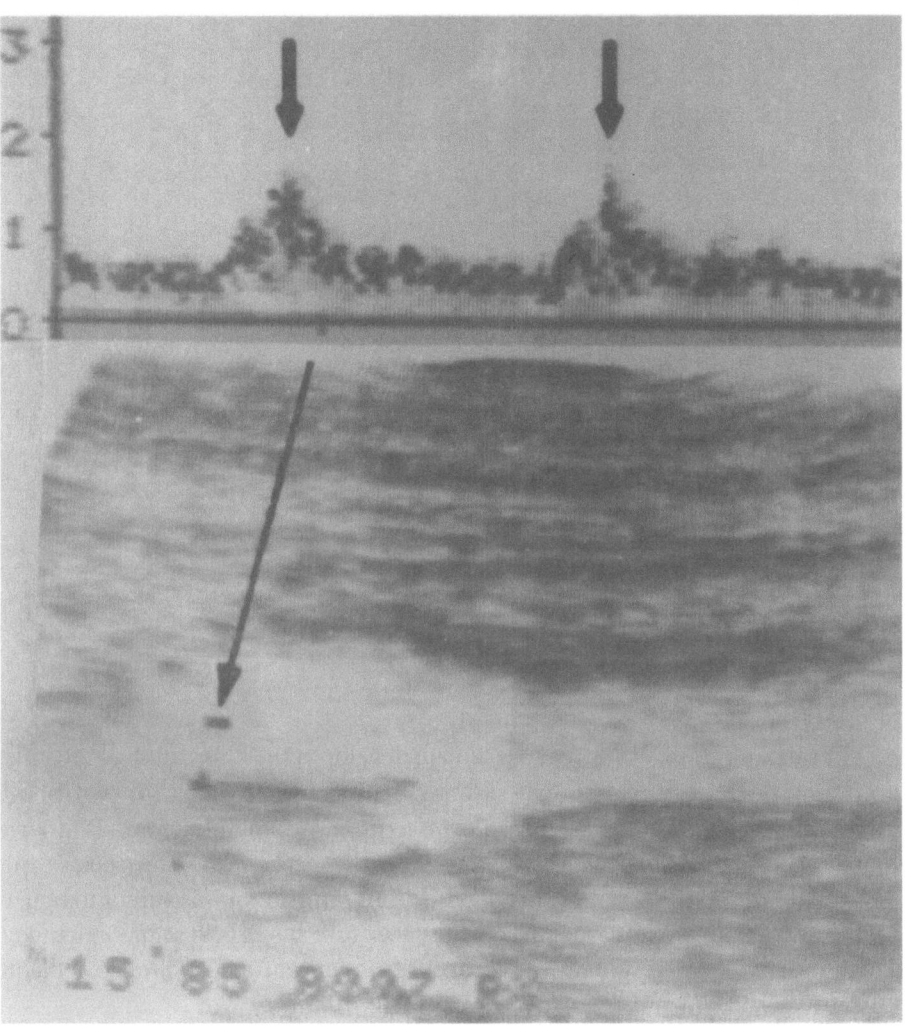

Figure 17. B-mode 5 MHz ultrasonic image of the bifurcation of the normal common carotid artery (C) demonstrating the wide diameter (B) measured across the beginning of the carotid sinus and origin of the external carotid artery (E). I_1 and I_2 represent the carotid sinus on the origin of the internal carotid artery. The widening of the carotid at its bifurcation provides a condition of increased wall tension which may be a mechanical factor in the site predilection for atherosclerosis.

When a bulb is present a special feature is seen on the continuous wave Doppler frequency spectrum called 'whipping'. It appears in mid-systole producing a spike or dip on the maximum frequency edge, Fig. 17. The cause of this feature is not yet completely explained but may represent tangential flow streams as described by Bharadvaj *et al.* [13]. This mid-systolic whip appears near the distal end of the bulb and is not considered an abnormality as it occurs quite frequently in young, distensible arteries. It does not represent atherosclerotic plaquing or stenosis.

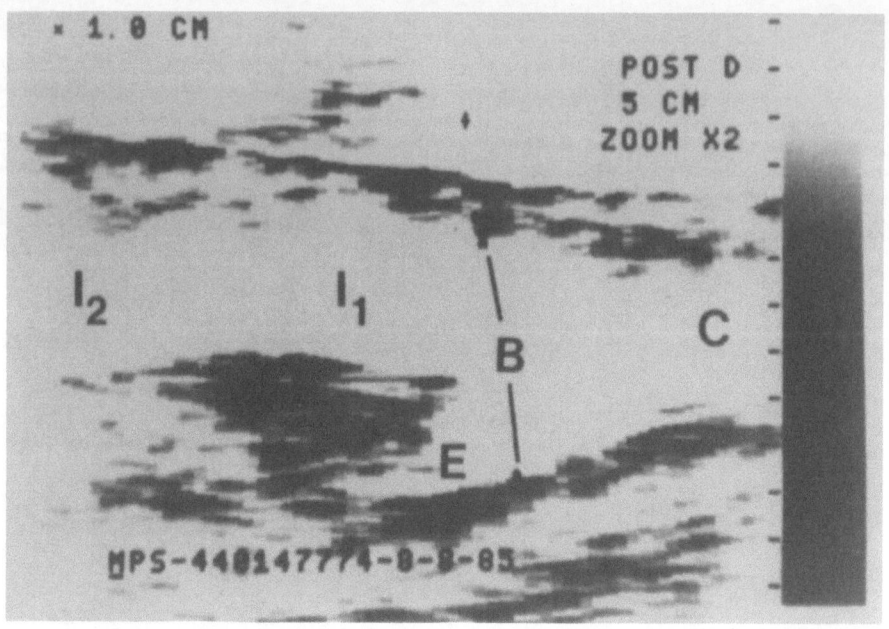

Because atherosclerotic plaques tend to develop at the bifurcation of the larger arteries, there is a widespread surmise that a mechanical factor works with biochemical and histological mechanisms to promote atherosclerosis. Bharadvaj and others propose low-wall shear stresses are the mechanical factor because they correlate with the locus of plaque deposits. It is difficult for this author to believe that artery walls would respond to an absence of shear stress. It seems more likely that the artery wall responds to a stress or strain concentrated at the site of plaque genesis.

An alternative hypothesis is presented here to provide the etiological mechanism for a predilection of plaquing at arterial bifurcations and in particular that of the common carotid bifurcation. It is proposed that the increased wall diameter at bifurcations increased tensions in the artery wall providing conditions for over-stretching of the endothelium to produce fractures. The histological processes leading to atherosclerosis are triggered as the repair and fracture process is repeated. Fig. 18 illustrates a normal common carotid bifurcation showing how the diameter just before the flow divider is greater than that of the common carotid or the bulb. The hypothesis set forth here assumes that wall tensions are greater at this location than lower in the common carotid or distal internal carotid. This follows from the La Place equation relating pressure in a vessel and its diameter to the tension in the wall. Such a hypothesis is also consistent with the apparent promotion of atherosclerosis by hypertension.

References

1. Green HD: Circulatory system: physical principles. In: Glasser (ed.), Medical Physics, Year Book Publ, Chicago, 2: 228–251, 1950.
2. Spencer MP *et al.:* Dynamics of the normal aorta: 'Inertiance' and 'Compliance' of the Arterial System which transforms the cardiac ejection pulse. Circ Res 6: 491, 1958.
3. Spencer MP, Denison AB: An explanation of the major features of the Arterial Pulse by Means of a Simple Analogy. Fed Proc *19* (1): 87, 1960.
4. Hamilton WF, Dow P: An experimental study of standing waves in the pulsed propogated through the aorta. Am J Physiol 125: 48, 1939.
5. Spencer MP: Frequency Spectrum Analysis in Doppler Diagnosis. In: Zwiebel WJ (ed.) Introduction to Vascular Ultrasonography, 2nd Edition. Grune and Stratton, New York, 1985.
6. Spencer MP, Denison A: In: Hamilton (ed) Pulsatile Blood Flow in the Vascular System. Handbook of Physiology – Circulation II, pp. 839–864, Chpt. 25, Am Physiol Soc, Publ, 1963.
7. Gosling RG, King DH: In: Reneman RS (ed) Continuous wave ultrasound as an alternative and complement to x-rays in vascular examinations, pp. 266–282. Cardiovascular Applications of Ultrasound, North-Holland, Amsterdam, 1974.
8. Pourcelot L: Applications cliniques de l'examen Doppler transcutane. Coloques de l'Institut National de la Sante' et de la Recherche Medicale. Inserm 34: pp. 213–240, 1974.
9. Mol JMF, Rijcken WJ: Doppler haematotachographic investigation in cerebral circulation disturbances. In: Reneman RS (ed), Cardiovascular applications of Ultrasound. North-Holland/American Elsevier, Amsterdam-London-NY, pp. 305–324, 1974.
10. Archie JP, Jr: A simple, non-dimensional, normalized common carotid Doppler velocity waveform index that identifies patients with carotid stenosis. Stroke 12: 3, pp. 322–324, May 1981.
11. Aaslid R, et al: Estimation of Cerebral Perfusion Pressure from Arterial Blood Pressure and Transcranial Doppler Recordings. Presented at the Sixth International Symposium on Intracranial Pressure, Glasgow 1985, Springer Verlag, Berlin, Heidelberg. In Press, 1986.
12. Roederer GO, Langlois YE, Chan AW, Primozich J, Lawrence RJ, Chikos PM, Strandness DE, Jr: Ultrasonic duplex scanning of the extracranial carotid arteries: improved accuracy using new features from the common carotid artery. J Cardiovascular Ultrasonography 1: 4, pp. 373–379, 1982.
13. Bharadvaj JB, Mabon RF and Giddens DP: Steady flow in a model of the human carotid bifurcation. Part II-Laser-Doppler anemometer measurements. J Biomech 15: 363–378, 1982.

Normal physiology and pathophysiology of human cerebral blood flow

P.C.M. Mosmans and E.J. Jonkman

The literature about physiology of the cerebral circulation is quite extensive since the study of the physiology of the cerebral circulation started in the latter half of the 19th century [1]. The possibility of studying human cerebral circulation *in vivo* by the use of radioactive isotopes has been an advance which has led to a large number of publications in this field. The studies of the physiology and pathology of the cerebral circulation have been published in many articles from numerous research groups. The reports are often overlapping in subject and results. Discrepancies in results and interpretation are frequently encountered and observations in normal volunteers have been relatively scarce. Our personal views of the subject only are presented in this chapter in order not to burden the reader with confusing discrepancies which arise when all the relevant literature is taken into consideration. This implies that a complete list of relevant literature will not be given and only a list of articles which can be considered as review articles or as representative papers for important topics is given at the end of this chapter.

Relevant Doppler problems and possibilities will be mentioned briefly; for details we may refer to the following chapters in this book.

Physiology of the cerebral circulation

Compared with other tissues the brain has remarkable high metabolic needs. The mean brain metabolism is only slightly enhanced when cerebral activation is present [2]. Cerebral glucose utilization is about 70% of the resting glucose output (while the brain comprises only 2% of the average body weight). The normal average blood flow through the brain is approximately 60 ml/min/100 gram. For the average brain weight this amounts to 900–1100 ml/min, which is 12–15% of the resting cardiac output. The cerebral blood flow value mentioned above is, however, a mean value. Blood flow through the white matter is considerably lower, blood flow through the grey matter is considerably higher. Moreover, regional differences are also present. With increasing age mean cerebral blood flow decreases [3].

The metabolism of brain tissue is extremely dependent on continuous and adequate supply of oxygen and glucose. Enhancement or diminution of the cerebral circulation does not, within certain limits, produce subjective or objective alterations in the clinical state; but, if circulation falls below a certain level (15–20 ml/min/100 gram) reversible impairment of cerebral function occurs; below a lower level irreversible brain damage is certain to occur. From animal experiments it is known that flow reduction below a certain threshold is accompanied by changes in the EEG pattern and a decrease in evoked potentials [4]. Among others [5], could demonstrate in animals a penumbra existing between functional and structural neuronal damage in regional cerebral blood flow disturbances. In the ischemic penumbra the neurons remain structurally intact but functionally inactive. An increase in blood flow, if sufficient, can restore electrical activity of the neurons. Blood flow below the lower limit of the penumbra resulted in massive release of intracellular potassium and cell death. It is likely that in human beings the same pathophysiologic mechanisms exists in case of regional disturbances of blood flow.

The total blood flow reaching the brain is divided between the two carotid arteries and the two vertebral arteries. In normals asymmetries occur (at least up to 30%) in the flow through both carotid arteries and sometimes these asymmetries are even larger for the flow through both vertebral arteries. Moreover, the watershed between the area of the carotid arteries and the vertebral arteries can differ from person to person. This implies that if one tries to measure the total cerebral blood flow (e.g. by ultrasound methods) one always has to measure all four cerebropetal vessels.

Blood pressure and the mechanism of autoregulation

The cerebral blood flow through the brain is determined by the pressure gradient between input and output of the system and the cerebrovascular resistance. In animal experiments no essential differences could be found between pulsating flow and non-pulsating flow [6]. It can be assumed that in man a continuous (non-pulsating) flow is well tolerated (extracorporal circulation in open-heart surgery) and is subject to the same regulation mechanisms existing for the pulsating flow. The pressure at the output of the system in man is rather low, the normal venous pressure in the skull about equals the tissue pressure (= intracranial pressure). The values show oscillations with the respiration and the heart rate but the normal values (20–40 mm H20 positive with respect to the right auricle) are very low compared with the input pressure. So the perfusion is determined mainly by the mean arterial blood pressure (MABP).

The cerebrovascular resistance is partially determined by the resistance in the brain capillaries (the term 'cerebrovascular resistance' instead of perhaps more appropriate 'cerebrovascular impedance' is still general use). This resistance can be assumed to be a constant because in the brain there are no possibilities to shut off or open important parts of the capillary system. Such a system could not exist because of the constant high metabolic need of the neurons. The most important determinant of cerebrovascular resistance is the resistance in the arterioles. This resistance, in series with capillary resistance, is not a constant. The arterioles have the ability to narrow or to dilate within a certain range. The effect being that the total cerebrovascular resistance can vary between certain limits.

The variability in cerebrovascular resistance makes it possible for the brain to maintain a constant cerebral blood flow which is to a large degree independent of the mean arterial blood pressure: if mean arterial blood pressure goes up, so does the cerebrovascular resistance, lowering of the mean arterial blood pressure results in a dilatation of the arterioles, resulting in a decrease in cerebrovascular resistance. This regulatory mechanism is called autoregulation, it plays the main part in maintaining a constant cerebral blood flow but can be easily disturbed by cerebral disorders. Autoregulation, however, is limited. There is a maximum possible dilatation of the arterioles and also the narrowing of these vessels has an obvious limit. In other words, the range of variations of cerebrovascular resistance has an upper and lower limit. Between these limits blood flow through the brain is independent of variations in MABP and the mechanism of autoregulation protects the brain against changes in systemic blood pressure [7]. Outside these limits the blood flow is passively pressure dependent. It will be clear that surpassing the lower and upper limits of autoregulation will be hazardous for the patient. In patients with chronic hypertension cerebral blood flow autoregulation is adapted to levels above those in normals.

There are 3 hypotheses for the underlying mechanisms of autoregulation:
– the neurogenic theory. The arteries in the brain are supplied by small nerve-fibres, probably originating in the upper brainstem. Neurohistological techniques have demonstrated several cerebral vascular neuro-effector mechanisms [8].
– the myogenic theory. The smooth muscle fibres in the arteriolar wall react directly to transmural pressure changes.
– metabolic theory. According to this theory changes in blood flow induced by changes in perfusion pressure are immediately followed by changes in metabolism and therefore by changes of brain tissue pH.
A decrease in pH produces a dilatation of the arterioles, an increase in pH a constriction.

The mechanisms which are involved in autoregulation are not completely understood; however, it is obvious from animal experiments that many factors play a role; for example, the influence of prostaglandines and neurotransmitters [9].

It should be pointed out that an increase in blood pressure does not necessarily have an influence on the diameter of larger arteries. This results in a constancy of the flow velocity e.g. in the carotid artery during modest increases or decreases of

MABP (the cerebral blood flow and the vessel diameter both being maintained at a fixed level). Besides the factors mentioned above another factor is of importance concerning blood flow. According to Poiseuille's law vascular resistance is not only influenced by the diameter of the lumen of the blood vessels and their length but to a certain degree also by blood viscosity [10]. From several studies it is clear that an increase of blood viscosity results in a decrease of blood flow. However, the influence on brain metabolism under these circumstances is not yet clear [11].

Influence of arterial pCO2 and pO2 on Cerebral blood flow

Hypercapnia causes a dilatation of the cerebral arterioles while hypocapnia produces a vasoconstriction. In normals there exists an almost linear relationship between changes in arterial pCO2 and cerebral blood flow (1% change in arterial pCO2 giving a change of about 2.2% of the resting value in cerebral blood flow [12]. The physiological meaning might be that acidosis caused by insufficient metabolism gives a vasodilatation and a better perfusion of the tissue. This seems to be the same mechanism as described under 'metabolic theory of autoregulation'. In brain disease, however, autoregulation can be impaired without disturbances of the CO2 response or vice versa [13]. The influence of arterial pCO2 can be important in Doppler flow velocity measurements. Changes in pCO2 results in changes in cerebral blood flow but do not influence the diameter of the larger arteries. An increase in pCO2 results in an increase in the flow velocity in the carotid arteries as can be measured with Doppler ultrasound techniques [14]. It is assumed that an increase of arterial pO2 results in a decrease, and a decrease of arterial pO2 results in an increase of the cerebral blood flow.

Regulation by metabolism

The assurance of an adequate blood supply meaning a correspondence between the actual rate of capillary blood flow and the metabolic demands is the most important of all regulatory mechanisms [15, 16].

In clinical practice it will be difficult to predict the overall result on cerebral blood flow after changes in blood pressure, ApCO2 and ApO2. One of the reasons is that there exists a very complicated inter-relationship between the effects of changes of aterial pO2, arterial pCO2 and blood pressure [8].

Pathophysiology of cerebral blood flow

Cerebrovascular diseases can be described and studied from many points of view.

The Ad Hoc Committee on Cerebrovascular Disease published a survey about the different aspects of cerebrovascular disease in 1975 [17]. Several pathophysiological mechanisms may play a role in the development of symptoms in patients suffering from a cerebrovascular accident. In part, these mechanisms are due to disturbances in the regulation mechanisms existing under physiological conditions like autoregulation and reactivity to changes in arterial pCO_2 and pO_2. To a certain degree these mechanisms protect the brain from inadequate blood and inadequate substrate supply. However, another protecting system should be mentioned: the collateral vascular system discussed later. This system can protect the brain from insufficient blood supply. Moreover, some other phenomena appear under pathological circumstances, e.g. the luxury perfusion syndrome and the steal syndromes.

Loss of normally regulating mechanisms

Autoregulation can be changed or abolished by cerebral or generalized disease. In the literature we can find references indicating that autoregulation can be lost globally or focally in patients with for example cerebral tumors, cerebral hemorrhage, ischemic cerebral disease, cerebral trauma, meningitis, encephalitis, subarachnoidal bleeding, hydrocephalus, during induced seizures, under hypercapnia, in Shy Drager syndrome [18] and in diabetes [19]. Especially in patients suffering from an acute severe cerebral lesion one should assume autoregulation to be diminished or lost until proven otherwise. Repeated blood flow measurements are hardly feasible in severely ill neurological patients so it is difficult to prove a disturbance of autoregulation. Doppler measurements however are innocuous. Changes in flow velocity with changes in MABP can put the clinician to the track of an impairment in autoregulation. This knowledge can be of importance in handling problems concerning blood pressure in patients suffering from diseases as mentioned above.

Abnormal reactions to changes in arterial pCO_2 and pO_2 result in a redistribution of blood flow, producing steal and inversed steal syndromes. It was already mentioned that hypercapnia (increase in arterial pCO_2) causes dilatation of cerebral arteries. This is a useful mechanism in cases with increased metabolic needs. However, generalized hypercapnia in patients with localized ischemia sometimes produces a deterioration of the cerebral blood flow conditions rather than an improvement. The study of the cerebral blood flow in animals with artifically induced local ischemia presented the solution of this problem: the arterioles in the ischemic brain area are already maximally dilated, probably partially by the fall of tissue pH in the ischemic region. When the vascular bed in the non-ischemic area is dilated by induced hypercapnia, a redistribution of the blood supply takes in favor of the healthy parts of the brain and at the cost of the already ischemic areas. This phenomenon is called 'intracerebral steal': the blood is 'stolen' from the ischemic area and supplied to the healthy brain tissue [20]. Hypocapnia on the contrary, can produce vasoconstriction of arteries in the non-ischemic brain area and has no effect on the maximally dilated arteries in the ischemic area where CO_2 responsiveness is lost. In this situation redistribution of the blood supply is now in favor of the ischemic brain tissue. This is called 'inversed steal'. This mechanism could have clinical implications.

Nevertheless, the clinical beneficiary effect of hypocapnia (induced by artificial hyperventilation) has never been proven in larger series of patients with ischemic brain disease [21]. It should be pointed out that 'intracranial steal' and 'reversed steal' have no influence on the total cerebral blood flow and cannot be detected by flow velocity studies of the large arteries. The same applies to a seldom encountered phenomenon: the so-called interhemispheric steal [22]. This is a situation where one hemisphere (e.g. after occlusion of the supplying carotid artery) steals blood from the contralateral hemisphere (e.g. through the circle of Willis). If a partial vascular occlusion is also present in the deprived hemisphere, neurological symptoms may rise originating from the side contralateral to the occlusion of the carotid artery.

Influence of hypoxia. Severe hypoxia (pO_2 in the arterial blood <55 mmHg) produces a dilatation of the arterioles. This is an example of an adequate defense mechanism, trying to prevent brain ischemia. The vasodilatation is probably caused in part by a fall of pH in the ischemic brain tissue. The change from aerobic to anaerobic metabolism, where lactate is produced, is responsible for this fall in pH.

The collateral vascular system

Though most focal ischemic cerebrovascular disease symptoms are due to emboli, an ischemia due to hemodynamic insufficiency does occur. In most cases, this is due to a severe stenosis in one of the major supplying arteries to the brain. Although a stenosis of 50% or more can produce a measurable pressure gradient over the stenosis, in most cases a reduction in cerebral blood flow is only measurable when the lumen diameter of the supplying artery is less than 1.5 mm [23].

Vasodilatation of the vascular tree distal to the stenosis can compensate to a large degree for diminished input pressure. This makes an early diagnosis of arterial stenosis difficult. Some patients show their first neurological deficit only when a vessel is either totally occluded or almost totally occluded.

The collateral system may play an important role in maintaining cerebral circulation. Several connections exist between the arterial systems which supply blood to the brain. These connections can serve as a defense mechanism for the brain in the case of failure of one of the major supplying arteries. The most important of these anastomoses are:

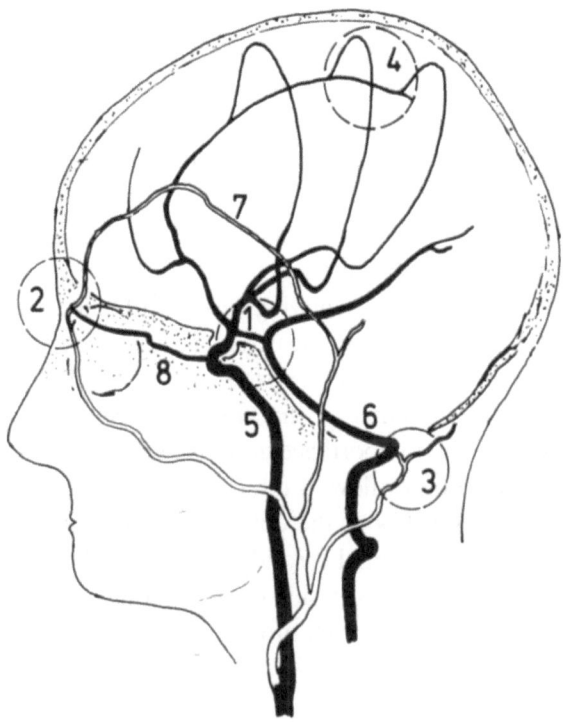

Figure 1.

Main anastomoses:
1. Circle of Willis; 2. Connection between ophthalmic artery and branches of external carotid artery; 3. Anastomoses between vertebral artery and branches of the external carotid artery; 4. Leptomeningeal anastomoses.

Main arteries:
5. Internal carotid artery; 6. Vertebral/basilar artery; 7. Superficial temporal artery (branch of the external carotid artery); 8. Ophthalmic artery.

Territories of the internal carotid and vertebral arteries are indicated in black. The external carotid artery and its branches are indicated in white.

- the circle of Willis, which forms the main anastomosis between the internal carotid arteries (and their main branches) and the vertebro basilar artery system, Fig. 1, (1)
- connections of several branches of the external carotid artery with branches of the ophthalmic artery thus forming an anastomosis between the external and internal carotid arteries, Fig. 1, (2)
- branches of the external carotid artery which are connected with branches of the vertebral artery, Fig. 1, (3)
- the so called 'leptomeningeal anastomosis', interconnections between the cortical branches of the anterior, middle and posterior cerebral arteries, Fig. 1, (4)

Anatomicaly and angiographically the presence of other anastomoses has been established. However, it is doubtful that these can have a real function in cases of vessel occlusion [24]. Via these anastomosis collateral circulation can take place. Fields [25] defines collateral circulation as follows: 'Collateral circulation is a term assigned to the subsidiary vascular channels, present throughout the circulatory network, which provide a secondary defense mechanism against failure of the primary blood vessels.'

The collateral vascular system is not of benefit in all patients with an occlusion of one of the major supplying arteries to the brain. For example, in some cases extensive steal mechaninisms, depriving the brain of blood, can develop resulting in the subclavian steal syndrome, the external carotid artery steal syndrome, and so on. In these cases, the collateral system may play a detrimental role [26].

Estimation of the direction of the blood flow with a directional Doppler apparatus can be of great importance in cases of collateral such as estimation of magnitude and direction of flow in the branches of the ophthalmic artery. An inward flow in the branches of the ophthalmic artery indicates an insufficient supply of the ipsilateral internal carotid artery. An enhanced outward flow can indicate a severe stenosis or occlusion of the internal carotid artery distal to the branching of the ophthalmic artery or an increased intracranial pressure.

Effect of increased intracranial pressure

Reconstructive surgery of the major arteries should be considered in patients with ischemic disease due to a local obstruction of one of these arteries. Early detection of these operable stenoses is the most important and most rewarding task for Doppler flow velocity measurement techniques. Another possibility in vascular surgery is the so called 'bypass technique.' A branch of the external carotid artery is connected (through a burr hole in the skull) with a branch of the internal carotid artery (middle cerebral artery in most cases), thus creating a normally non-existent anastomosis which 'bypasses' an obstruction in the internal carotid artery or one of its primary branches.

From the point of view of Doppler technology it might be worthwhile to note that this artificial anastomosis can be easily studied by ultrasound techniques. This is a simple way to prove the patency of such anastomosis.

Under physiological conditions the perfusion pressure of the brain is mainly determined by the MABP, both the intracranial pressure and venous pressure having a low value. Under pathological conditions (especially space occupying lesions like cerebral edema, intracranial hemorrhage, tumors etc.) intracranial pressure may slowly or abruptly rise to high values. This rise causes a diminished perfusion pressure when mean arterial blood pressure remains constant. As long as the difference between MABP and intracranial pressure equals at least 50 mmHg and autoregulation is intact; i.e., a rise in intracranial pressure does not always diminish cerebral blood flow. In clinical practice, however, increased intracranial pressure often leads to decreased cerebral blood flow. This decrease in cerebral blood flow resulting in a decrease of flow velocity can be demonstrated in patients with hydrocephalus, subarachnoidal bleeding or cerebral tumors in whom a short lasting increase in intracranial pressure was artificially induced or occurred spontaneously [14]. It will be apparent that a disastrous situation arises when the intracranial pressure raises to such heights that the perfusion pressure gets very low and ultimately equals zero. At this point no cerebral circulation is possible any longer and the brain dies. In this situation the flow through the common carotid artery mainly represents the flow through the external carotid artery only. This situation can be evaluated by Doppler flow velocity measurements (disappearance of diastolic flow in the common carotid artery and a short lasting reversal of flow velocity after the systole).

Sometimes when intracranial pressure reaches very high levels and comes close to the diastolic arterial blood pressure a very interesting reaction is set into action by the body: the MABP increases to prevent a complete abolition of the perfusion pressure. This mechanism, the Cushing reflex, is probably one of the defense mechanisms of the body but, unfortunately, it is usually the beginning of a disastrous viscious circle. When perfusion pressure is very low, all arterioles become maximally dilated. This dilatation, which means an increase in intracranial blood volume, implies an increase in intracranial pressure. The intracranial pressure may be further increased by cerebral edema. This increase in intracranial pressure is once again a stimulus to increase blood pressure and a viscious cycle occurs.

Luxury perfusion syndrome

This syndrome, for the first time described by Lassen [27], is an acute disturbance of the cerebral circulation associated with severe brain damage. The syndrome is characterized by an excessive blood supply as related to the abnormally low metabolic needs of the brain tissue. Because the uptake of oxygen is low, the difference in pO2 between arteria and venous blood is abnormally small in these circumstances. The syndrome can appear in a whole hemisphere, but also more locally. The syndrome occurs particularly in acute cerebral disburbances such as vascular accidents and brain injuries.

Diaschisis

Following the acute onset of unilateral cerebral infarction, the blood flow in the contralateral hemisphere may be reduced. The pathogenesis of this well known phenomenon is not clearly understood. Over the weeks following regional infarction, the blood flow returns to normal in the noninvolved hemisphere. The flow in the infarcted area remains reduced [28]. Studies with the positron emitting scan

(PET scan) have demonstrated that not only blood flow but also the metabolic rate is lowered in the contralateral hemisphere as well [29].

Vasospasms and arteriovenous malformations

Two principally different conditions will be described here, both leading to ischemia in smaller or larger areas of brain tissue. Severe vascular spasms may result in an insufficient blood supply of (part of) the brain. The benign forms of vascular spasms e.g. as encountered in migraine, rarely lead to permanent neurological deficit but in isolated cases this is possible [30].

The most severe spasms, often resulting in severe impairment of cerebral circulation, are encountered in patients with subarachnoidal hemorrhage. This is a bleeding from an abnormal congenital or acquired outpouching of the arterial wall (aneurysm) in most cases. Such bleeding may in itself have disastrous results or even cause sudden death. If the patient survives for several days, cerebral arterial spasms may occur, probably induced by the blood around the cerebral arteries. These spasms are sometimes more important to the clinical outcome than the bleeding itself [31].

Arteriovenous malformations are a developmental or traumatic disorder in which direct connections exist between the arterial and venous system without the normal system of small arteries, capillaries and small veins. These pathological connections can be quite large. Moreover, the vessel wall of these structures has often an abnormal structure prone to rupture and bleeding. Apart from this, the locally diminished cerebrovascular resistance gives rise to shunting of the blood from the arterial to the venous system without any participation of this blood in the normal metabolic process. This shunting of the blood may attain such proportions that the blood is withdrawn from neighboring areas leading to ischemic disturbances in a smaller or larger part of the surrounding brain tissue. It will be understandable that this kind of ischemic brain disease is the only one where blood flow velocity in the common carotid artery, as measured by Doppler techniques is not diminished but normal or even enhanced.

References

1. Purves MJ: The Physiology of the Cerebral Circulation. Cambridge University Press, 1972.
2. Ingvar DH: Patterns of brain activity revealed by measurements of regional cerebral blood flow. In: Benzon A (ed.) Brain Work, Symposium VIII pp. 397–413, Munksgaard, Copenhagen, 1975.
3. Naritomi H, Meyer JS, Sakai F, Yamaguchi F, Shaw T: Effects of advancing age on regional cerebral blood flow. Arch. Neurol. 36: 410–416, 1979.
4. Branston NM, Symon L, Crockard HA: Recovery of the cortical evoked response following temporary middle cerebral artery occlusion in baboons: relation to local blood flow and pO2. Stroke 7: 151–157, 1976.

5. Astrup J, Siesjö BK, Symon L: Thresholds in cerebral ischemia – The ischemic penumbra. Stroke 12: 723–725, 1981.

6. Held K, Gottstein U, Niedermeyer W: CBF in non-pulsatile perfusion. In: Cerebral Blood Flow. (Brock M, Fieschi C, Ingvar DH, Lassen NA, Schürmann K eds), pp. 94–95, Springer Verlag, Berlin Heidelberg New York, 1969.

7. Strandgaard S, Paulson OB: Cerebral autoregulation. Stroke 15: 413–416, 1984.

8. Mchedlishvilli G: Physiological mechanisms controlling cerebral blood flow. Stroke 11: 240–248, 1980.

9. Pickard JD: Prostaglandin mechanisms and the relationship between local glucose utilization and local blood flow. J Cereb. Blood Flow Metabol. 1: S291–S292, 1981.

10. Häggendall E, Norback B: Effect of viscosity on cerebral blood flow. Acta Chir. Scand. Suppl. 364: 13–22, 1966.

11. Marshall J: The viscosity factor in cerebral ischemia. J. Cer. Blood Flow Metabol. S47–S49, 1982.

12. Reivich M: Arterial pCO2 and cerebral hemodynamics. Am. J. Physiol. 206: 25–35, 1964.

13. Fieschi C, Agnoli A, Battistini N, Bozzao L: Derangement of regional cerebral blood flow and of its regulatory mechanisms in acute cerebrovascular lesions. Neurology 18: 1166–1179, 1968.

14. Jonkman EJ, Tans JTJ, Mosmans PCM: Doppler flow velocity measurements in patients with intracranial hypertension. J. Neurol. 218: 1157–169, 1978.

15. Betz E: Cerebral blood flow: its measurement and regulation. Physiol. Rev. 52: 595–630, 1972.

16. Raichle ME, Grubb RL, Gado MH, Eichling JO, Ter-Pogossian MM: Correlation between regional blood flow and oxidative metabolism. Arch. Neurol. 33: 523–526, 1976.

17. Millikan CH et al: A Classification and Outline of Cerebrovascular Disease II. Stroke 6, 565–616, 1975.

18. Depresseux JC, Rousseau JJ, Franck G: The autoregulation of cerebral blood flow, the cerebrovascular reactivity and their interaction in the Shy-Drager syndrome. Europ. Neurol. 18: 295–301, 1979.

19. Dandona P,.James IM, Newbury PA, Woollard ML, Beckett AG: Cerebral blood flow in diabetes mellitus: evidences of abnormal cerebrovascular reactivity. Brit. Med. Journal 2: 325–326, 1978.

20. Lassen NA, Palvölgyi R: Cerebral steal during hypercapnia and the inverse reaction during hypocapnia observed by the 133-Xenon technique in man. Scand. J. Clin. Lab. Invest. Suppl. 102 sect. XIII: D, 1968.

21. Christensen MS, Paulson OB: Prolonged artificial hyperventilation in severe cerebral apoplexy. Europ. Neurol. 8: 137–141, 1972.

22. Zulch KJ, Eschbach O: The interhemispheric steal syndromes. Neuroradiol. 4: 179–184, 1972.

23. Spencer MP, Reid JM: Quantitation of carotid stenosis with continuous-wave (CW) Doppler ultrasound. Stroke 10: 326–330, 1979.

24. Fields WS, Weibel J: Collateral circulation of the brain. The Williams and Wilkins Comp. Publishers, Springfield, Illinois, 1965.

25. Fields WS: Arteriography collateral circulation in cerebrovascular disease. In: Zulch KJ (ed.) Cerebral Circulation and Stroke pp. 100–105. Springer Verlag, Berlin Heidelberg New York, 1971.

26. Mosmans PCM, Jonkman EJ: The significance of the collateral vascular system of the brain in shunt and steal syndromes. Clin. Neurol. Neurosurg. 82: 145–155, 1980.

27. Lassen NA: The luxury perfusion syndrome and its possible relation to acute metabolic acidosis localised within the brain. Lancet ii: 1113–1115, 1966.

28. Meyer JS, Naritomi H, Sakai F, Ishihara A, Ishihara N, Grant P: Regional cerebral blood flow, diaschisis and steal after stroke. Neurol. Res. 1: 101–119, 1977.

29. Kuhl DE, Phelps ME, Kowell AP, et al: Effects of stroke on local metabolism and perfusion: Mapping by emission computed tomography of 18FDG and 13NH3. Ann. Neurol. 8: 47–60, 1980.

30. Bousser MG, Baron JC, Iba-Zizen IT: Migrainous cerebral infarction: a tomographic study of

CBF and oxygen extraction with the 15 oxygen inhalation technique. Stroke 11: 145–148, 1980.

31. Du Boulay G, Marshall J, Merory J, Symon L: The location of spasm and its relation to symptoms. In: Wilkins RH, (ed.) Cerebral Arterial Spasms pp. 394–396. Williams and Wilkins, Baltimore, 1980.

Cranial blood flow measurement by means of Doppler ultrasound

H.R. Muller, E.W. Radue and M. Buser

Ultrasonic Doppler techniques for transcutaneously measuring blood flow can be divided in two types. With one type of instrument the blood vessel is uniformly insonated with either continuous or single-gated pulsed wave ultrasound, and velocity is determined from the mixture of Doppler frequencies arising. The cross-sectional area, by which mean velocity must be multiplicated to compute volume flow, is either calculated from the internal vessel diameter, as measured with the impulse echo technique [1, 2] or by moving a single gate across the vessel for detecting the borders of the blood column from the Doppler signal [3, 4].

With another category of Doppler flowmeter, multi-gated pulsed wave systems are used, and flow is calculated from the velocity profiles recorded by this means [5, 6].

With both groups of techniques a circular shape of the cross-section is assumed. The multi-gated systems additionally make the assumption that the velocity profiles are symmetrical. While at many sites of the arterial system both requirements may be sufficiently fulfilled, they are certainly not with veins, which therefore have appeared to be excluded from ultrasonic flow measurement. Only recently we have been tentatively measuring internal jugular venous flow using a CW technique for assessing mean flow velocity and a linear array scanner for computing the cross-sectional area [7]. Our series of measurements must be further extended before a final conclusion of their reliability can be drawn from these experiences. If the subject of jugular venous flow measurement is still under investigation, much data has accumulated over the last few years on the cranial arterial circulation.

Arterial data are mostly confined to the common carotid artery (Table I) since it has been found that for anatomical and rheological reasons (superpositions of other vessels contaminating the CW Doppler signal, asymmetry of the velocity profile at the sites accessible to multigated techniques) flow measurements at the internal carotid and the vertebral artery cannot reliably be made using currently available equipment.

Measurements on the common carotid artery have so far received little clinical attention; one of the reasons being that the normal values obtained vary considerably according to the techniques used.

Table 1 shows that with continuous wave and single gated methods mean common carotid flow was in the order of 400–500 ml/min, while the measurements with multigated techniques resulted in considerably lower values of about 300 ml/min. A comparative study which we carried out on the same 100 volunteers using the (cw) QFM-system [10] and the (multigated) MAVIS scanner [14] in a mean value of 282 ml/min obtained with this latter which was 38% lower than the one determined with the QFM-system (464 ml/min).

Comparison of the two values with those obtained with electromagnetic [15] and densitometric [16] measurements as well as with a volumetric contrast medium injection method [17] showed a much better agreement with the QFM than with the MAVIS values (Table 2).

The same is true, if total hemispheric flow is estimated based on a normal mean regional blood flow of 54 ml/100 g/min [14, 15]. With the assumption that the mean hemisphere weight be 600 g, that 20% of the hemisphere be perfused by the posterior cerebral artery, originating in some 20% from the internal carotid, and that the ratio of external to internal carotid flow be about 2 : 1 [15, 16], common carotid flow calculated from these data is 408 ml/min. This value is exceeded by only 13% by the QFM measurements, while the deviation by the MAVIS measurements is as much as − 31%. Based on these comparisons and the excellent *in vitro* correlation of the QFM measurements to timed collection of pulsatile flow [10], we have been limiting our further investigations to the use of the QFM system.

Table 1. Normal values of common carotid flow, as measured with ultrasonic flowmeters.

Equipment and authors			n	age, y	ml/min
contin. wave	QFM Hayashi Denki	Uematsu *et al.*, 1983 (8)	16	21–40	479 ± 90
			14	41–69	433 ± 69
		Fujishiro, Yoshimura, 1982 (9)	120	21–70	486–570
		Müller *et al.*, 1984 (10)	100	16–65	464 ± 75
single gated	Alvar	Payen *et al.*, 1982 (4)	11	20–56	387 ± 183
		Simon *et al.*, 1982 (11)	11	?	428 ± 32
	Octoson	Ackroyd *et al.*, 1984 (2)	53	?	461 ± 107
multi-gated	SFIT*	Keller *et al.*, 1976 (6)	22	23–45	300–480
		Hirschl *et al.*, 1980 (12)	24	?	294 ± 42
	MAVIS	Weiss *et al.*, 1983 (13)	14	36–78	296 ± 33
		Müller *et al.*, 1983 (14)	100	16–65	282 ± 76

* prototypes Swiss Federal Institute of Technology.

Measurement principle of the QFM-system

With this instrument, an A-mode transducer transmitting a frequency of 6 MHz is used for measuring the internal diameter of the vessel. A tracking gate is adjusted to the echoes arising from the interfaces between the blood column and the vessel wall, and follows their excentrical pulsations. Velocity is simultaneously measured by means of a double beam CW technique using three transducers; one is transmitting at a frequency of 5 MHz at an angle of 65° and the other two transducers receiving the reflected waves at 55° and 65° respectively. This allows an 'angle-independent' measurement of true velocity. Measurement of both diameter and velocity are made every 2 m/sec, and flow is computed and averaged over 5 pulse cycles. The printout of the system, which is available some 5 seconds after termination of measurement (Fig. 1) also included digital and analog velocity and diameter data.

Normal values of common carotid flow as measured with the QFM-system

QFM values of common carotid flow measured in 100 healthy volunteers 16 to 65 years of age have been published in an earlier paper [10]. In order to study the flow evolution over a wider age range we have extended our normal series to comprise 140 subjects ages 11 to 80 years (5 males and 5 females in each age group of 5 years). On each of the subjects three consecutive measurements were made and averaged bilaterally. The 95% confidence interval for immediate reproducibility of the measurement was ± 11%. In 10 of the volunteers four QFM investigations were done at intervals of one week. The 95% confidence interval for the means of the four measurements was M ± 22%. Normal reference values for clinical use were additionally determined, based on the 95% confidence interval, in the subgroup of our material consisting of the 60 subjects ages 41 to 70 years. These values are compiled on Table 3. Table 4 shows data of the entire material.

Mean unilateral common carotid flow as measured in our volunteers ages 41 to

Table 2. Comparison of mean common carotid flow as measured with the QFM system and the MAVIS scanner to values obtained with other methods.

Method	Authors	flow ml/min
Electromagnetic	Kristiansen, Krog, 1962 (15)	535
Densitometry	Hilal, 1966 (16)	516
Angiogr. volumetr.	Klingler, 1959 (17)	360–480
Doppler, QFM	Müller et al., 1983 (10)	464
Doppler, MAVIS	Müller et al., 1984 (14)	282

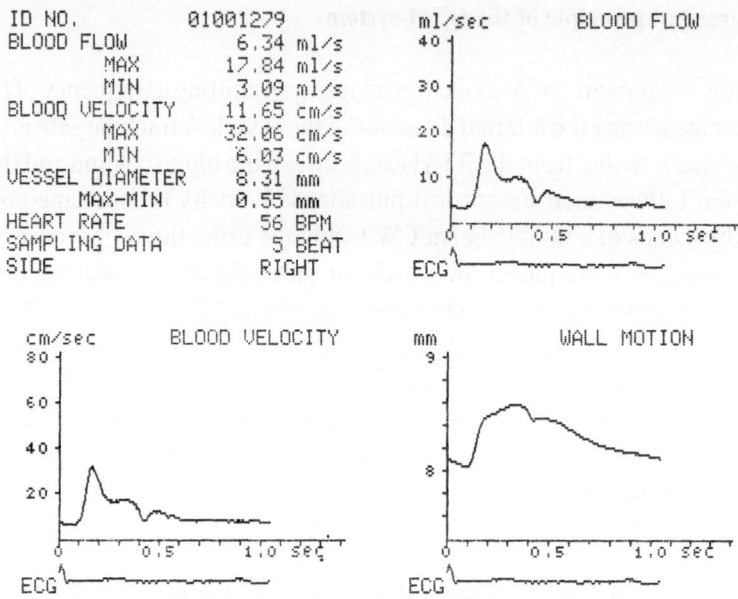

Figure 1. Printout of the QFM-system. Right common carotid of a normal subject.

70 years (7.65 ± 1.33 ml/sec) is in good accordance with the data obtained in a similar age group by Uematsu *et al.* [8], i.e. 7.21 ± 1.15 ml/sec on the right and 7.48 ± 1.10 ml/sec on the left side. The normal range of 5.0 to 10.3 ml/sec, based on the mean ± 2 sd is somewhat lower than the one published in our earlier paper [16] for subjects ages 16 to 65 years (6 to 11 ml/sec). The normal range of side difference (≤19.2% of R + L flow) was about the same in the two studies which was to be expected, assuming that side differences are due to variations of the circle of Willis [10].

The evaluation of the entire group of 140 volunteers confirmed the sex difference of common carotid flow. As in our earlier study, flow was about 5% lower in females than in men (p<0.001), which is in accordance with the difference in brain weight between the two sexes [13]. Within the male and female group there was, however, no significant correlation to body size. The correlation of flow to this parameter which we had found in our previous study [16] must therefore be attributed to the sex difference of body size (males 175 ± 7.1 cm, females 165 ± 6.8 cm in the present material, p<0.001).

Table 3. Normal values of common carotid flow, age group 41 to 70 years.

unilateral flow	R + L flow	side difference
5.0–10.3 ml/sec	10.9–19.2 ml/sec	≥19.2% of R + L

On studying the evolution with age (Table 4) we found a drop in flow, significant in either sex (p<0.001) between the age groups of 11 to 20 years and 21 to 30 years, which was more marked in males than in females. After the age of 30 years, flow remained rather constant up to the fifth decennium in men and to the sixth decennium in females. Thereafter, female flow decreased with a marked step occurring on the left side between the seventh and eighth decennium. On the contrary, a considerable increase occurred on the right side in men after the age of

Table 4. Common carotid flow, internal carotid diameter and maximal mean velocity in 280 common carotids of 140 healthy subjects ages 11 to 80 years. (5 males and 5 females in each age group.)

age y	males, flow ml/sec		females, flow ml/sec	
	R	L	R	L
11–20	8.7 ± 1.0	9.6 ± 1.3	7.9 ± 1.4	7.9 ± 1.4
21–30	7.6 ± 1.4	7.9 ± 0.9	7.5 ± 1.1	7.2 ± 1.0
31–40	7.6 ± 1.1	7.8 ± 1.4	7.6 ± 0.8	7.5 ± 1.0
41–50	7.6 ± 1.3	7.5 ± 1.0	7.8 ± 1.5	7.5 ± 1.2
51–60	8.5 ± 1.4	7.8 ± 0.9	7.6 ± 0.7	7.5 ± 1.1
61–70	8.2 ± 1.6	7.7 ± 1.5	7.1 ± 1.5	7.2 ± 1.2
71–80	7.4 ± 1.3	7.7 ± 1.1	7.1 ± 1.6	6.2 ± 1.0

	males, diameter mm		females, diameter mm	
	R	L	R	L
11–20	6.5 ± 0.5	6.6 ± 0.3	6.1 ± 1.1	6.2 ± 0.4
21–30	6.5 ± 0.6	6.4 ± 0.3	6.2 ± 0.4	6.3 ± 0.5
31–40	7.1 ± 0.5	7.0 ± 0.5	6.5 ± 0.5	6.4 ± 0.6
41–50	7.2 ± 0.6	7.2 ± 0.9	6.4 ± 0.5	6.4 ± 0.6
51–60	7.3 ± 0.5	6.9 ± 0.6	6.6 ± 0.7	6.7 ± 0.6
61–70	8.4 ± 1.2	8.6 ± 1.3	7.1 ± 0.7	7.1 ± 0.8
71–80	8.8 ± 1.4	8.3 ± 1.4	7.9 ± 0.8	7.7 ± 0.8

	males, v_{max}, cm/sec		females, v_{max}, cm/sec	
	R	L	R	L
11–20	63.3 ± 10.1	66.5 ± 8.5	61.5 ± 9.2	64.1 ± 8.9
21–30	67.0 ± 10.9	68.8 ± 10.0	60.7 ± 10.1	58.1 ± 13.6
31–40	50.7 ± 8.4	52.7 ± 12.0	51.3 ± 7.5	50.9 ± 11.1
41–50	46.1 ± 6.2	44.1 ± 8.7	47.7 ± 10.8	45.0 ± 13.6
51–60	43.1 ± 6.7	43.6 ± 9.5	44.1 ± 10.4	40.5 ± 10.0
61–70	33.8 ± 10.4	28.9 ± 8.2	35.9 ± 8.9	34.3 ± 7.7
71–80	28.3 ± 12.0	32.6 ± 12.0	33.0 ± 9.7	29.2 ± 6.3

50 years. The flow in men decreased again between the seventh and eighth decennium reaching values which are little below those observed in the twenties.

This age evolution is quite different from that observed by Fujishiro and Yoshimura [9] These authors found, in accordance to reports on regional cerebral blood flow [19, 20], a rather linear decrease of flow from the twenties to the sixties, and a more marked drop thereafter. Differences between our findings and those of the Japanese authors also include the data on vessel diameter. The increase of this parameter occurring after the age of 20 years was much more continuous in Fujishiro and Yoshimura's series than in ours, where in males there was a definite step of caliber increase from the twenties to the thirties. Furthermore, the increase in diameter from the sixties to the seventies observed in either series was considerably larger (+ 13.5%) in our series than in that of Fujishiro and Yoshimura (+ 6.5%). Mean diameter increase from the third to eighth decennium was only 10% in the Japanese study and as much as 29% in ours.

Considering both the difference of age evolution of flow found in our study to that anticipated from Xenon[133] studies [19, 20] and the difference of evolution observed within our own material between the two sexes, one must bear in mind that common carotid flow also includes flow to the external carotid territory. This latter may well be in the opposite direction compared to flow evolution in the internal carotid artery, and also may be different in males and in females. Any conclusion to the evolution of brain circulation can therefore be drawn from our data but with great reserve. Obviously, there may also be differences in external carotid flow evolution between the Japanese and Europeans, and this might well account for part of the difference of our results to those of Fujishiro and Yoshimura.

Common carotid flow, controlled study in patients

We checked the hypothesis that side differences of common carotid flow in normals are due to variations of the circle of Willis. In 50 patients having had flow measurements, as well as bilateral carotid angiography, without evidence of carotid or middle cerebral artery stenosis of more than 10% linear narrowing of the vessel lumen, the angiograms were blindly reevaluated, grading the filling of the individual cerebral arteries in percent of full perfusion, according to a rigid set of neuroradiological criteria. These percent values were then normalized according to an estimation based on the weights of the individual arterial territories as dissected from 5 normal cadaver brains, based on the relative weight of blood flow distribution to the hemispheres. The perfusion of one anterior and one middle cerebral artery was thereby set to be 100%. From this data a 100% angiographical filling was normalized to 29.6% for the anterior, to 70.4% for the middle, and to 23.0% for the posterior cerebral artery.

The sum of these normalized values (angiographical filling index in Figs. 2 and

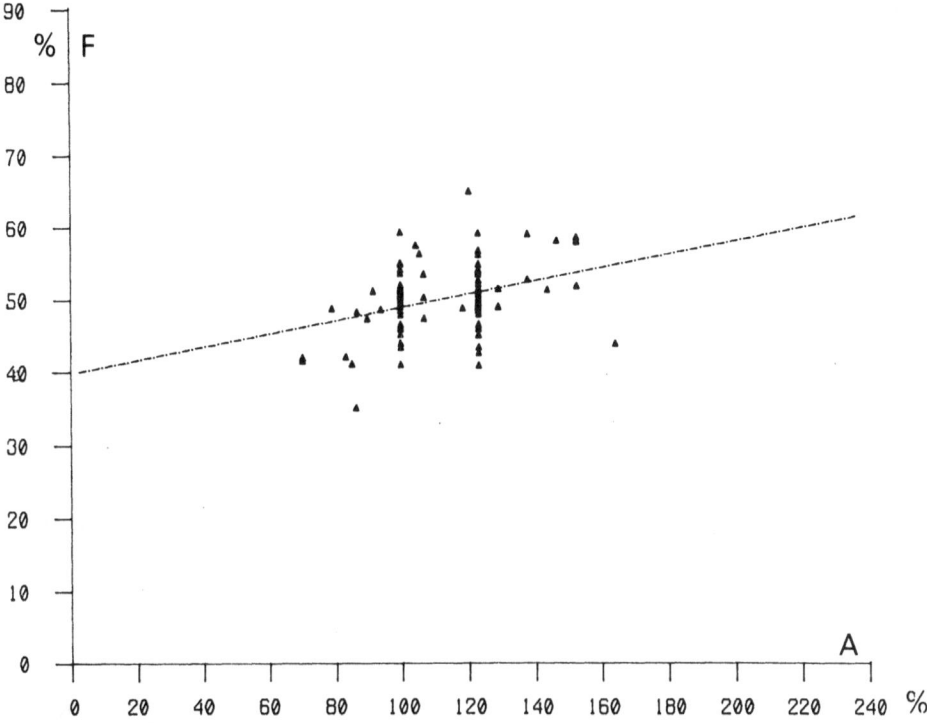

Figure 2. Correlation of flow index (F) to angiographical filling index (A) in 50 patients not having obstructive carotid pathology.

3) was then compared to the respective common carotid flow and to the fraction it represented of bilateral flow (flow index in Figs. 2 and 3). While the level of significance was just missed for the former correlation (p = 0.038), there was a significant linear correlation between flow index and angiographical filling index (p<0.01) proving the hypothesis that side differences of carotid flow are due to variations of the circle of Willis (Fig. 2).

The same was done in 100 consecutively investigated patients suffering from angiographically demonstrated obstructive or occlusive carotid disease, and an equally strong correlation (p<0.01) was found between the two parameters (Fig. 3). The large spread of the values in this latter series (Fig. 3) compared to the former (Fig. 2) is obviously due to carotid cross flow, which in conjunction with the homolateral flow reduction, in many cases, considerably increased the side difference in size of the carotid tree.

For assessing the diagnostic value of common carotid flow measurement, the 100 cases having occlusive or obstructive pathology (Fig. 3 and 4) were then reviewed considering the range of normal values of Table 3. One or more parameters were not within normal limits in 72% of the entire material, in 100% of the bilateral occlusions, in 90% of the unilateral occlusions, 53% of the

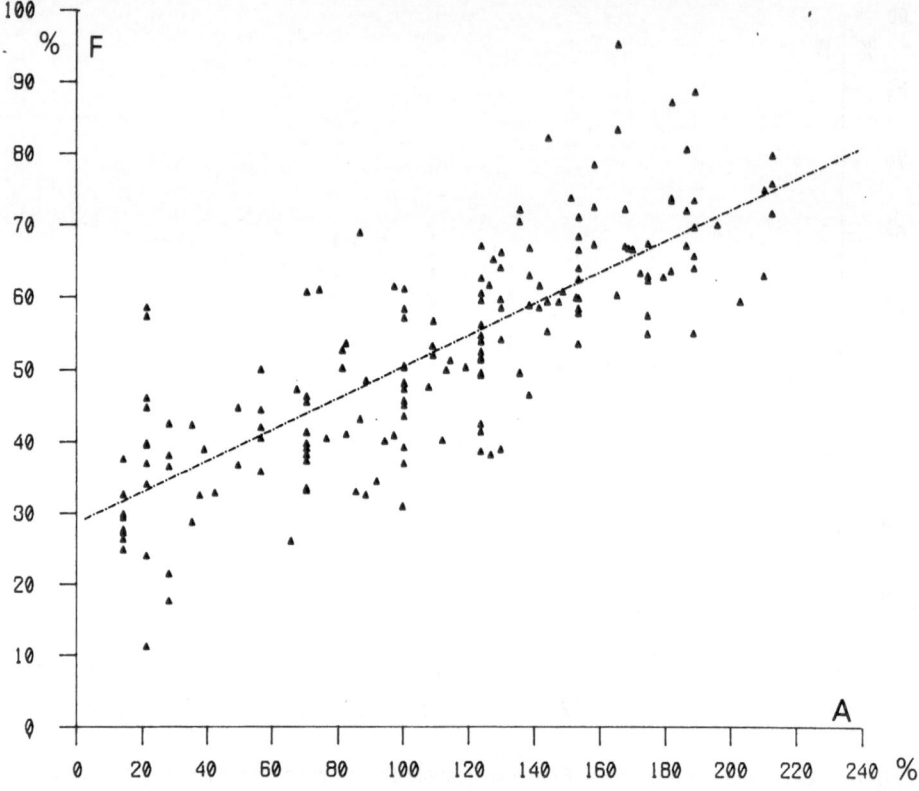

Figure 3. Correlation of flow index (F) to angiographical filling index (A) in 100 patients having obstructive carotid pathology.

bilateral stenoses, and 52% of the unilateral stenoses of the internal carotid artery.

In a further study the reasons were investigated why homolateral common carotid flow remained within normal in as much as 28% of all internal carotid occlusions. This was done by correlating flow to a number of angiographical parameters (Fig. 5). Contrary to our expectation [16] there was no significant correlation to the presence of an ophthalmic collateral. There was, however, a strong correlation of flow to both the diameter of the external carotid trunk (p<0.0001), as well as to the sum of cross-sectional areas of the main branches of this artery (p<0.0001). Both correlations remained significant even after the cases having an ophthalmic collateral were excluded.

Neither in the group of unilateral nor in bilateral internal carotid stenoses (Fig. 5) was there a significant correlation of common carotid flow to the degree of luminar narrowing as measured on the lateral view angiograms. Moreover, it is obvious from this figure that with contralateral high grade stenosis or occlusion of the internal carotid artery flow may be in the upper half of the normal range or

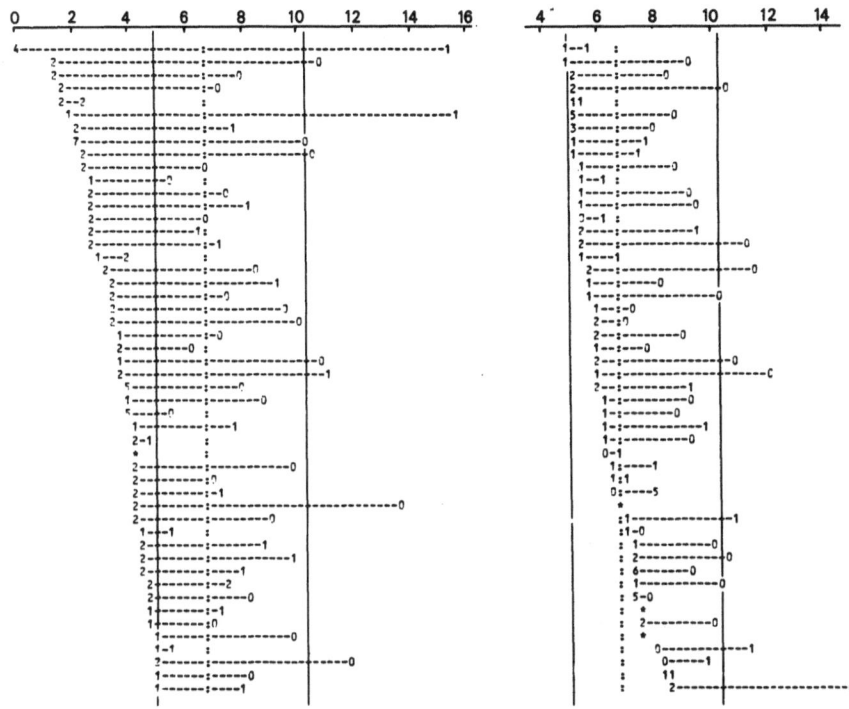

Figure 4. Common carotid flow in 100 patients having obstructive or occlusive carotid pathology. A blood flow scale in ml/sec is shown at the top of the two groups. Vertical lines represent normal range. Dotted lines represent the difference in blood flow between the right and left carotids. The numbers at the end of each line represent the severity of arterial disease. 0 = normal carotid, 1 = internal carotid stenosis, 2 = internal carotid occlusion, 3 = common carotid stenosis, 4 = common carotid occlusion, 5 = middle cerebral artery stenosis, 6 = compression of internal carotid through aneurysm, 7 = hypoplastic internal carotid artery.

above it even with stenoses generally considered as hemodynamically significant. This obviously indicates collateral cross flow over the circle of Willis as demonstrated on Fig. 6 with a typical case example.

On Table 5, in which the mean flow values are listed according to the grade of stenosis and to the nature of contralateral pathology, as well as on Table 6 where the percent difference to mean normal flow (reference value I) is indicated, it can clearly be seen that with contralateral stenosis mean flow is situated above the normal mean in the group of less than 30% stenosis and with contralateral occlusion this is the case even with all stenoses up to 70%. For recognizing the true hemodynamic effect of a carotid stenosis associated to contralateral obstructive pathology it is, therefore, necessary to compare flow to the mean value determined in normal carotids having the same contralateral pathology (ref. II, III).

On evaluating our material in this way, we found that mean flow reduction of more than 10%, as observed in unilateral stenoses of more than 50%, occurred in

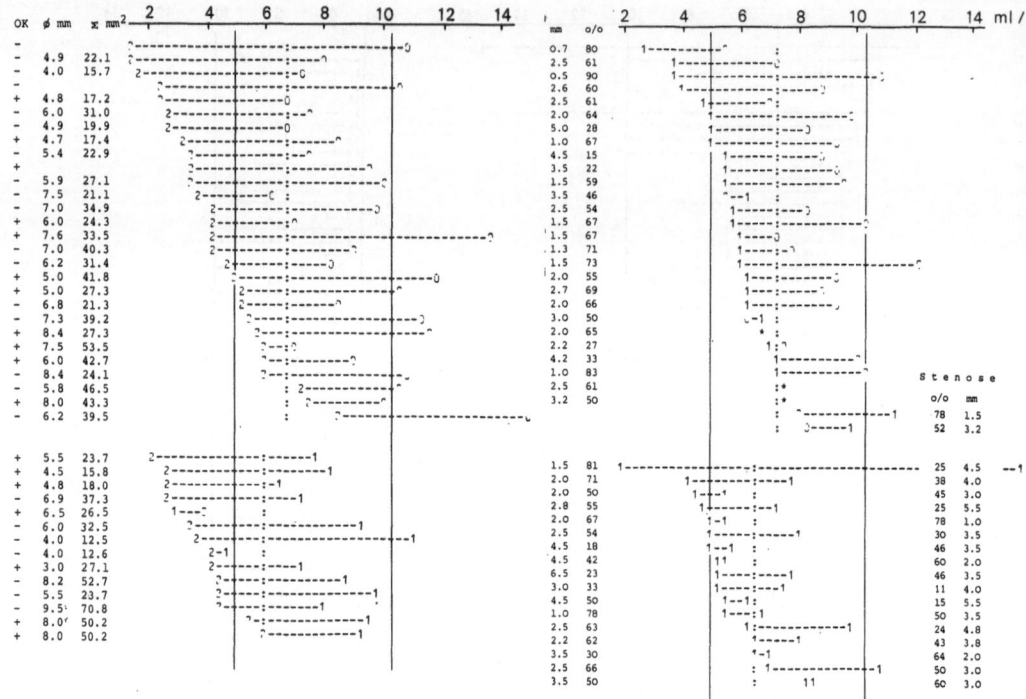

Figure 5. Synopsis of carotid flow findings in carotid arteries according to the severity of internal carotid obstruction. The patients are divided into four groups. The upper left hand group (n = 28) lists those cases having unilateral internal carotid occlusion with normal contralateral carotid. The lower left hand group (n = 14) consists of the cases of unilateral occlusion with contralateral stenosis. The upper right group (n = 29) of those having unilateral stenosis. Lower right hand group (n = 17) bilateral internal carotid stenosis. For coding 0, 1, 2 see legend to Fig. 4. Also tabulated is the presence or absence of ophthalmic collateral ('OK' in the left hand column). In the second column '0 mm' indicates the diameter of the external carotid trunk and '$\sum mm^2$' in the 3rd column indicates the sum of the cross-sectional areas of the superior thyroid, facial, maxillary, superficial temporal, and occipital arteries. The paired column of figures represents severity of stenosis in millimeters.

Table 5. Common carotid flow in 77 internal carotid stenoses according to grade and contralateral pathology.

grade of stenosis		≤30%	31–50%	51–70%	>70%
unilat. stenosis	ml/sec	(5.9 ± 0.9*)	6.9 ± 0.6	5.9 ± 1.2	5.2 ± 1.9
	n	4	4	15	6
bilat. stenosis	ml/sec	8.1 ± 3.2	6.9 ± 1.8	6.3 ± 1.2	4.4 ± 1.7
	n	9	12	9	4
sten. with contra-lat. occlusion	ml/sec	8.3	8.4 ± 2.2	8.3 ± 1.0	7.3 ± 2.9
	n	1	7	3	3

* This group, comprising two cases with the stenotic carotid feeding only the middle cerebral artery, was not further evaluated.

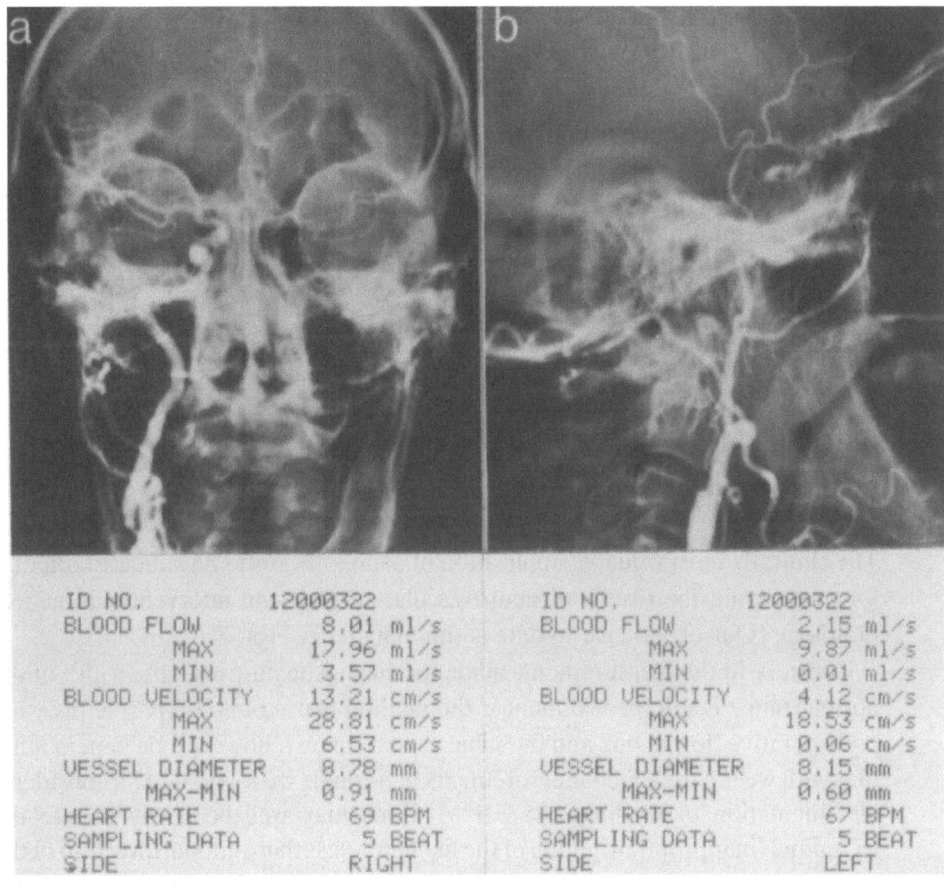

ID NO.	12000322		ID NO.	12000322	
BLOOD FLOW	8.01	ml/s	BLOOD FLOW	2.15	ml/s
MAX	17.96	ml/s	MAX	9.87	ml/s
MIN	3.57	ml/s	MIN	0.01	ml/s
BLOOD VELOCITY	13.21	cm/s	BLOOD VELOCITY	4.12	cm/s
MAX	28.81	cm/s	MAX	18.53	cm/s
MIN	6.53	cm/s	MIN	0.06	cm/s
VESSEL DIAMETER	8.78	mm	VESSEL DIAMETER	8.15	mm
MAX-MIN	0.91	mm	MAX-MIN	0.60	mm
HEART RATE	69	BPM	HEART RATE	67	BPM
SAMPLING DATA	5	BEAT	SAMPLING DATA	5	BEAT
SIDE	RIGHT		SIDE	LEFT	

Figure 6. a) High grade internal carotid stenosis on the right side with cross flow to the left side due to b) left internal carotid occlusion. At the bottom of the figure printouts of the QFM meter indicating common carotid flow.

stenoses of more than 30% if a contralateral stenosis was present, and even in the single case having a stenosis of less than 30% associated to a contralateral internal carotid occlusion. This is in good accordance with the hemodynamic principle that a stenosis becomes a flow obstacle if its resistance approaches the one in the peripheral vascular bed, this latter obviously being the highest in unilateral stenoses and the lowest in stenoses associated to contralateral occlusion. Our results also show that the concept of critical carotid stenosis [21] must be revised considering that flow reduction through a carotid stenosis is not solely dependent on the degree of vessel narrowing. Flow may rather vary substantially with the peripheral resistance which may be considerably reduced by contralateral obstructive pathology.

Diagnostic use of common carotid flow measurement

It is obvious that with the wide range of normal values the sensitivity of the method for detecting pathology of the cerebral circulation is rather limited. Moreover, the method if used on its own lacks sufficient diagnostic specificity even in those cases having clear abnormal findings. There is no means from flow values to differentiate between internal carotid occlusion or high grade stenoses at any site along the internal carotid. Also, with cases having a normal flow value on one side and a moderate increase on the other side, the question remains whether this side difference is due to obstructive carotid disease or to an AV shunt. The use of common carotid flow measurement as a diagnostic tool should therefore be limited to an adjunct of conventional Doppler sonography and/or angiography, the results of which it adds valuable information.

Common carotid flow measurement in neurovascular surgery

The clinically most valuable application of common carotid flow measurement is for quantifying the results of neurovascular surgery and interventional neuro-radiology (Our experience to date is summarized in Figs. 7 and 8).

Contrary to the measurements made for diagnostic purposes, the width of the normal range is not inconvenient if the method is used for comparing pre- and postoperative flow in one and the same vessel. It must, however, be kept in mind that with weekly repeated measurements in normals we found quite a considerable fluctuation of readings $(M \pm 11\%)$ which may well be partly due to the technique (inappropriate gating of the diameter, less than optimal direction of the transmitted beam of the Doppler system) but almost certainly also reflects

Table 6. % difference of common carotid flow to various reference values in 73 internal carotid stenoses according to grade and contralateral pathology. Reference values: I = mean normal flow $(7.6 \pm 1.4\,\text{ml/sec})$. II = mean flow in normal artery with contralateral internal carotid stenosis $(8.6 \pm 1.5\,\text{ml/sec})$. III = mean flow in normal artery with contralateral internal carotid occlusion $(9.6 \pm 2.1\,\text{ml/sec})$. In unilateral stenoses all differences to reference I were significant $(p<0.05)$. Difference to reference II was only significant for the mean calculated from all stenoses of more than 30% $(p = 0.0001)$. Significance was just missed for the respective mean as compared to reference III.

grade of stenosis		≤30%	31–50%	51–70%	>70%
unilat. stenosis	% diff. to I		− 9.2%	− 22.4%	− 31.6%
bilat. stenosis	% diff. to I	+ 6.6%	− 9.2%	− 17.1%	− 42.2%
	% diff. to II	− 5.8%	− 19.8%	− 26.8%	− 48.8%
sten. with contra-	% diff. to I	+ 9.2%	+ 10.5%	+ 9.2%	− 4.0%
lat. occlusion	% diff. to III	− 13.5%	− 12.5%	− 13.5%	− 24.0%

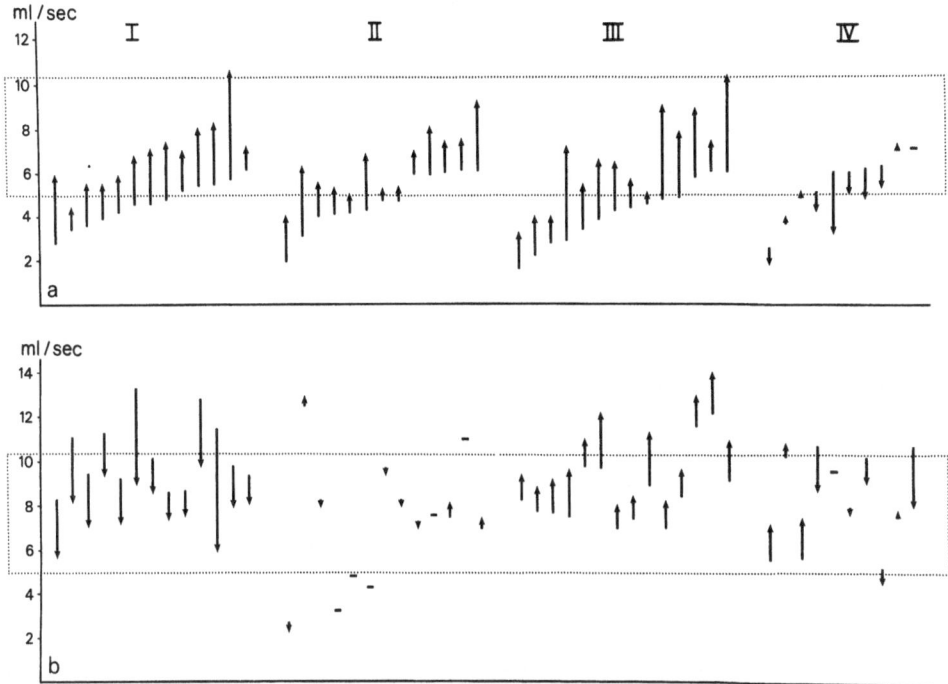

Figure 7. Common carotid flow in 50 patients having an unilateral EC/IC bypass. a) side of operation. b) contralateral side. Postoperative measurements were made between 2 weeks and 12 months (mean 4 months) after the operation. Arrows indicate evolution from pre- to postoperative flow. Dotted lines indicate normal range. I = cases with reversal of carotid cross flow as evident from flow evolution on the contralateral side. II = cases without change in flow on the contralateral side. III = cases where the bypass appeared to produce a steal from the contralateral external carotid. IV = cases without a significant increase or with a decrease in homolateral flow.

physiological variation of flow. Therefore, minor flow differences between a single pair of measurements must be interpreted with reserve, as demonstrated with Figs. 7 and 8. The flow evolution on the contralateral side helps in many cases to verify the hemodynamic effect of the surgical or neuroradiological intervention as the true or at least the dominant reason for a change in flow observed.

Further, with EC/IC bypass operations it is important to always additionally investigate the donor vessel using the conventional Doppler technique[22] in order to assess the patency of the bypass. This is particularly essential if there is no significant difference between pre- and postoperative common carotid flow, or if early postoperative flow is lower than preoperatively. Thus, in all but one case of group IV, Fig. 7, the bypass proved to be patent on direct examination in spite of the minimal increase or even decrease between the pre- and postoperative common carotid flow.

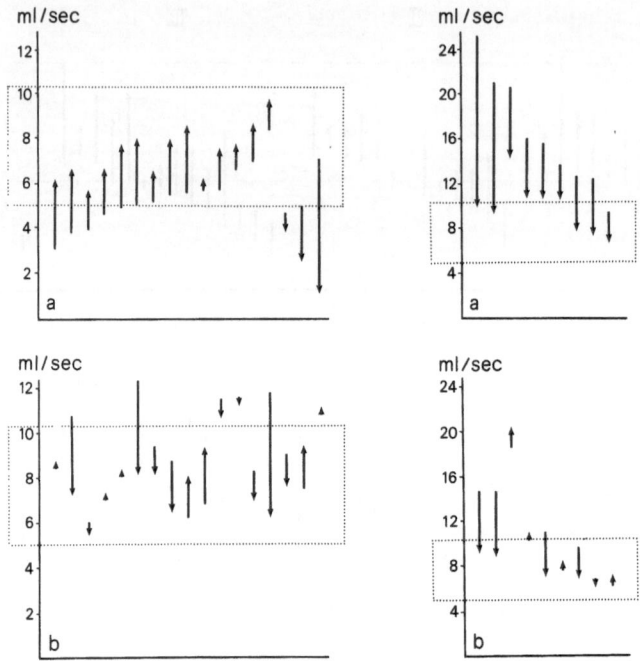

Figure 8. Common carotid flow in 17 patients having endarterectomy for internal or common carotid stenosis, including 3 cases with clinically silent postoperative internal carotid occlusion (left diagram) and in 9 patients treated with surgery or embolization for AV malformations or AV fistulae in the carotid territory (right diagram). Postoperative measurements were made between 1 week and 6 months (mean 3 months) after the endarterectomies and within 24 hours after the (last) intervention in the majority of cases with AV shunt pathology. Arrows indicate evolution from pre- to postoperative measurements. Dotted lines indicate normal range.

Conclusion

The results of our study clearly show that the normal range of common carotid flow is too large to use ultrasonic flow measurement at this vessel as a diagnostic tool on its own. The method is most valuable, however, as an adjunct to conventional Doppler sonography and angiography and particularly helpful for assessing the hemodynamic results of neurovascular surgery and neuroradiological interventions in the carotid territory.

Common carotid flow measurement using the QFM-system has additionally provided us with new data both on the evolution of carotid flow with age and on the hemodynamic effects of carotid stenoses. From our data it is obvious that flow through stenoses not only depends on the residual cross-sectional area but also very strongly on the presence and grade of contralateral obstructive carotid lesions.

References

1. Furuhata H, Kanno R, Kodaira K, Aoyagi T, Hayashi J, Matsumoto H, Yoshimura S: An ultrasonic blood flow measuring system to detect the absolute volume flow. Jpn J Med Electron Biol Engrng 16, Suppl: 334, 1978.
2. Ackroyd N, Gill RW, Griffiths M, Appleberg M, Kossoff G: Pulsed Doppler ultrasound measurement of carotid artery blood flow before and after endarterectomy. 5th Congr Europ Fed Soc for Ultrasound in Med and Biol, Strasbourg, May 7–11, 1984. Abstract Book, p 21, 1984.
3. Peronneau P, Hinglais J, Pellett M, Leger F: Vélocimètre sanguin par éffet Doppler à émission ultra-sonore pulsée. L'onde électrique 50: 369–389, 1970.
4. Payen DM, Levy BI, Menegalli DJ, Layat YI, Levenson JA, Nicolas FM: Evaluation of human hemispheric blood flow based on non-invasive carotid blood flow measurements using the range-gated Doppler technique. Stroke 13: 392–398, 1982.
5. Fish PJ: A method for transentaneous blood flow measurement-accuracy considerations. In: Kurjak A, Kratochwil A (eds) Recent Advances in Ultrasound Diagnosis, Vol 3, pp 110–115. Excerpta Medica, Amsterdam, Oxford, Princeton, 1981.
6. Keller HM, Meier WE, Anliker M, Kumpe DA: Noninvasive measurement of velocity profiles and blood flow in the common carotid artery by pulsed ultrasound, Stroke 7: 370–377, 1976.
7. Muller HR: Quantitative Bestimmung des Blutflusses in der Vena jugularis interna mittels Ultraschall 6, 51–54, 1985.
8. Uematsu S, Yang A, Preziosi TJ, Kouba R, Toung TJK: Measurement of carotid blood flow in man and its clinical application, Stroke 14: 256–266, 1983.
9. Fujishiro K, Yoshimura S: Hemodynamic changes in carotid blood flow with age. Jikeikai Med J 29: 125–138, 1982.
10. Muller HR, Radue EW, Pallotti C, Gratzl O: Common carotid CW Doppler flow measurement in neurovascular surgery. Recent Advances in Ultrasound Diagnosis (Kurjak A, Kossoff G, eds), Vol 4, pp 17–36. Elsevier, Amsterdam, 1984.
11. Simon A, Levenson J, Safar M, Diebold B, Peronneau P: Noninvasive pulsed Doppler measurement of blood flow: Investigation of internal carotid stenosis. Abstr 3rd meeting of WFUMB. Ultrasound in Med and Biol 8, Suppl 1, p 180, 1980.
12. Hirschl M, Ehringer H, Marosi L: Flussmessung der A. carotis communis mit einem viel-kanaligen gepulsten Doppler-Ultraschallgerät. In: Müller-Wiefel H, (ed), Mikrozirkulation und Blutrheologie pp 436–440. Witzstrock, Baden-Baden, Köln, New York, 1980.
13. Weiss H, Haass A, Schimrigk K, Wenzel E: Measurement of blood flow by ultrasound in healthy subjects and in patients with cerebrovascular disease. Internat Symp on Measurement on Cerebral Blood Flow and Cerebral Metabolism in Man. Heidelberg, 29 Sep-1 Oct, 1983. In: Hartmann H (ed) Proceedings in press, 1983.
14. Muller HR, Radue EW, Saia A, Pallotti C: Doppler ultrasonic measurement of carotid blood flow (Letter to the Editor). Ultrasound in Med and Biol 9: L91–L95, 1983.
15. Kristiansen K, Krog J: Electromagnetic studies on the blood flow through the carotid system in man. Neurology 12: 20–22, 1962.
16. Hilal SK: Human carotid artery flow determination using a radiographic technique. Invest Radiol 1: 113–122, 1966.
17. Klingler M: Angiographische Messung der Carotisdurchblutung. II. Messung der Carotisdurch-blutung beim Menschen durch Beobachtung des Refluxes von Kontrastmittel. Acta Neurochir 7: 333–343, 1959.
18. Ho K, Roessmann U, Straumfjord V, Monroe G: Analysis of brain weight. I. Adult brain weight in relation to sex, race and age. Arch Pathol Lab Med 104: 635–639, 1980.
19. Melamed E, Lavy S, Bentin S, Cooper G, Rinot Y: Reduction in regional cerebral blood flow during normal aging in man. Stroke 11: 31–35.

20. Meyer JS, Ishihara N, Deshmukh VD, Naritomi H, Sakai F, Hsu MCh, Pollack P: Improved method for noninvasive measurement of regional cerebral blood flow by [133]Xenon inhalation. Part I: Description of method and normal values obtained in healthy volunteers. Stroke 9: 195–205, 1978.
21. Brice JG, Dowsett DJ, Lowe RD: Hemodynamic effects of carotid artery stenosis. Brit Med J II: 1363–1366, 1964.
22. Muller HR, Gratzl O: Continuous-wave Doppler sonography in EC/IC bypass surgery. Ultrasound in Medicine and Biology. Proc and Meeting WFUMB (Wagai T, Omoto R, eds) pp 240–246. Excerpa Medica, Amsterdam, Oxford, 1980.

Early carotid lesions and flow disturbances

R.S. Reneman and A.P.G. Hoeks

Introduction

With most of the Doppler techniques, presently available to diagnose cerebrovascular disease, vascular lesions associated with substantial narrowing of the carotid arteries (more than 50–60% diameter reduction) can be detected accurately, while they can distinguish between tight stenosis and total occlusion [1]. The latter is important because in tight stenosis high shear stresses are considered to induce thrombus formation causing, for example, transient ischemic attacks (TIA's) due to emboli. Accurate diagnosis of lesser degrees of stenosis, however, is still problematic.

The detection of lesions in the internal carotid artery without or with slight narrowing of the vessel, may be important because they may cause cerebral disturbances through emboli [2]. Moreover, the diagnosis of vascular lesions at an early stage of the disease will be helpful in epidemiological studies [3] as well as in obtaining more insight into the natural course of the disease.

Since disturbances in the flow pattern do occur at relatively slight degrees of artery narrowing [4, 5, 6] the detection of these disturbances is commonly used to diagnose arterial lesions at an early stage of the disease. In the clinic disturbances in the flow pattern are generally detected and quantified by estimating the degree of broadening of the Doppler audio spectrum, using either continuous wave (CW) [7, 8, 9, 10] or pulsed Doppler systems [11, 12, 13, 14]. Spectral broadening, however, does not necessarily mean pathology, because it may be induced by several other factors [15].

More recently multi-channel pulsed Doppler systems have been developed which theoretically provide more detailed information about the flow pattern in arteries (Chapter 3). This detailed information may be necessary to be able to distinguish in the carotid artery bulb flow disturbances, as induced by minor atherosclerotic lesions, from the complicated flow pattern normally occurring at this site in the arterial system [16, 17].

In this chapter we will discuss some approaches to the diagnosis of athe-

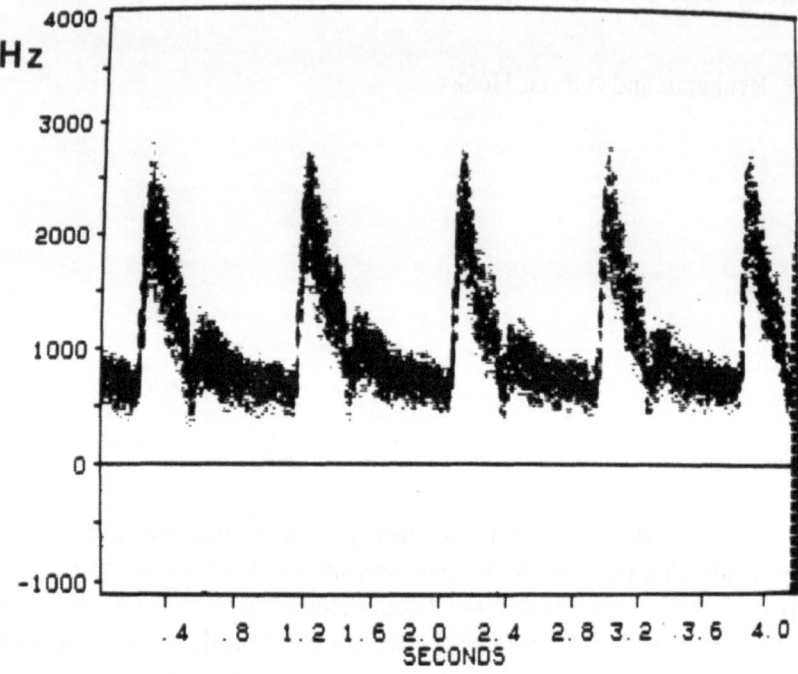

Figure 1. Doppler audio spectrum as recorded in the common carotid artery of a healthy volunteer (age: 55 years) with a multi-channel pulsed Doppler instrument. In this spectrum frequency is depicted as an instantaneous function of time, while the intensity of the pattern represents the amplitude of the frequencies, indicating the number of red blood cells moving at a given velocity. Note the spectral window, that is the open area in the spectrum, representing velocities at which practically no red blood cells are travelling.

rosclerotic lesions at an early stage of the disease. We limit ourselves to the methods based upon the detection of flow disturbances as induced by these lesions, because the remaining approaches will be dealt with in other chapters of this book.

The use of spectral broadening to detect disturbances in the flow pattern

In Doppler audio spectrum analysis frequencies are presented as an instantaneous function of time, while the intensity of the pattern represents the amplitude of the frequencies, indicating the number of red blood cells moving at a given velocity (Fig. 1; Chapter 2). Doppler audio spectrum analysis yields information about the maximum blood flow velocities and the velocity distribution of the red blood cells, giving insight into the flow pattern. In laminar flow the outline of the audio spectrum, defined as the line following the maximum frequencies during the cardiac cycle, is regular (Fig. 1). Because of the relatively flat velocity profiles [17, 18, 19], (Chapter 3) most of the red blood cells are travelling near the maximum velocity, resulting in a narrow Doppler audio spectrum, provided that

10 kHz

0

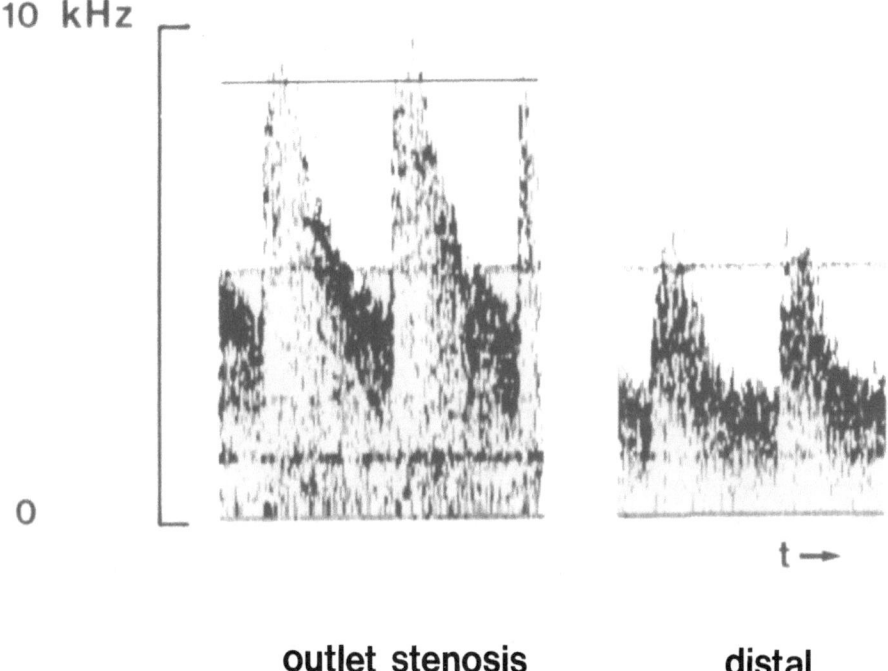

t →

outlet stenosis   distal

Figure 2. Doppler audio spectra as recorded in the internal carotid artery at the outlet of a stenosis and more distally in the artery with a multi-channel pulsed Doppler instrument. Estimated degree of carotid artery narrowing at the angiogram: 65% (diameter reduction). Note the spectral broadening and the disappearance of the spectral window (cf Fig. 1).

small sample volumes are used and sampling occurs in the center of the vessel (see below). In turbulent flow the spectrum broadens and the outline of the spectrum becomes irregular due to random changes in flow velocities occurring at any time during the cardiac cycle (Fig. 2).

In general atherosclerotic lesions associated with limited narrowing of the carotid arteries (e.g. less than 30% diameter reduction) induce flow disturbances which lead to only minimal broadening of the Doppler audio spectrum. CW Doppler instruments are unsuitable to detect this degree of spectral broadening because in these systems velocities are sampled along the whole cross-section of the artery so that the lower velocities near the vessel wall are presented in the Doppler audio spectrum as well. Hence, the audio spectra as recorded with CW Doppler instruments are broader (Fig. 3) than those recorded with pulsed Doppler systems in which samples are generally taken from the center of the vessel. To detect the flow disturbances as induced by minor atherosclerotic lesions, audio spectrum analysis should therefore be combined with pulsed Doppler systems. Although promising results have been obtained with this approach [11, 12, 13, 14], this method has its limitations.

Spectral broadening also occurs when in the sample volume the velocity profile is parabolic rather than flat, the sound beam is non-homogeneous or divergence

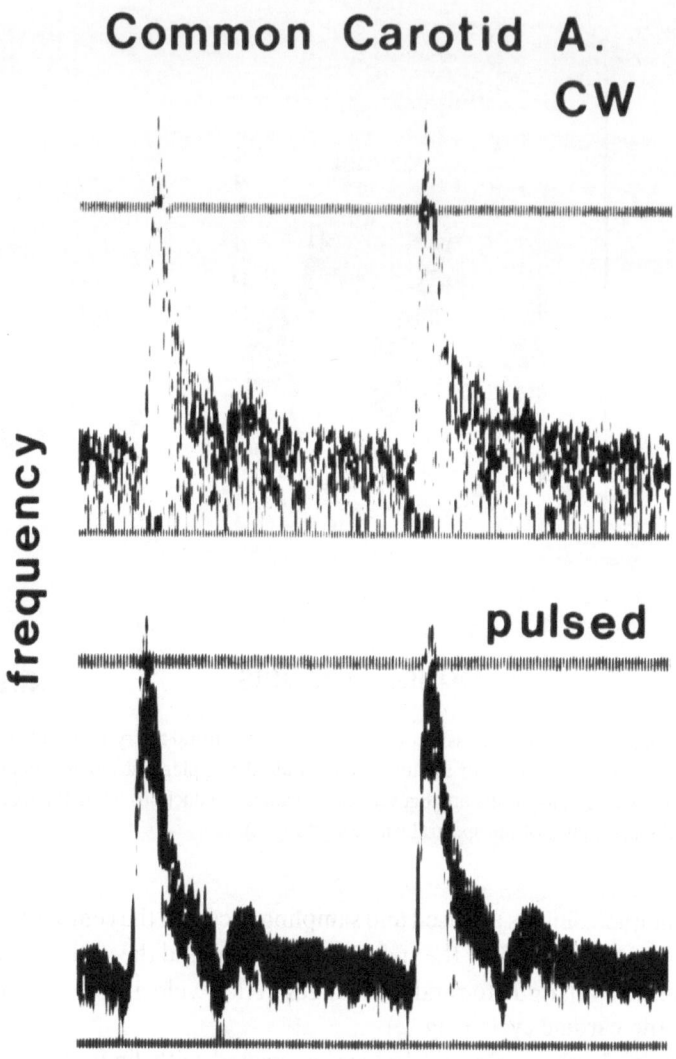

Figure 3. Doppler audio spectra as recorded with a continuous wave and a multi-channel pulsed Doppler system at the same site in the common carotid artery of a healthy volunteer.

of the beam occurs. The latter may be induced by vessel wall calcifications without narrowing of the arteries [20].

To avoid the recording of lower velocities near the vessel wall, the sample volume of the pulsed Doppler instrument used has to be small, relative to the artery diameter. Besides, sampling should occur in the middle of the blood-stream. In pulsed Doppler systems the size of the sample volume depends on both the beamwidth and the effective sample duration. This duration is set by the duration of emission combined with the bandwidth of the receiver section and the gate-width [21]. Increasing the bandwidth and shortening the duration of emission (high emission frequency) and the gate-width will reduce the sample volume, but decreases the signal-to-noise ratio. A complicating factor in pulsed Doppler

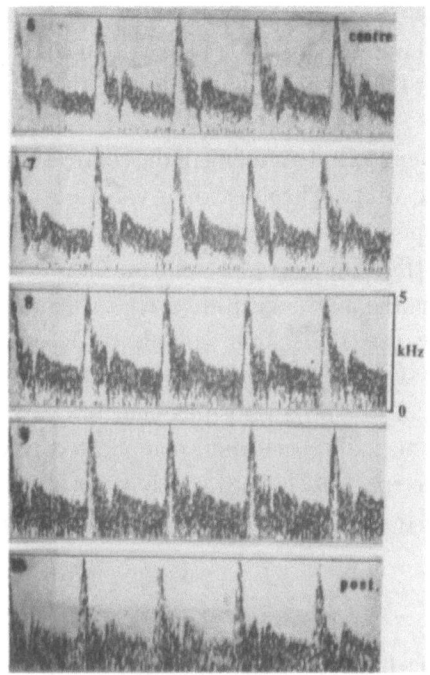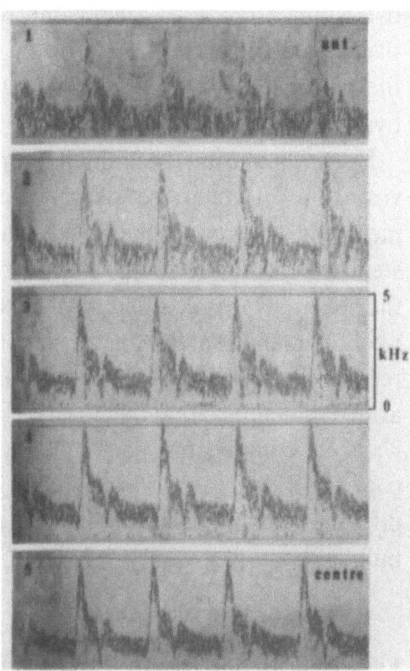

Figure 4. Doppler audio spectra as recorded in the common carotid artery of a healthy volunteer (age: 23 years) at successive sites along the ultrasound beam during consecutive cardiac cycles with a multi-channel pulsed Doppler system without changing the position of the probe. Note that normal spectra are only observed in the most central gates. Ant = anterior wall; post = posterior wall.

devices is that spectral broadening will be introduced by the finite dimensions of the sample volume (transit time effect). The smaller the dimensions are, the larger the effect will be. Therefore, this phenomenon is more pronounced in high resolution pulsed Doppler systems. The velocity component of scatterers along the ultrasound beam induces spectral broadening proportional to the average Doppler frequency, which means that the ratio of spectral broadening and average frequency is constant for a given system [22]. On the other hand scatterers moving perpendicular to the ultrasound beam induce spectral broadening proportional to the lateral velocity component (the average Doppler frequency induced by this velocity component is zero). Under normal circumstances, when the scatterers are moving under an angle of, for example, 60°, both effects will be present simultaneously.

The importance of a small sample volume and sampling in the middle of the bloodstream in the use of spectral broadening to detect minor lesions is illustrated in Fig. 4. In this figure the Doppler audio spectra, as recorded in the common carotid artery at successive sites along the ultrasound beam with a high resolution multi-channel pulsed Doppler system (Chapter 3), are depicted. Even with a sample volume of 1.2–1.7 mm^3 and a sample distance along the ultrasound beam of 0.5 mm, normal spectra are only found in the middle of the bloodstream, i.e. in the most central gates. Towards the vessel wall spectral broadening occurs due to the presence of velocity gradients within the sample volume, despite the relatively flat profile in these arteries.

Even when using these small sample volumes and sampling in the centre of the vessel is ascertained, in the internal carotid artery of healthy young volunteers the incidence of Doppler audio spectra, supposed to be associated with low grade stenosis, was found to be relatively high [15]. This was especially the case when the spectra were recorded more distally in the internal carotid artery. The most likely explanation for this observation is that the sample volume of the high resolution multi-channel pulsed Doppler system is still too large, relative to the artery diameter, to avoid the recording of low flow velocities near the vessel walls. A complicating factor is that the normally occurring, complicated flow patterns in the carotid artery bulb induce spectral changes which are probably difficult to distinguish from those induced by minor atherosclerotic lesions in this bulb [17].

Flow velocity patterns in the carotid artery bulb

In a recent study [17] it was found that in the carotid artery bulb of healthy volunteers the axial blood flow velocities are highest on the side of the flow divider (Fig. 5). This skewness is most pronounced early in systole and can be considered as a curvature effect because the internal carotid artery branches from the common carotid artery at an angle. In younger subjects (age 20–30 years) regions of flow separation and recirculation are observed on the side opposite to this divider. Flow separation is not continuously present throughout the cardiac cycle, but starts during the deceleration phase (Fig. 6). Flow separation and recirculation were less pronounced and less common in older subjects (age 50–60 years).

The flow patterns as found in the carotid artery bulb of young volunteers are similar to those observed in model bifurcations [23, 24, 25, 26] and in excised human carotid artery bifurcations [27]. The diminished flow separation and recirculation in older volunteers can probably not be ascribed to geometrical factors, but likely results from alterations in arterial distensibility at the transition from common to internal carotid artery with increasing age [17].

Spectral changes as induced by the normally occurring, complicated flow patterns in the carotid artery bulb, are shown in Fig. 7. The Doppler audio spectrum as depicted in this figure is similar to the spectra recently reported by Philips and his colleagues [16]. These spectra are probably difficult to distinguish from those induced by minor atherosclerotic lesions. Since in asymptomatic volunteers the velocity pattern is undisturbed in the internal carotid artery 3–4 cm distal to the flow divider (Fig. 5), one may argue that disturbances in the flow

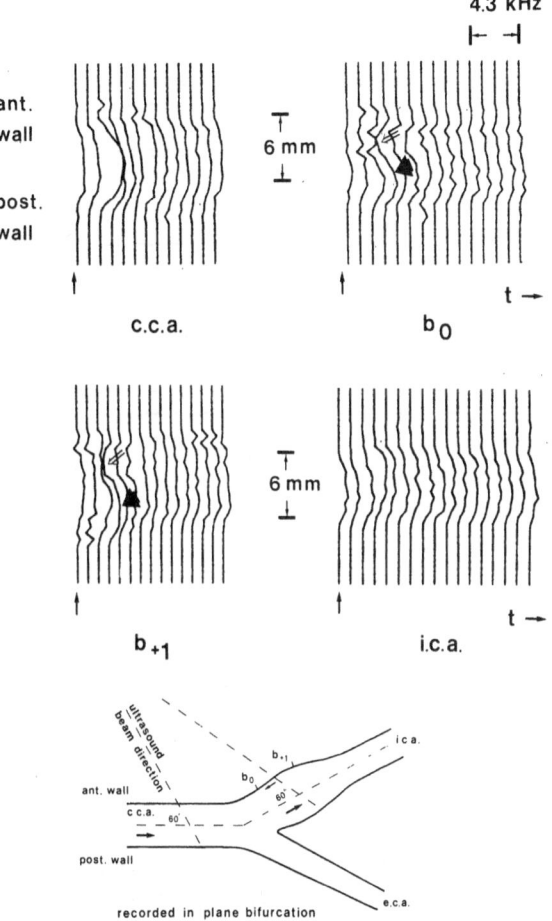

Figure 5. The velocity profiles at discrete time intervals during the cardiac cycle as recorded in the common (CCA) and internal carotid (ICA) arteries and proximally (bo) and more distally (b + 1) in the bulb of a healthy subject (age: 27 years) with a multi-channel pulsed Doppler instrument. The arrow represents the trigger derived from the R-wave of the ECG. Note the skewed velocity profile (arrow head) towards the flow divider and retrograde flow (open arrow) on the opposite side in systole at both levels in the bulb. The velocity profiles in the common and internal carotid arteries are symmetric and no retrograde flow is observed in these arteries. The arrows in the schematical drawing indicate the direction of flow. From Reneman *et al.*, 1985; with permission of the American Heart Association.

pattern as induced by vascular lesions in the carotid artery bulb, can be diagnosed at the former site. One should realize, however, that so far downstream to a lesion flow disturbances, even those induced by lesions associated with more than 60% diameter reduction, have disappeared [7]. An additional problem is that the sample volume cannot be made sufficiently small to distinguish normal from slightly diseased arteries on the basis of spectral broadening when measuring at this site in the internal carotid artery (see above).

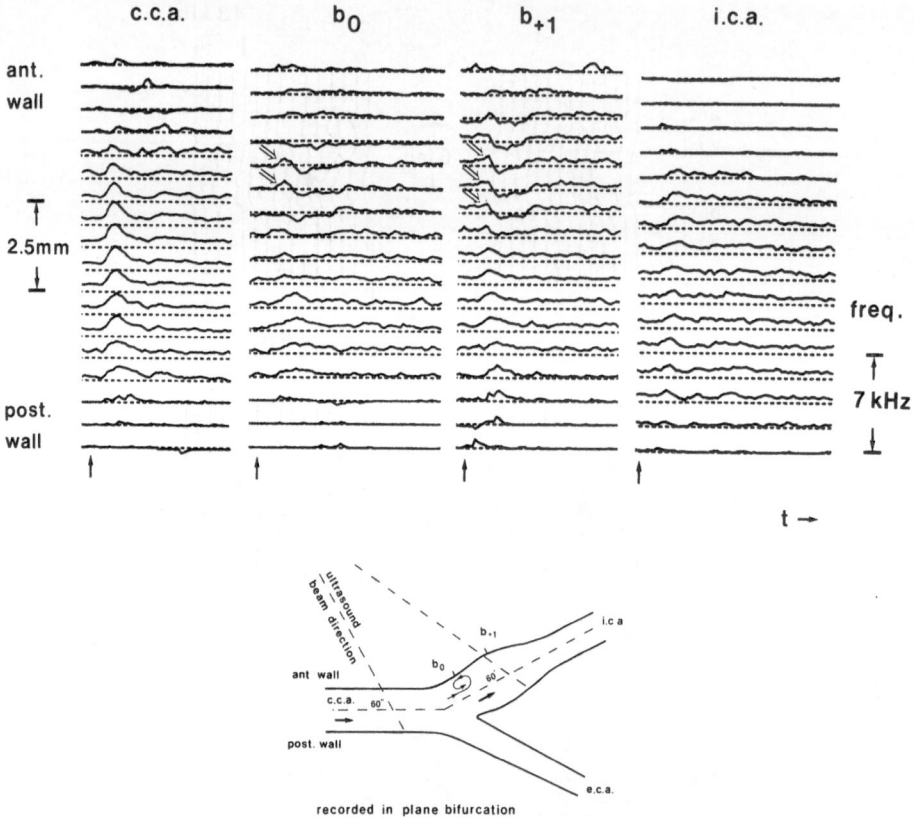

Figure 6. The mean instantaneous velocities as recorded simultaneously at various sites along the ultrasound beam with a multi-channel pulsed Doppler instrument at the same sites and in the same subject as in Fig. 5. The arrow represents the trigger derived from the R-wave of the ECG. Note the triphasic pattern of the velocity waveform in the bulb on the side opposite to the flow divider (open arrow) with forward flow early in systole followed by retrograde flow, starting during the deceleration phase, and forward flow again later during the cardiac cycle. This pattern is indicative of flow separation and recirculation as depicted in the schematical drawing. In this drawing recirculation is only shown at the level of bo. The arrows in the schematical drawing indicate the main direction of flow. From Reneman *et al.,* 1985; with permission of the American Heart Association.

The use of multi-channel pulsed Doppler instruments to detect disturbances in the flow pattern

As discussed in chapter 4, multi-channel pulsed Doppler systems allow the on-line recording of (1) the mean instantaneous velocity, simultaneously measured at various sites along the ultrasound beam, (2) velocity profiles at discrete time intervals during the cardiac cycle and (3) the relative diameter changes of an artery during the cardiac cycle. In healthy adults the mean instantaneous velocity tracings along the ultrasound beam in the common and internal carotid arteries

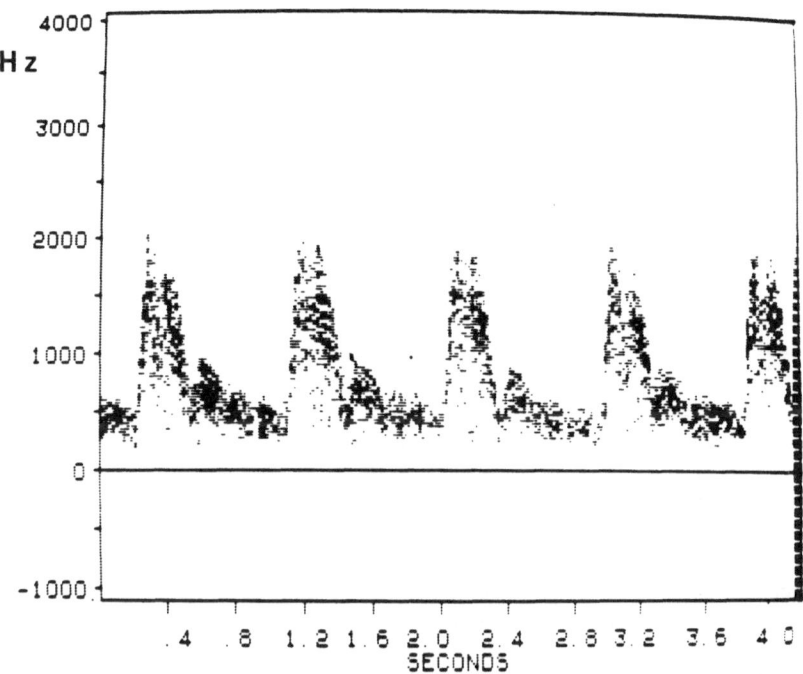

Figure 7. Doppler audio spectra as recorded proximally in the carotid artery bulb of a volunteer (age: 57 years). Note the absence of retrograde flow during the deceleration phase at this age (see text).

are similar in shape, resulting in a symmetric velocity profile. In these arteries the velocity profile is generally flat (Fig. 5), which is representative of plug flow. The widening of the velocity profile during systole is generally symmetric because the anterior and posterior walls of the cervical carotid arteries are contributing equally to the increase in diameter. It should be noted, however, that the widening of the velocity profile is less pronounced in older subjects because the relative increase in carotid artery diameter during systole diminishes with age [17, 28].

In a preliminary study we found that information about the presence and localization of lesions can be derived from data provided by the multi-channel pulsed Doppler system. Indicative of vascular lesions are:
– distortion of the mean velocity waveforms and oscillations on these tracings locally in the artery or along its cross-section, representing the presence of turbulence
– asymmetry of the velocity profile at sites where the profile is symmetric under normal circumstances
– a narrow velocity profile in combination with high peak velocities during systole.

Local distortion of the mean instantaneous waveform near the posterior wall of the common carotid artery (Fig. 8) could be caused by a small lesion, barely

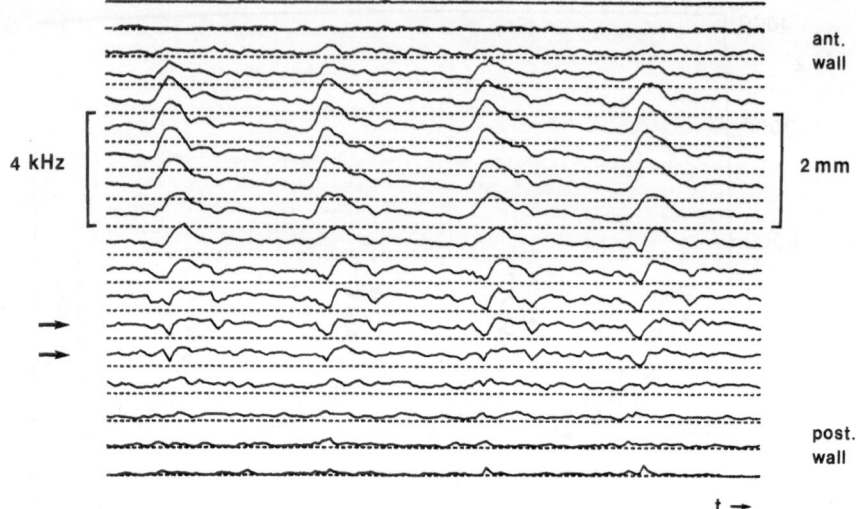

Figure 8. The mean instantaneous velocities as recorded simultaneously at various sites along the ultrasound beam in the common carotid artery of a patient with TIA's. Four cardiac cycles are depicted. Note the distorted velocity waveforms near the posterior wall (arrows).

visible on the angiogram, but troubling the patient with T.I.A.'s. Just proximal to a low grade stenosis (less than 30% diameter reduction) in the internal carotid artery the velocity profile showed asymmetry as compared with the non-diseased side (Fig. 9). This asymmetry probably results from reflections or local contraction of the bloodstream or both. In this case the asymmetry was most pronounced near the posterior wall, indicating that the lesion was located at this site of the vessel which was confirmed by contrast arteriography.

In a preliminary prospective study on 50 cervical carotid arteries in 34 subjects, combining audio spectrum analysis according to Langlois and co-investigators [14] and Breslau [13] and the above mentioned criteria, lesions with a degree of artery narrowing of less than 50% (diameter reduction) could be diagnosed with a sensitivity of 89%, a specificity of 83% and an accuracy of 87% as compared to contrast arteriography. Although these results are promising several problems are encountered in this approach:
– quantification of the disturbances in the velocity profile is difficult
– the maximum velocity that can be detected unambiguously is limited (Chapter 3) so that information about lesions has to be derived from recordings proximal to and distal to the lesion
– positioning and maintenance of the sample volume within a tight stenosis are difficult, especially when narrow sound beams are used.

Further clinical studies are required to investigate whether the detailed velocity information which can be obtained with multi-channel pulsed Doppler instruments allows the distinction between the flow disturbances induced by low grade vascular lesions and those normally occurring at the carotid artery bifurcation.

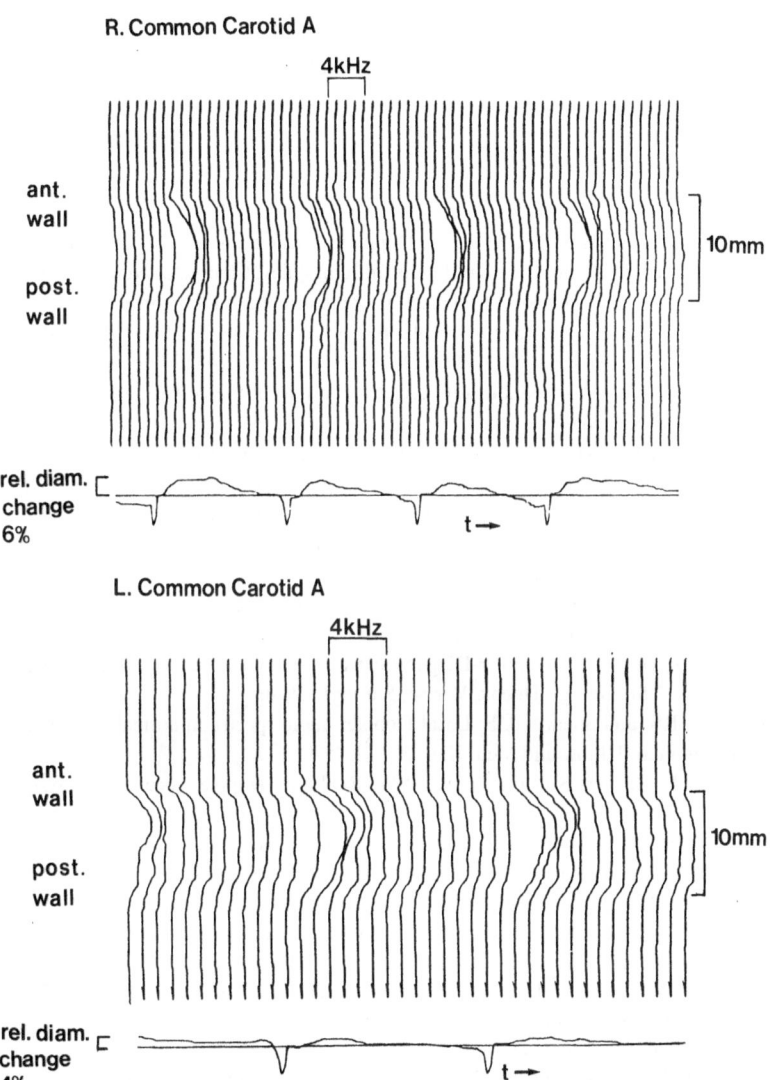

Figure 9. The velocity profiles at discrete time intervals during the cardiac cycle as recorded in the left and right common carotid arteries of a patient (age: 66 years) with a stenosis (<30% diameter reduction) proximal in the left carotid artery bulb. Note the asymmetric velocity profile at the diseased side. At this side the relative increase in artery diameter during systole is diminished. An increase of 6% is normal for this age. The negative deflection coincides with the R-wave of the ECG. From Reneman et al, 1982; with permission of the J. Cereb. Blood Flow Metabol.

Acknowledgements

The authors are indebted to Mariet de Groot and Jos Heemskerk for typing the manuscript and to Paul Hick for making the illustrations. The investigations were supported by the Dutch Heart Foundation and FUNGO, which is subsidized by the Netherlands Organization for the Advancement of Pure Research.

References

1. Reneman RS, and Hoeks APG (eds.): Doppler ultrasound in the diagnosis of cerebrovascular disease. Research Studies Press – A division of John Wiley, Chichester-New York-Toronto, 1982.
2. Thiele BL, Young JV, Chikos PM, Hirsch JH, and Strandness DE: Correlation of arteriographic findings and symptoms in cerebrovascular disease. Neurology 30: 1041–1046, 1980.
3. Van Merode T, Hick P, Hoeks APG, and Reneman RS: Serum HDL/total cholesterol ratio and blood pressure in asymptomatic atherosclerotic lesions of the cervical carotid arteries in men. Stroke 16: 34–38, 1985.
4. Giddens DP, Mabon RF, and Cassanova RA: Measurements of disordered flows distal to subtotal vascular stenoses in the thoracic aortas of dogs. Circ. Res. 39: 112–119, 1976.
5. Barnes RW, Bone GE, Reinertson J, Slaymaker EE, Hokanson DE, and Strandness DE: Non-invasive ultrasonic carotid angiography: prospective validation by contrast arteriography. Surgery 80: 328–335, 1976.
6. Sandmann W, Peronneau PA, Schweins G, Bournat J, and Hinglais J: Turbulenzmessung mit dem Doppler-Ultraschallverfahren: Eine neue Methode der Qualitatskontrolle in der Arterienchirurgie. In Ultraschall-Doppler-Diagnostik in der Angiologie. (Kriesmann A. and Bollinger A, eds.), pp. 77–81. George Thieme Verlag, Stuttgart, 1978.
7. Reneman RS, and Spencer MP: Local Doppler audio spectra in normal and stenosed carotid arteries in man. Ultrasound Med. Biol. 5: 1–11, 1979.
8. Barnes RW, Rittgers SE, and Putney WW: Real-time Doppler spectrum analysis: predictive value in defining operable carotid artery disease. Arch. Surg. 117: 52–57, 1982.
9. Van Baalen JM, Jakimowicz JJ, and Reneman RS: Noninvasive evaluation of carotid artery stenosis – Comparison of direct and indirect techniques. Vasc. Surg. 18: 88–95, 1984.
10. Arbeille Ph, Lapierre F, Benhamou AC, Salez F, Lagueyrie M, and Pourcelot L: L'echotomographie et l'analyse spectral du signal Doppler dans le bilan des lesions carotidiennes. J. Maladies Vasc. 9: 171–178, 1984.
11. Blackshear WM, Phillips DJ, Thiele BL, Hirsch JH, Chikos PM, Marinelli MR, Ward CJ, and Strandness DE: Detection of carotid occlusive disease by ultrasonic imaging and pulsed Doppler spectrum analysis. Surgery 86: 698–706, 1979.
12. Fell G, Phillips DJ, Chikos PM, Harley JD, Thiele BL, and Strandness DE: Ultrasonic Duplex scanning for disease of the carotid artery. Circulation 64: 1191–1195, 1981.
13. Breslau PJ: Ultrasonic duplex scanning in the evaluation of carotid artery disease. Thesis, University of Limburg, Maastricht, The Netherlands, 1982.
14. Langlois Y, Roederer GO, Chan A, Phillips DJ, Beach KW, Martin D, Chikos PM, and Strandness DE: Evaluating carotid artery disease – The concordance between pulsed Doppler/spectrum analysis and angiography. Ultrasound Med Biol 9: 51–63, 1983.
15. Van Merode T, Hick P, Hoeks APG, and Reneman RS: Limitations of Doppler spectral broadening in the early detection of carotid artery disease due to the size of the sample volume. Ultrasound Med Biol 9: 581–586, 1983.
16. Phillips DJ, Greene FM, Langlois Y, Roederer GO, and Strandness DE: Flow velocity patterns in the carotid bifurcations of young, presumed normal subjects. Ultrasound Med Biol 9: 39–49, 1983.
17. Reneman RS, Van Merode T, Hick P, and Hoeks APG: Flow velocity patterns in and distensibility of the carotid artery bulb in volunteers of varying age. Circulation 71: 500–509, 1985.
18. Reneman RS: What measurements are necessary for a comprehensive evaluation of the peripheral arterial circulation. Cardiovasc. Dis. 8: 435–454, 1981.

19. Reneman RS, Van Merode T, Hick P, and Hoeks APG: Noninvasive detection of atherosclerotic lesions in cervical carotid arteries at an early stage of the disease. J. Cereb Blood Flow Metabol 2, Suppl. 1: 32–34, 1982.

20. Spencer, MP: Ultrasonic detection of the non-stenotic plaque. In Cerebrovascular evaluation with Doppler ultrasound (Spencer MP, and Reid JM, eds), p. 164. Martinus Nijhoff, The Hague-Boston-London, 1981.

21. Peronneau PA, Bournat JP, Bugnon A, Barbet A, and Xhaard M: Theoretical and practical aspects of pulsed Doppler flowmetry: real-time application to the measure of instantaneous velocity profiles *in vitro* and *in vivo*. In: Reneman RS (ed.) Cardiovascular applications of ultrasound pp. 66–84. North-Holland/American Elsevier, Amsterdam-London-New York, 1974.

22. Hoeks APG: On the development of a multi-gate pulsed Doppler system with serial data-processing. Thesis, University of Limburg, Maastricht, The Netherlands, 1982.

23. Bharadvaj BK, Mabon RF, and Giddens DP: Steady flow in a model of the human carotid bifurcation. Part I-Flow visualization. J Biomech 15: 349–362, 1982.

24. Bharadvaj BK, Mabon RF, and Giddens DP: Steady flow in a model of the human carotid bifurcation. Part II-Laser-Doppler anemometer measurements. J Biomech 15: 363–378, 1982.

25. Zarins CK, Giddens DP, Bharadvaj BK, Sottiurai VS, Mabon RF, and Glagov S: Carotid bifurcation atherosclerosis – Quantitative correlation of plaque localization with flow velocity profiles and wall shear stress. Circ Res 53: 502–514, 1983.

26. Ku DN, and Giddens DP: Pulsatile flow in a model carotid bifurcation. Arteriosclerosis 3: 31–39, 1983.

27. Motomiya M, and Karino T: Flow patterns in the human carotid artery bifurcation. Stroke 15: 50–56, 1984.

28. Reneman RS, Van Merode T, Hoeks APG, and Hick P: The on-line recording of velocity profiles and diameter changes in normal and stenosed cervical carotid arteries in man. Ultrasound Med Biol 8, Suppl 1: 166, 1982.

Hemodynamics of arterial stenosis

M.P. Spencer

The adverse consequences of carotid atherosclerotic plaques are manifest through two effects on brain perfusion: 1) embolism from intimal ulcerations to the brain and eye, and 2) a reduction in hemispheric flow. The purpose of this chapter is to understand the local Doppler velocity signals and the local pressure-flow relationships associated with stenosis of the carotid arteries in order to quantitate the degree of carotid narrowing and its effect on brain perfusion.

Definitions

Stenosis is defined as a narrowing or constriction in the otherwise normal diameter of a flow channel. It is usually limited to a short segment (less than 10 mm) along the axis of the vessel, beyond which there is a return towards the normal luminal dimensions. In the case of the carotid bifurcation, the definition must be further refined since there is normally a broadening of the common carotid at its bifurcation which includes the first 2 cm of the internal carotid artery. In the strictest sense, any encroachment on this 'bulb' of the carotid is a stenosis and this definition is useful if the object is to quantitate the mass of atherosclerotic plaque with real-time B-mode ultrasound. If hemodynamic consequences, so far as blood flow through the internal carotid is the object of study, then stenosis may be defined in terms of the lumen beyond the bulb which is usually of constant dimensions from the carotid bulb to the base of the skull (Fig. 1). This later definition is often used in comparing radiologic determined diameters with blood velocity as indexed by continuous-wave Doppler examinations, since neither of these methods can visualize the original diameter when the bulb is encroached upon. For the purposes of this chapter, the later definition of stenosis is used. Other definitions of terms used in this chapter include: 'occlusion' which represents total obliteration of the vessel lumen and 'obstruction' representing either stenosis or occlusion.

Various quantifications of morphological degrees of carotid stenosis have been

118

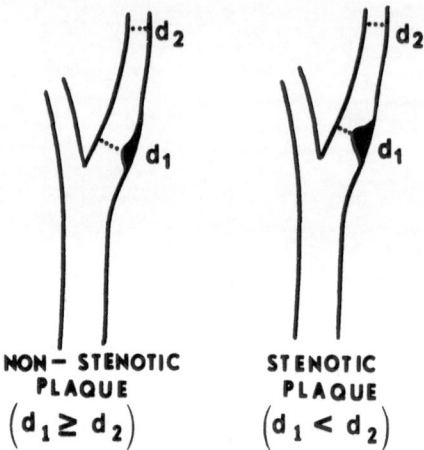

NON-STENOTIC
PLAQUE
$$\left(d_1 \geq d_2\right)$$

STENOTIC
PLAQUE
$$\left(d_1 < d_2\right)$$

Figure 1. A definition of stenosis in terms of using the downstream distal internal carotid as a reference. This definition works well for angiography where there are various magnification factors.

reviewed [1]. Presently the best overall standard for degree of stenosis comes from angiography but varying uncalibrated magnifications, especially compounded by digital subtraction techniques, make it difficult to find an absolute determination. Brown and Johnston [1] recommend an absolute measurement of minimal residual diameter corrected for arteriographic magnification. Imaging of the arterial lumen with injections of radiation opaque media produces a silhouette of the lumen projected by the x-rays on photographic film. Thus the fundamental measurement represents diameter of the projected plane. Several factors distort this diameter information including magnification and resolution limits. In addition, several projections may be necessary to characterize the residual lumen which may not be circular. The best practical method we have found is to calculate the percent reduction in diameter by measuring with a micrometer the smallest diameter found on the x-ray film at the stenosis site, dividing it by the downstream diameter near the jaw, subtracting the fraction from one and multiplying by 100. Such a procedure obviates the effects of magnification and minimizes the resolution problem. To be objective each measurement should be accompanied by a range of confidence and the measurement method must be stated. Another objective measure of degree of stenosis is to use at the time of endarterectomy a calibrated probe inserted through the common carotid. Certainly all methods have their advantages and limitations but contrast radiography still provide the best opportunity for checking the accuracy of noninvasive estimates of morphological severity of arterial stenosis.

Hemodynamic significance is a term which is often used with regard to arterial stenosis with different intents and usually with no clear definition. There are actually several levels of significance to arterial obstructions. As atherosclerotic plaque growth fills in the bulb, there results various grades of stenosis proceeding to total occlusion. The various levels of significance may be described as in Table 1.

All these effects of progressive stenosis in various forms may be said to be hemodynamically significant. The most common intent for 'hemodynamically significant' probably refers to the evoking of collateral effects around the branches of the ophthalmic artery. The phenomenon of collateral around the orbit, and various detectable aspects of it, formed the basis for the first noninvasive test for carotid artery obstruction. These included: infrared detection of skin temperatures of the forehead, modifications of cutaneous capillary pulsations, pneumatic and liquid methods of studying pulsations of the orbital globe [2, 3], ophthalmodynometry and continuous-wave Doppler interrogation of the periorbital arteries [4, 5, 6, 7, 8]. Most of these modalities were used in conjunction with compressions of the common carotid and temporal and facial arteries. The underlying principle of these methods is when collateral effects are demonstrated it can be concluded that there is a 'hemodynamically significant' obstruction of the internal carotid artery. These methods have shown a high degree of sensitivity but, unfortunately, negative tests can often be obtained in the face of high grades of stenosis and total occlusion of the internal carotid probably because of adequacy of intracranial collateral channels. Also, when positive, these tests do not separate between high grade stenosis and total occlusion.

Primary, secondary and tertiary hemodynamic effects

For the purposes of Doppler evaluation of the definitions of arterial hemodynamic significance, the information available may be classified into primary, secondary and tertiary effects. These are listed in Table 2.

Table 1. Definitions of hemodynamic significance.

I. Arterial Significant
1. Modification of the normal flow disturbances in the bulb
2. Local increase in velocity
3. Local turbulence
4. Production of a drop in pressure
5. Reduction in volume flow through the stenotic artery
6. Modification of pulsatile flow and velocity waveform
7. Evoking of collateral effects

II. Tissue Significant
8. Reduction of tissue perfusion
9. Production of embolus to the terminal arteries
10. Reduction of oxygen and substrate delivery to the tissues
11. Production of symptoms and functional incapacity
12. Tissue death and infarction

Primary effects

The primary effects of arterial obstruction are found within the stenotic channel itself and when blood is flowing through a stenotic channel, all of these effects are observable with Doppler ultrasound. With continuous-wave Doppler the most useful effect in diagnosis and quantitation of stenosis is the acceleration and increased velocity at the site of stenosis as compared to the normal range of velocities found there (Fig. 2). Fig. 3 illustrates how the velocity of blood increases with progressive increase in severity of stenosis. In spite of the dependence of Doppler frequency shift on the angle of the ultrasonic beam clinical routines generally limit the problem of not knowing the angle accurately. For example, with free hand interrogation of the carotid bifurcation, the strongest signals are generally found at an angle of 50 degrees. When this interrogation is attempted routinely, a range of normal velocities for the origin of the internal carotid artery can be compiled and compared to increased velocities produced by stenosis. The effect of increased velocity does not significantly rise beyond the normal variations until stenoses greater than 50 percent are present.

Table 2. Effects of arterial obstruction detectable with Doppler ultrasound

---

I. Primary: Within the Stenotic Channel
A. Acceleration and Increased Blood Velocity
    compared to normal at same site
    compared to downstream sites in same artery
    compared to upstream in parent artery
B. Flattened velocity profile
C. Loss of normal bulb flow patterns

II. Secondary: Immediately Below and Above the Stenotic Segment
A. Downstream Effects
    1.   Turbulence immediately downstream
       a) flow patterns, whipping, fluttering and whispering
       b) bruit qualities from wall vibrations
    2.   Damping – diminished velocity, slow acceleration and decreased pulsatility
B. Upstream Effects
    1.   Decreased Velocity
    2.   Increased Pulsatility

III. Tertiary: Collateral Channels
A. Adjacent Branches
    1.   Increased Flow and Velocity
    2.   Decreased Pulsatility
B. Distant Interconnecting Collaterals
    1.   Decreased Velocity
    2.   Reversed Direction
    3.   Alternating Flow
    4.   Turbulence at Branch Points

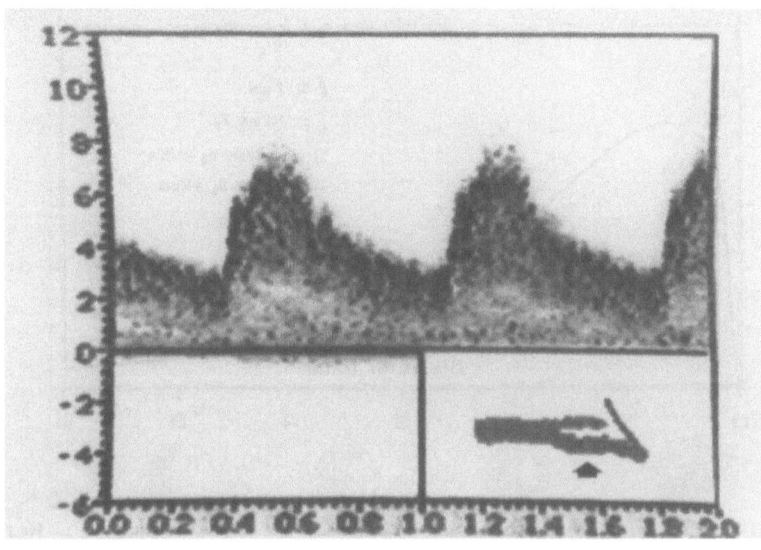

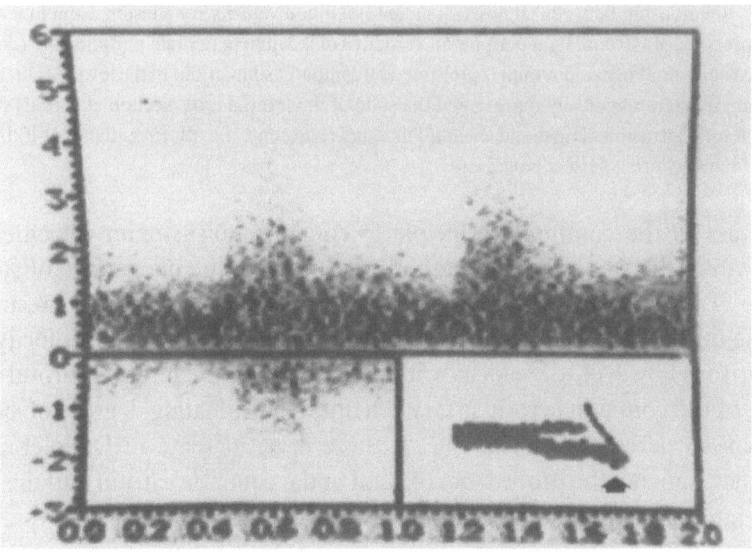

Figure 2A. Doppler frequency spectrum using 5 MHz ultrasound obtained on the origin of the internal carotid artery where there is a 50% of stenosis. Normal peak systolic frequencies should range from 1 to 3 kHz at this level. A concentration of energies near the upper f_{max} border of the time varying spectrum indicates laminar flow within the stenosis.

Figure 2B. Doppler frequency spectrum in the same patient and internal carotid artery as from Figure 2A. Here the ultrasonic beam is directed downstream beyond the stenosis and elevated frequencies of stenosis. Spectrum indicates considerable broadening and uncertain margin on the upper edge of the spectrum as well as inverted reverse spectral representations all of which represent turbulence in the downstream segment.

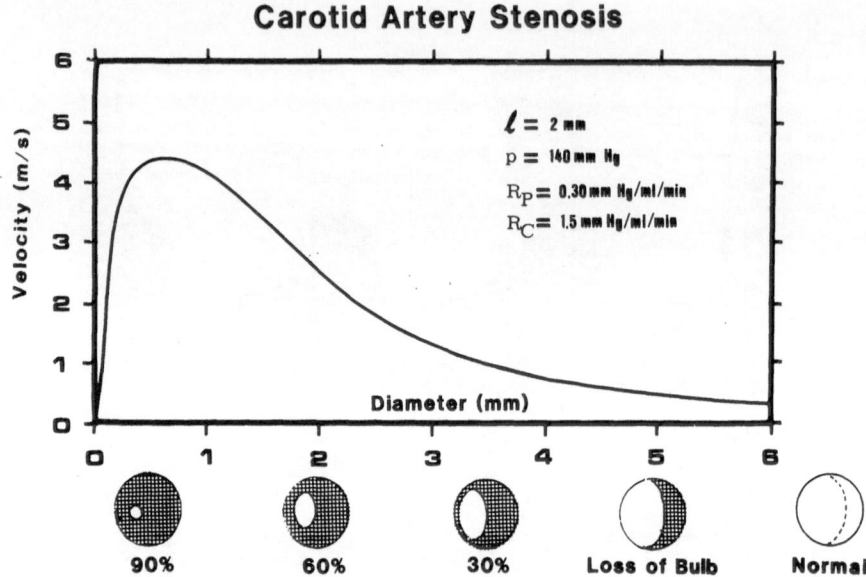

Figure 3. Relationship between stenosis diameter and blood velocity for a lesion 2 mm in length, an arterial pressure of 140 mmHg, a peripheral resistance of 0.3 mmHg per mm per/min and a collateral resistance of 1.5 mmHg per mm/min, represented by computer simulation. In the lower segment of the illustration it diagrammatically represented the state of the arterial cross-section at various stages of atherosclerotic intrusion. The diameter in millimeters represents the effective diameter if the cross-sectional lumen were a perfect circle.

The use of the continuity principle to compare downstream velocities with those within the stenosis, as a method of estimating the percentage of stenosis compared to downstream dimensions, has not worked in practice, presumably because turbulence effects makes it difficult to measure the mean velocity. The comparison, however, of velocity within the origin of the internal carotid artery to that of the common carotid artery is helpful in estimating degrees of stenosis less than 50 percent. For example, if there is an increase in Doppler shifted frequency, moving the probe from the end of the common carotid into the origin of the internal carotid, then one can be sure there is a loss of the vessel bulb diameter and some degree of stenosis is present. If this shift in frequency is a low degree, such as from 2 kHz in the common to 3 kHz in the internal carotid, one may conclude there is some degree of stenosis less than 50 percent on the origin of the internal carotid artery. Normally, the velocities in the end of the common carotid are comparable, or higher than those found in the normal bulb on the origin of the internal carotid.

Secondary effects

The secondary effects of arterial stenosis, which are detectable by Doppler,

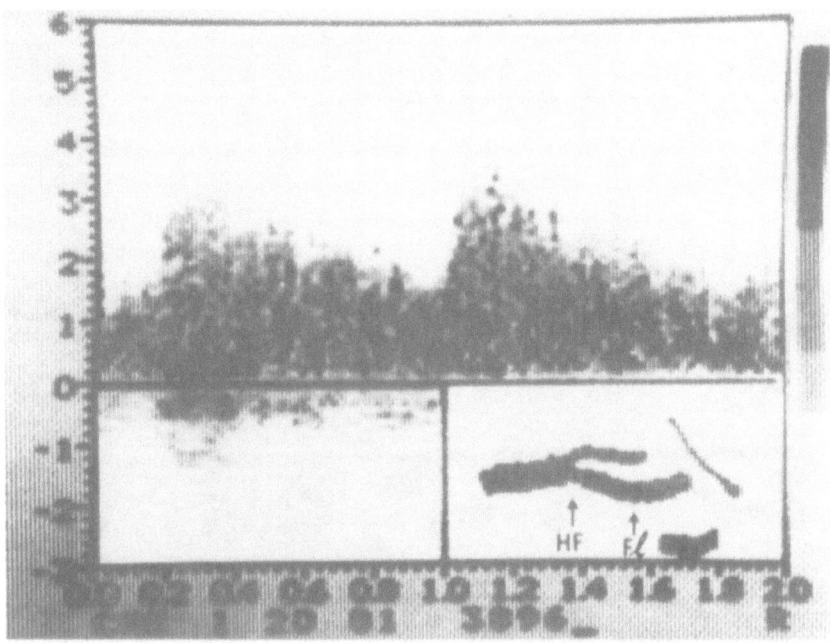

Figure 4. Doppler frequency spectrum representation of 'fluttering' downstream to high frequency of a stenosis on the origin of the internal carotid artery. This spectrum represents extreme turbulence producing a 'stuttering' effect. Lower righthand panel indicates a continuous wave Doppler image of the carotid bifurcation. HF represents the site of high frequency in stenosis. The F indicates the site of the sample in the Doppler frequency spectrum. Also represented is a segment of the vertebral artery posterior to the angle of the jaw represented by a line.

include both upstream and downstream effects. The downstream 'turbulence' phenomena must be separately understood from 'disturbed' flow in the normal carotid bulb. These disturbed flow patterns of flow separation, static zones, reverse flow and helical flow are discussed in Chapter 5 on normal carotid flow and in Chapter 8 on early detection of atherosclerotic plaques. When the plaque has grown to fill the bulb and leave a lumen diameter equal to the normal downstream diameter the disturbed flow effects largely disappear.

True turbulence effects are most prominent in moderate degrees of stenosis between 50–70 percent when there is sufficient blood flow to release greatest turbulent energies. The turbulence produces several manifestations on the Doppler frequency spectrum and are also recognized by hearing various qualities in the Doppler sounds. The audio qualities have been defined as 'fluttering' or 'stuttering' produced by interaction between the high velocity jet, emerging from the stenotic segment, and the slower moving blood downstream (Fig. 2B and 4). Also we recognize 'gruffness' or 'coarseness' and harmonic 'moaning', 'seagull' sounds representing motion of the arterial wall driven by the underlying turbulent flow. Fig. 5. These arterial wall motions representing bruit qualities may be heard with the stethoscope or recorded with a microphone and are not produced by the Doppler effect. Rather they are produced by phase modulation of the ultrasonic

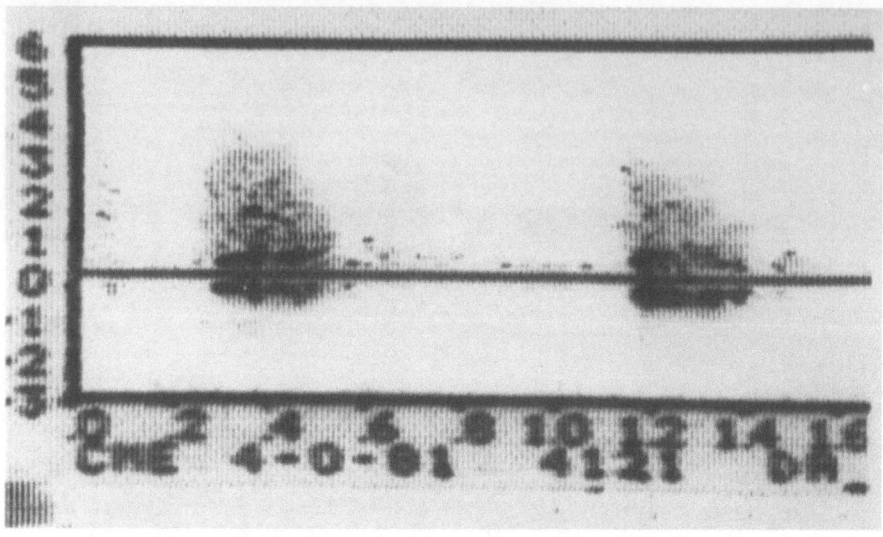

Figure 5. Doppler frequency spectrum representation of a moaning (harmonic) bruit arising from stenosis in the external carotid artery. The 'Doppler bruit' is seen as two dark horizontal bars during two systolic intervals immediately above and below the zero line between +1 and −1 kHz.

wave. In this role Doppler may be considered a directional ultrasonic microphone.

Spectral broadening is a term applied to the pulsed Doppler spectrum when turbulence widens the normally narrow spectral band representing an unobstructed artery. Spectral broadening has been used to diagnose lower grades of stenosis from 1 to 50 percent (Fig. 6A & B). In using this parameter one must be careful to integrate the axis of the flow streams and not near the wall as the velocity gradient near the wall produces a broader spectrum than in the center. Also to use this parameter one must be careful of the effects of disturbed flow in the normal carotid bulb. Chapter 8 also discusses the effects in early carotid lesions. The velocities detectable in the bulb of the normal internal carotid artery do not fully reflect the enlarged diameter, probably because of the effects explained by Giddens [9]. The disturbed flows described by these workers may produce an effect on the continuous-wave Doppler called 'whipping' as discussed in Chapter 5.

Dampening of the downstream Doppler effect develops with severe degrees of stenosis unless the volume of blood flowing through the stenosis is low. The Doppler features of dampening are low velocity, particularly in systole, slow acceleration during systole, delayed peak systolic frequency and lower pulsatility. The lower pulsatility results from the greater lowering of systolic velocities than of diastolic velocities. This feature represents critical upstream stenosis often accompanied by minimal turbulence and no audible bruits by auscultation. It is an

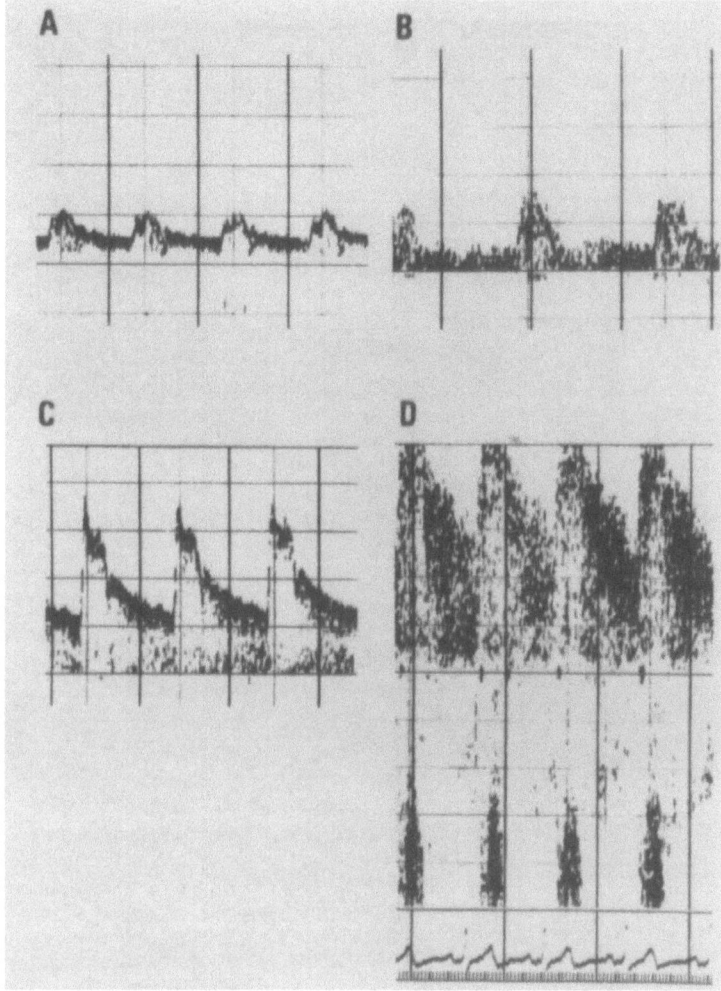

Figure 6A. Spectral characteristics for four grades of stenosis of the internal carotid artery using the spectral broadening concept. A) – represents 16–49% stenosis, B) represents 50–75% stenosis and C & D) represent 76–99% stenosis.

important diagnostic sign which should be carefully sought. Dampening in the common carotid flow streams suggests stenosis at its origin from the aortic arch and may be the only sign of this lesion in the cervical common carotid artery. When found in the internal carotid artery preocclusive stenosis may be present.

Upstream to an obstruction of the internal carotid artery one often finds diminished velocities. If collateral up the external carotid is strong, this effect may not be present. However, when there is an asymmetry in the pulsatility and velocities between the two common carotid arteries, increased pulsatility indicates severe obstruction of the homolateral internal carotid artery.

126

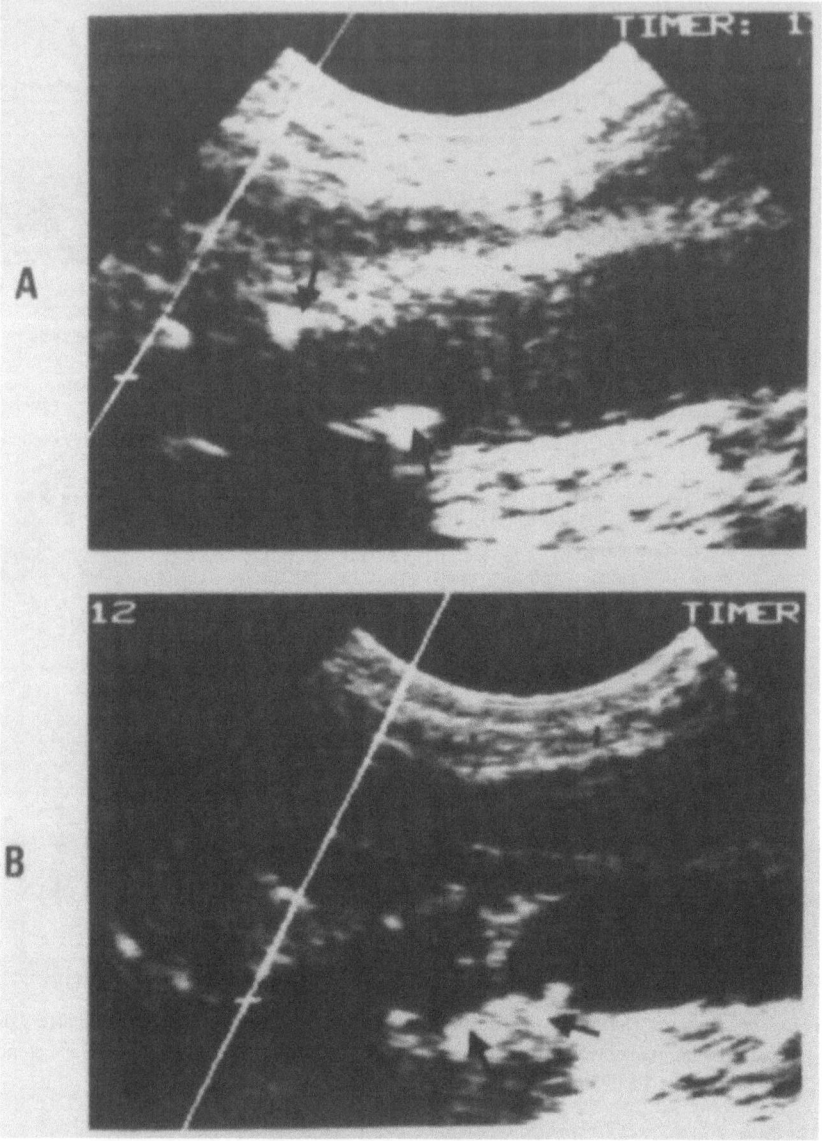

Figure 6B. B-mode imaging generated at the time of Duplex scanning of two minor grades of internal carotid artery stenosis. A – image corresponding to the spectrum of 6A A). B – image generated at the time of the spectrum shown in Figure 6A B).

Tertiary effects

The arterial branches adjacent to an obstructed artery which carry blood or support the pressure in the vascular territory of the unobstructed artery are termed 'collaterals' (Fig. 7). They develop because the pressure gradients of

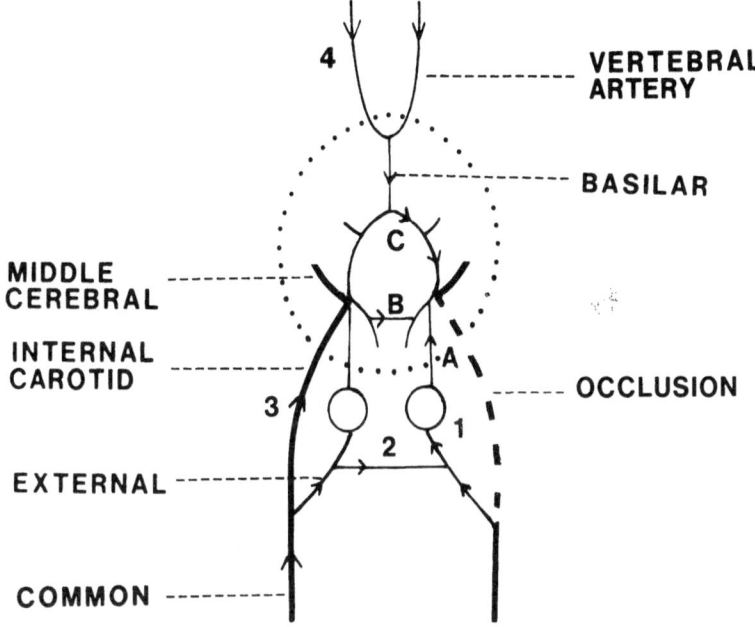

Figure 7. Diagram of major collateral pathways when there is occlusion of an internal carotid artery. Extracranial pathways are: 1 = homolateral external carotid branches, 2 = cross midline communications of the external carotid arteries, 3 = contralateral internal carotid and 4 = vertebral arteries. Intracranial pathways are: A = ophthalmic artery, B = anterior cerebral arteries via the anterior communicating artery and C = basilar-posterior cerebral and posterior communicating arteries. Leptomeningeal arteries serve the surface of the brain [10].

interconnecting branches are in their favor. The initial and persistent effect is to increase velocities in the nearest branches of the parent artery common to the obstructed one. This increased velocity is accompanied by decreased pulsatility expressing the lowered peripheral resistance now supplied by the collateral artery. The more distant collaterals however nearer the territory of the obstructed artery have a reversed flow which may be of higher velocity than they normally carry (Fig. 8). Between the immediately adjacent branches and the more distant ones, there may be connections which carry an 'alternating' flow (Fig. 9). Alternating flow moves blood first in one direction and then the other during the same heart cycle. The ophthalmic artery in the case of the carotid artery obstruction and the vertebral artery at the base of the skull in the case of subclavian artery stenosis are typical locations for alternating flow.

Where reversed high velocities form a collateral into its former parent artery, conditions for turbulence are present (Fig. 10). This situation producing high Doppler frequencies with spectral broadening and low frequency bruit energies must be differentiated from stenosis. This differentiation is particularly important when examining the intracranial arteries with transcranial pulsed Doppler. The

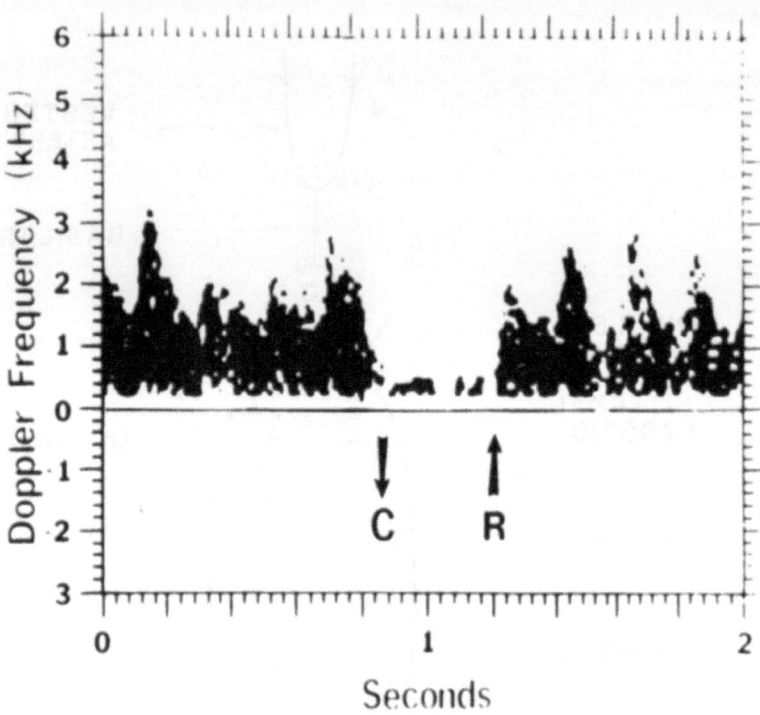

Figure 8. Doppler frequency spectrum of reversed flow in the ophthalmic artery on the side of occlusion of the internal carotid artery. Normal direction of flow is anterior towards 5 MHz CW transducer placed over the eyelid producing a negative 5 MHz CW spectrum below the zero line. Between 'C' and 'R' the homolateral common carotid artery is compressed producing severe reduction in flow through the external carotid and periorbital communicating branches.

Vertebral Arteries

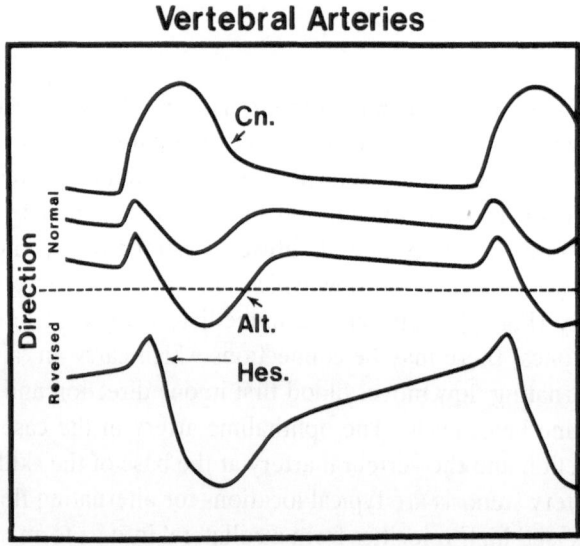

Figure 9. Representative blood flow waveforms seen in the vertebral arteries during various stages of subclavian steal. The upper curve represents the normal 'continuous' waveform. The lower curve represents a complete steal with a slight hesitation (Hes) in early systole. 'Alt.' represents an alternating waveform which may be converted to a complete steal if reactive hyperemia is produced in the homolateral arm.

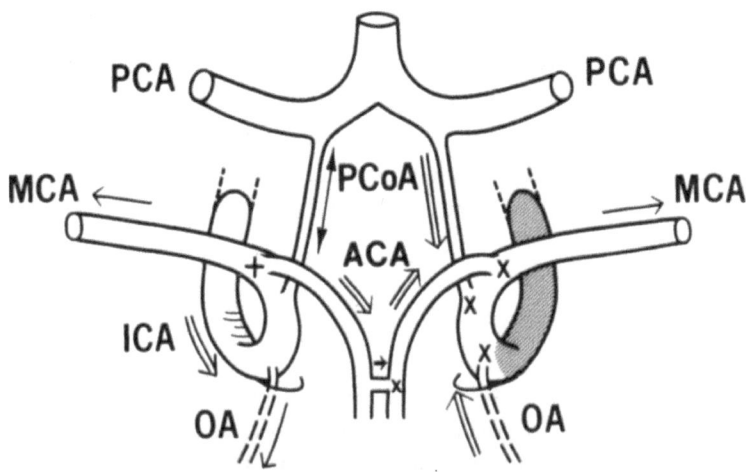

Figure 10. Diagram of the major basal arteries of the brain and intracranial collateral channels. Elevated Doppler frequencies may be expected where the double shafted arrows are shown. Sites for turbulence in the flow streams are indicated by an 'X' where the elevated velocities jet into a wider channel. A + indicates a site for turbulence where elevated internal carotid blood velocities change direction to enter the anterior cerebral artery. PCA = posterior cerebral artery, MCA = middle cerebral artery, PCoA = posterior communicating artery, ACA = anterior cerebral artery, ICA = internal carotid artery and OA = ophthalmic artery.

presence of extracranial carotid artery obstruction alerts the observer of the possibilities of this confusion in the components of the circle of Willis.

Compression of the various extracranial arteries is helpful in confirming and sorting out collateral effects. Two types of compression may be used, total occlusion or rapid oscillating imcomplete. The proper techniques for these two types of compression are described in the Chapter 11 on Free Hand Doppler techniques. When, for example, obstruction of one internal carotid artery is present, collateral effects accoss the interior communicating artery may be diminished by total contralateral compression, but collaterals from the posterior communicating artery may be enhanced by the same manner. Collateral channels around the periorbital arteries may be confined by ipsilateral temporal artery total compression because if the temporal artery is a collateral supply periorbital Doppler signals will be diminished, obliterated or reversed by compression.

Occlusion of an artery is an important diagnosis. Table 3 is provided to list the most important Doppler and B-scan imaging diagnostic features of occlusion of the internal carotid artery. All features are seldom found but sufficient numbers of the features are usually present to confidently differentiate between occlusion or not.

The orifice equation

In the chapter on Normal Blood Flow we discussed how blood viscosity explains resistance to blood flow and the velocity profile. Also blood density was shown to explain temporal acceleration effects between pressure drop and pulsation of the blood flow. When a stenosis develops in a vascular channel, two additional effects of density and viscosity come into play. These are termed the Bernoulli effect and the boundary layer effect. First we will discuss the Bernoulli effect.

Bernoulli effect

The drop in arterial pressure due to a stenosis in the larger arteries and of the heart valves is primarily governed by the convective acceleration of blood. This Bernoulli effect represents a term not entering the normal flow equation of the previous chapter. The Bernoulli Effect, so named because it was mathematically described by Bernoulli, explains the loss in pressure due to an orifice or partial obstruction of a flow channel. The principle is diagrammed in Fig. 10. The blood approaching the stenosis must accelerate to an increased velocity within the stenosis. This is called, 'convective acceleration' to separate it from the 'temporal' type of acceleration explained in the chapter on normal hemodynamics. The Bernoulli equation quantitating this pressure drop is shown in Fig. 11. In this equation, rho = the density of the blood, v_1 is the spatial maximum velocity upstream to the orifice and v_2 is the maximum velocity at the entrance of the orifice. For practical purposes this equation can be simplified for use in cardiac stenosis by eliminating the v_1 term because these velocities are relatively low and the squaring effect on v_2 makes v_2 far more important. Holen [11] has given the simplified cardiac formula as:

$$\triangle p = 4\, v_{max}^2$$

Table 3. Extracranial diagnostic features of internal carotid occlusion.

DOPPLER

No high frequencies or other primary effects found
No Doppler image of the internal carotid found
No signals in the parasellar siphon found with transcranial Doppler
Diminished common carotid frequencies and increased pulsatility compared to the opposite side
Greater than normal vertebral and basilar artery frequencies
Collateral effects found around the periorbital arteries and ophthalmic artery
Transmission of temporal artery manual oscillations down common carotid artery

B-MODE

Loss of pulsatility in artery image
Speckling in internal carotid artery
Headward thrusting of common carotid artery
No Doppler signal in internal carotid image

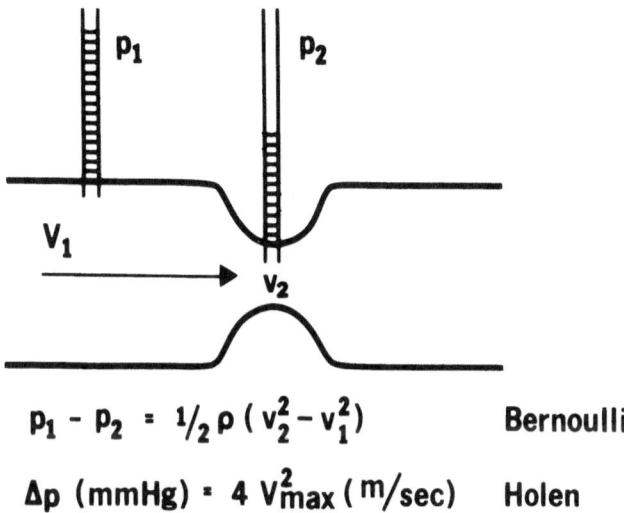

$$p_1 - p_2 = \frac{1}{2} \rho \left(v_2^2 - v_1^2 \right) \qquad \textbf{Bernoulli}$$

$$\Delta p \text{ (mmHg)} = 4 \, V_{max}^2 \text{ (m/sec)} \qquad \textbf{Holen}$$

Figure 11. Diagram of the hemodynamic situation where velocity (v) is accelerated into a stenotic channel from v_1 to v_2 producing a drop in pressure between p_1 and p_2. The Bernoulli equation relates the pressure drop to the blood density rho and the difference in the squared velocities. The Holen formula simplifies the Bernoulli equation for clinical purposes when the maximum velocity can be obtained from the Doppler spectrum.

where Δp is in mmHg and v is in meters/second. Doppler spectral analysis is particularly useful in calculating these pressure drops because it is the maximum velocity that is used in the equation and this is represented on the upper edge of the Doppler spectrum. In actual fact, in arterial stenoses, there may be a partial recovery in pressure downstream to the stenosis due to the confinement of the arterial walls on the flow stream as discussed by Clark [12]. In applying the equation to arterial stenosis, it is probably advisable to use the v_1 term or substitute for v_1 a nominal, normal velocity when no upstream determination can be made. This procedure avoids the overestimation of the pressure drop when some recovery takes place. In fact, the tighter the stenosis the less the recovery effects will have on the net pressure drop.

In order to use Doppler to calculate the pressure drop, it is important to use an angle of insonation less than 30° in order to estimate the true velocity. Angle correction techniques using B-mode to determine the angle between the sound beam and the vessel wall is not advisable because the jet direction may not be parallel to the vessel axis. The best technique is to move the probe around at different angles in free hand style to find the highest possible Doppler shift frequency. When this is found, a small change in angle of insonation will not produce a perceptible frequency shift. It is also important to use a high pass filter on the Doppler spectrum in order to reduce the low frequency turbulence effects which obscure the upper edge of the spectrum (Fig. 12A & B). Once the highest maximum frequency is found, the true maximum velocity can be calculated from

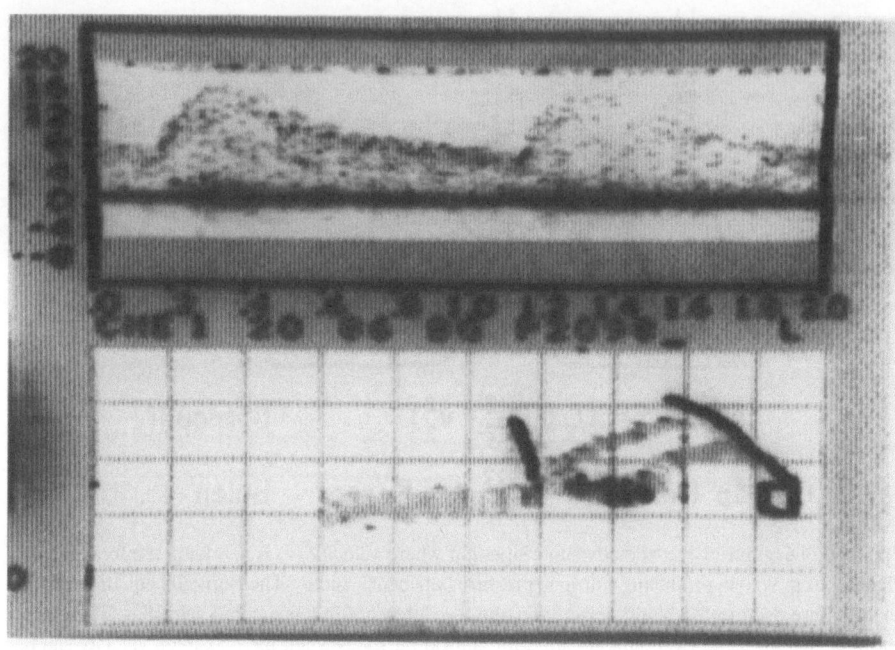

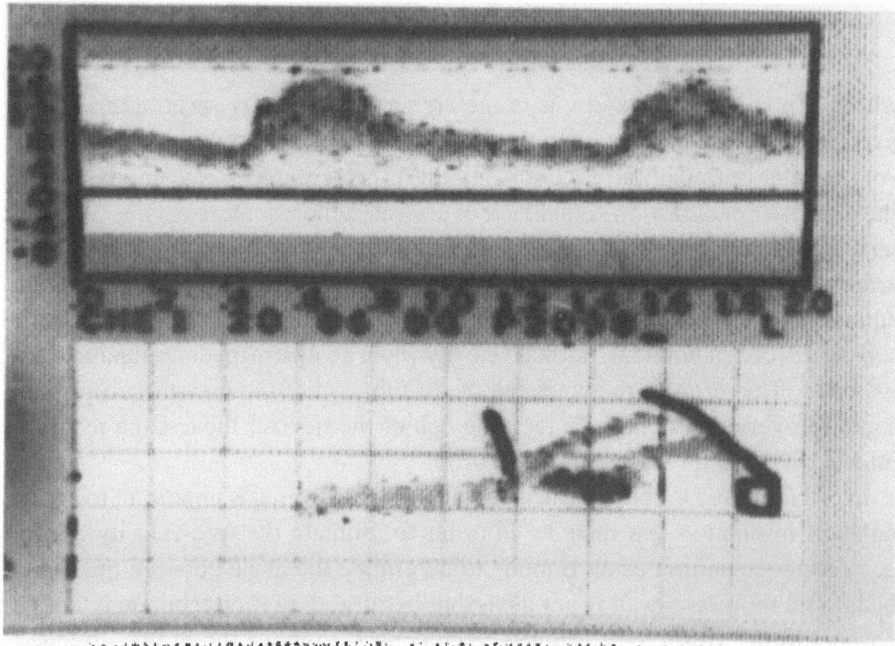

Figure 12A. High frequency and turbulence of internal carotid artery stenosis shown in upper panel. The CW Doppler image of the carotid bifurcation. Dark area representing the origin of the ICA represents region from which the spectrum was obtained.

Figure 12B. Effect of a high pass filter on the Doppler arterial stenosis frequency spectrum. High energy lower frequencies, which virtually attenuate the upper high frequency f_{max} are attenuated. An extra boost in amplitude of frequencies above 6 kHz is also provided. The upper f_{max} of the Doppler spectrum is enhanced.

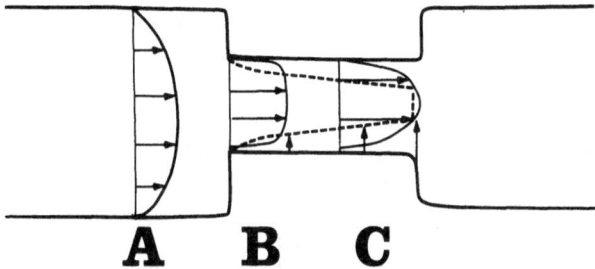

Figure 13. Diagrammatic representation of velocity profile changes occurring within a stenotic arterial segment. A = parabolic profile before stenosis, B = flat profile produced by acceleration at entrance of stenosis and C = return to parabolic profile in long stenosis.

the Doppler equation and subsequently the pressure drop is calculated with the Bernoulli equation.

The value of the pressure drop calculation lies in the fact that it better represents the arterial hemodynamic significance better than any of the other first seven parameters of Table 1. From the pressure drop and the brachial artery pressure one may make a good estimate of the brain perfusion pressure on the side of a carotid stenosis.

Boundary layer effect

As we follow the flow streams from the stenosis entrance along the stenotic channel, there is a gradual change from the flattened profile, produced by Bernoulli convective acceleration, towards a parabolic profile (Fig. 13). The change in shear-rate, producing this modification in profile, produces a pressure drop which is related to the length of the stenotic segment as well as its radius. This loss is in addition to the Bernoulli density loss but is usually small compared to the Bernoulli effect.

The boundary layer term of the flow equation, however, must be considered [13] and the viscous effects given special consideration as the velocity profile changes in long stenoses. Gravity effects may generally be ignored in short vascular segments. Temporal acceleration effects may be eliminated by averaging over a heart cycle or computing pressure drop only when temporal changes in velocity are minimal, such as at peak systole or during diastole.

Computer simulations

When the Bernoulli and the boundary layer Poiseuille effects are programmed in a computer, along with peripheral resistance, the relationship between various parameters may be studied in isolation. Fig. 14 illustrates the model of the orifice equation.

Modeling the Orifice Equation

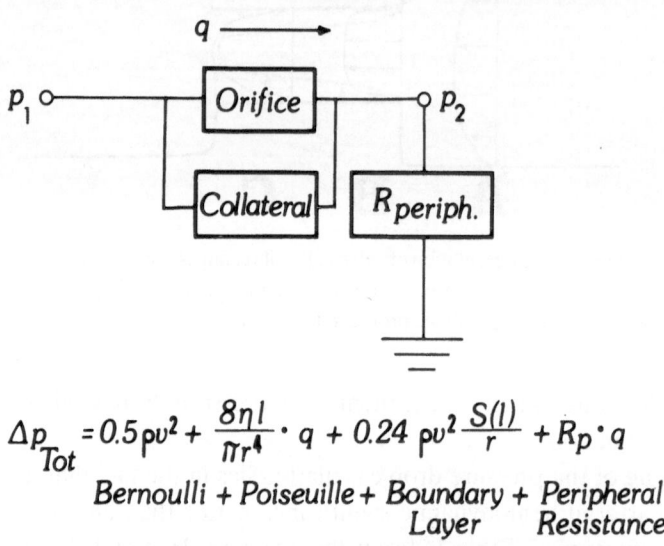

$$\Delta p_{Tot} = 0.5\rho v^2 + \frac{8\eta l}{\pi r^4} \cdot q + 0.24 \rho v^2 \frac{S(l)}{r} + R_p \cdot q$$

Bernoulli + Poiseuille + Boundary + Peripheral
                                    Layer   Resistance

Figure 14. Diagram and equation of the orifice (stenosis) equation. Δp_{tot} = pressure drop across the stenosis between p_1 and p_2, R_p = peripheral resistance, rho = blood density, eta = blood viscosity, v = maximum velocity with the stenosis, q = blood flow through the peripheral resistance (total of stenosis and collateral) l & r = length and radius of stenotic channel and S = change in velocity profile within stenosis.

Figs. 15A & B show what may be expected when the length of a carotid artery stenosis varies from 1 to 10 mm covering most of the clinically expected range. Fig. 16 illustrates how the arterial pressure affects the relationship between stenosis diameter and blood velocity.

The greatest f_{max} possible even with no collaterals available and an arterial pressure of 200 mm Hg does not reach 6 m/sec. Fig. 17 demonstrates how a low peripheral resistance is important to increase velocity and bring out the Bernoulli effect.

The largest single influence on the velocity-diameter relationship within a carotid stenosis is that of collateral channels. Fig. 18 demonstrates how changing the R_c/R_p ratio produces a wide range of velocities for a given degree of stenosis. Because of this there is limited ability of the Doppler frequency to accurately reflect the stenosis morphology. The pressure drop relationship to velocity is, however, a very stable relationship irrespective of the collaterals, thus pressure drop and Doppler f_{max} are reflections of hemodynamic severity of carotid stenosis.

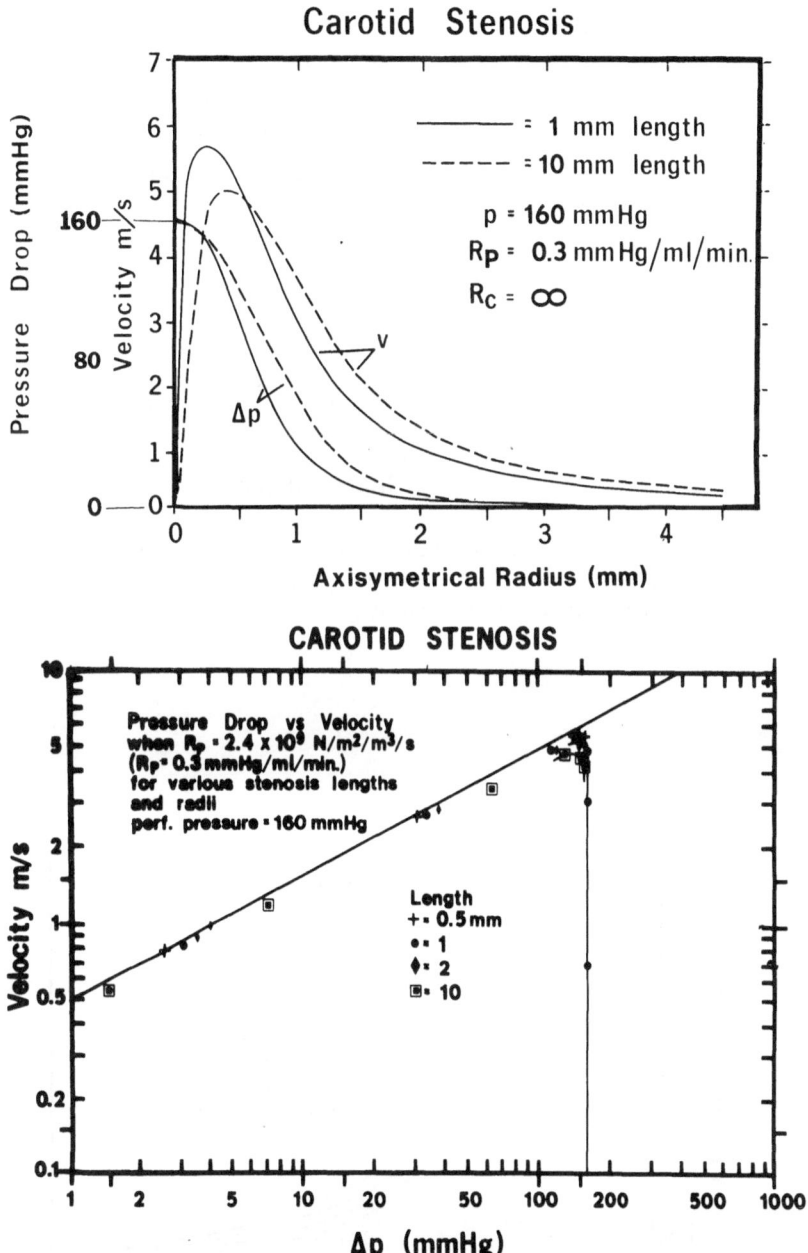

Figure 15A. Effect of changing length of stenosis on the relationships between stenosis radius, velocity (v) and pressure drop (△p). Two lengths are shown 1 mm solid line and 10 mm dashed line. Increasing length diminishes the highest velocity attainable in severe stenosis but in moderate degrees of stenosis increasing length elevates both velocity and pressure drop proportionately. p = arterial pressure, R_p = peripheral resistance and R_p = collateral resistance which is taken as infinite (no collateral) in this case.

Figure 15B. Demonstration of how length of a stenotic channel does not greatly affect the relationship between pressure drop and velocity until severe stenosis occurs. If a long stenotic channel is present, the pressure drop calculated from the Bernoulli effect (solid line) is slightly underestimated. Continuous wave Doppler imaging of the carotid bifurcation.

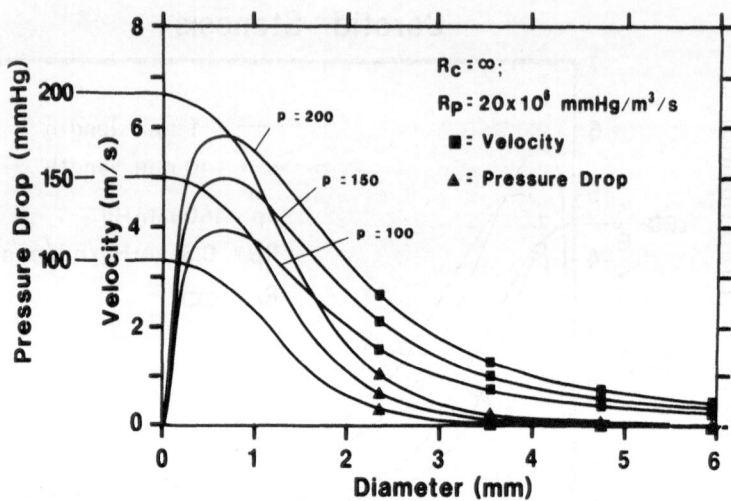

Figure 16. Effect of changing arterial pressure calculated from the orifice equation on blood velocity and pressure drop within carotid stenoses of various diameters. Three different arterial pressures are used and no collaterals in the model (R_C = infinity).

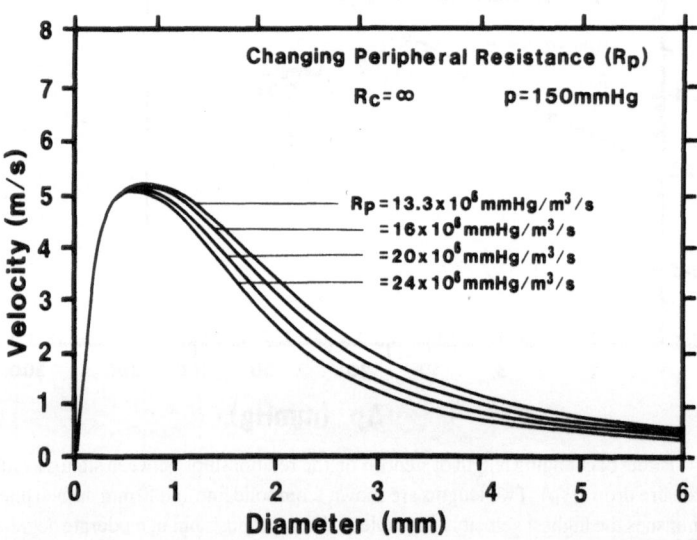

Figure 17. Effect of changing peripheral resistance (R_P) on the relationship between axisymmetric stenosis diameter and blood velocity. R_C = collateral resistance and p = arterial pressure. Peripheral resistance primarily affects the relationship in moderate degrees of stenosis.

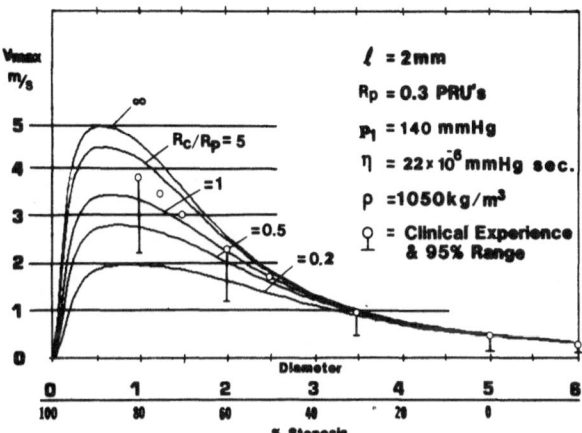

Figure 18. Effect of variations in collateral (R_C) on blood velocity through various degrees of carotid stenosis. Collateral is indicated as a ratio R_C/R_P while peripheral resistance is held constant. R_C/R_P ranges between 0.2 and 5 in most patients and clinical experience shows a wide variation in the Doppler frequency versus diameter relationship due in part to variations in collateral between patients. Mean values for clinical experience among 211 carotid arteries (circles) is superimposed for normal carotids and selected degrees of stenosis. Some of the variation is due both to the ultrasound beam angle variations and limitations of x-ray films.

Surgical and experimental measurements

Flow vs pressure drop in stenosis

Prior to the availability of the noninvasive transcutaneous Doppler ultrasonic velocity detector, the hemodynamics of carotid arterial stenosis in humans was investigated with measurements of blood flow and the pressure gradient. Such measurements required surgical exposure for the application of the electromagnetic flowmeter probes and the insertion of pressure measuring needles. The electromagnetic flowmeter measures the instantaneous volumetric flow across the artery lumen integrating the velocities of all the flow streams.

The occasion of surgical application of the Selverstone clamp for treatment of intracranial aneurysm allowed the opportunity for study of the local hemodynamic effects of graded carotid stenosis in humans. Fig. 19A illustrates the positioning of the Selverstone clamp on the common carotid at the bifurcation, the electromagnetic flow meter probe on the internal carotid artery, and pressure recording of needles inserted below and above the clamp. The interposition of the external carotid branch between the clamp and the internal carotid flow probe does not significantly affect the interpretation of the data presented.

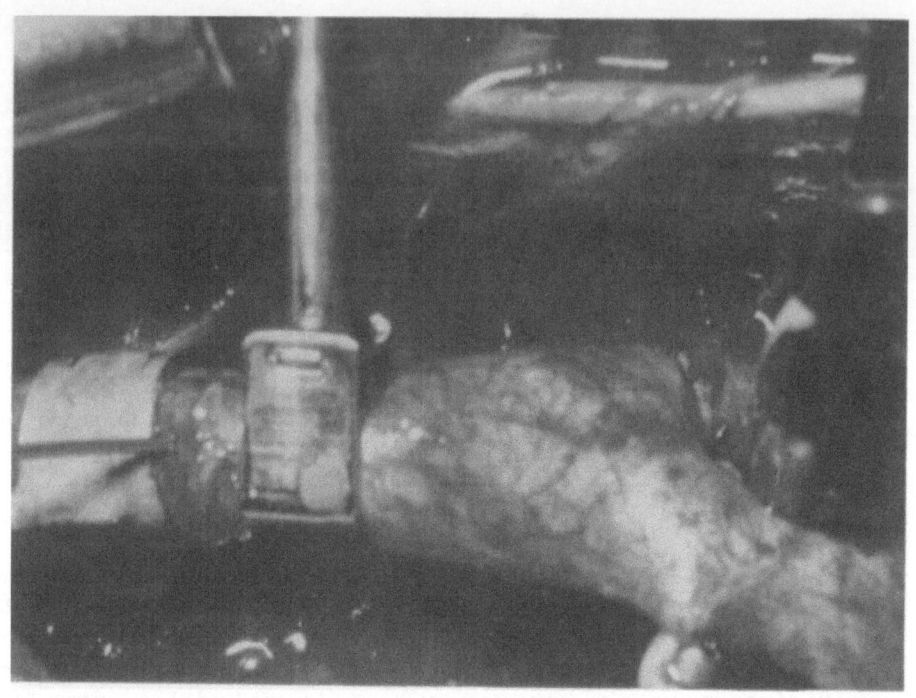

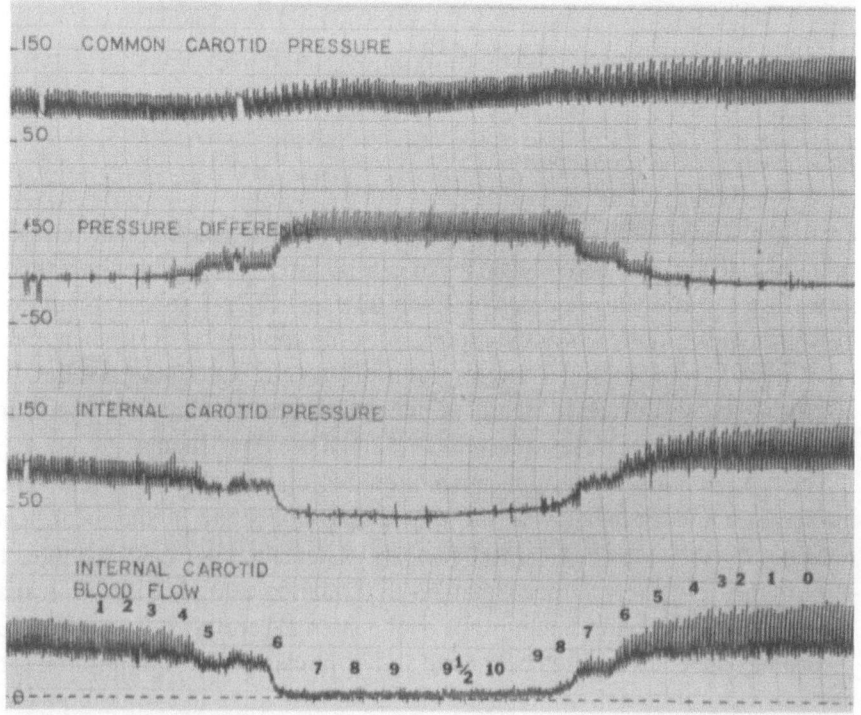

Fig. 19B illustrates typical progressive changes in the flow and pressure gradient in the artery during graded constriction and release of the clamp. The inverse proportional relationship between flow and pressure difference is seen. It is seen that considerable reduction in the vessel lumen is necessary before flow was significantly affected. Five turns of the clamp represents approximately a 50 percent reduction in the lumen and less than 10 percent reduction in flow. It is further noted that a critical stage occurs at this time when six turns produce a profound reduction in carotid flow. When the common carotid is completely obstructed, there is a residual pressure ('stump' pressure) in the distal carotid due to collaterals. Slight residual flow in the internal carotid is produced by minimal flow from the external carotid but most of the residual pressure arises from collaterals [14].

Fig. 20 illustrates a computer simulated relationship between peak systolic flow and velocity and perfusion pressure as the lumen of a stenosis becomes progressively narrowed. Nominal values are taken for all important parameters to simulate situations often found in patients. Several important observations can be made:

1. Carotid flow is not reduced below 20 percent of its initial value until the arterial diameter is less than 2.5 mm regardless of the initial unobstructed diameter. During this early phase of stenosis, the velocity increases with the inverse square of the diameter.

2. Velocity continues to increase rapidly as the stenosis diameter approaches 1 mm diameter. The increase in velocity cannot sustain flow which falls rapidly.

3. When the diameter (D) is reduced below 0.5 mm, a critical phase is reached where a small change in D produces a great decrease in velocity and consequent Doppler frequencies pass back through the same range produced by the early and lesser degrees of stenosis. In practice this apparent ambiguity of the velocity diameter relationship is not a problem probably because the channel is so narrow that the occlusion occurs rapidly when the diameter diminishes below 0.5 mm.

←

Figure 19A. Photographic view of bifurcation of the human common carotid artery at the time of surgical exposure for the purpose of placing a Selverstone occlusion clamp on the common carotid artery. During graded occlusion blood flow in the internal carotid artery as well as pressure above and below the clamp were continuously measured as in the next figure.

Figure 19B. Simultaneous monitoring of internal carotid blood flow (lower tracing) internal carotid pressure (3rd tracing from above) and common carotid pressure (upper tracing) during grade constriction of the common carotid artery with the arrangement shown in the previous figure. The second from the top tracing represents the pressure drop across the constricting clamp measured by subtracting internal carotid pressure from common carotid pressure. Numbers on lower tracing represent turns of the screw moving against a pressure plate within the clamp. Note when total occlusion occurs at time number 7 internal carotid pressure drops to a pressure of 45 mmHg. Slight residual brachial flow in the internal carotid is maintained by collateral from the branches of the external carotid.

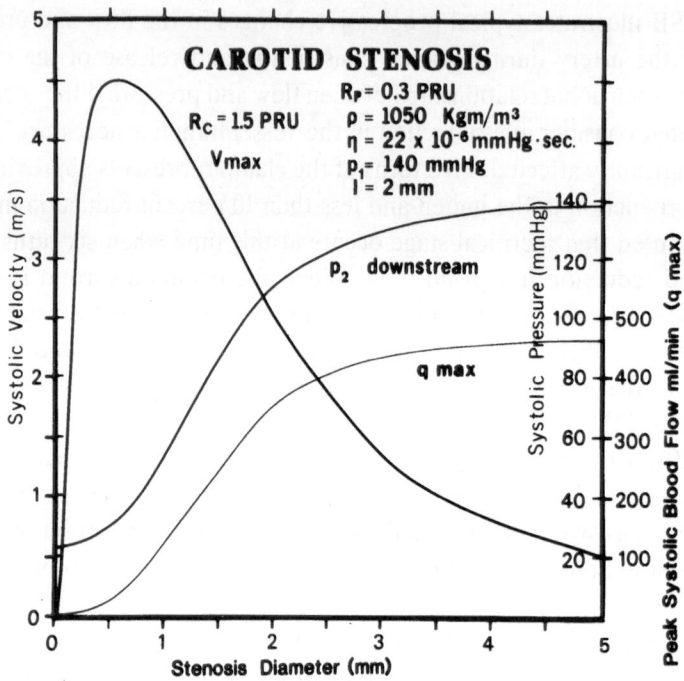

Figure 20. Internal carotid artery computer simulation of the orifice equation with R_C/R_P ratio of 5. Note flow is well maintained by increasing velocity with the stenosis diameter is reduced below 2.5 mm. Between 2 to 1 mm diameter flow diminishes precipitously. From number 6 of the previous figure probably constricted the artery through this critical phase. During this phase downstream pressure closely parallels blood flow but does not fall to zero because of support by collaterals.

Experimental stenosis

Experimental stenosis was produced in the abdominal aorta of dogs [20] while f_{max} and $\triangle p$ were measured with Doppler ultrasound and strain gauge manometry. Results are reproduced in Fig. 21. The correlation coefficient for the relationship between $\triangle p$ and v^2 was 0.98 though scattering indicated sometimes overestimation of $\triangle p$ and sometimes underestimation. Spencer and West [16] also found a high correlation between $\triangle p$ and f_{max}^2 in a human subject when the femoral artery was manually compressed with the finger and $\triangle p$ intermittently recorded by means of ankle pressure.

The sum of theoretical evidence and experiments in animals and man indicate that stenosis in arteries supplying peripheral resistance, such as the carotid and femoral arteries, produces pressure drops which are directly proportional to the square of the velocity within the stenosis and that the Bernoulli effect dominates over Poiseuille viscous resistance as the cause of the pressure drop, at least up to a stenosis severity of 0.5 mm. Direct measurements in pressure drop carotid artery stenosis of man is not yet available but there is excellent theoretical evidence and

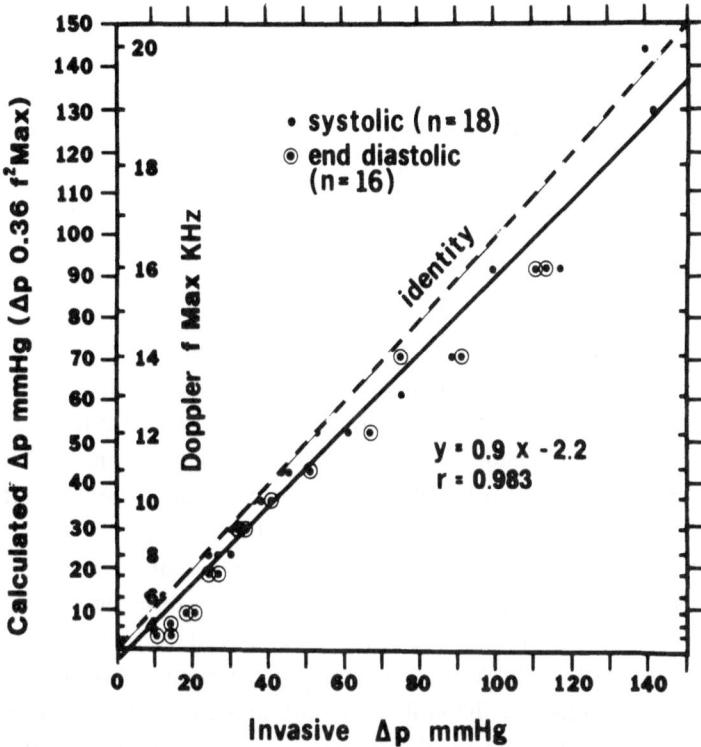

Figure 21. Experimental confirmation of the relationship between pressure drop measured and calculated from Doppler f_{max} in graded constriction of the dog's abdominal aorta. As in the computer simulation calculated pressure drop slightly underestimates the time pressure drop. By permission of Angiology, Westminster Publications, Inc., New York, Vol 36: 899, 1985.

experimental evidence in arteries of comparable size and peripheral resistance that the principle applies in the carotid arteries.

Carotid occlusion and collateral support

It may well be that the magnitude of stroke from carotid artery disease, whether embolic or thrombotic in origin, is related to the extent of collateral available in any given patient. Immediately following acute carotid occlusion, brain perfusion falls significantly, avaraging 50 percent of control in 19 patients [17] and falling to 35 percent in 45 patients of another study [18]. Internal carotid obstructions caused a greater decrease than did common carotid obstructions. However, in patients with longstanding complete occlusion of one or both carotids, cerebral blood flow (CBF) was reduced by an average of only 12 percent and the lowest CBF was 40 ml/min/100 gms, a reduction of 27 percent [19]. No statistically significant improvement in CBF results from carotid endarterectomy of stenotic lesions [19, 20]. Combined carotid-vertebral lesions or aortic arch lesions, however, do depress CBF.

In eight carotid Selverstone clamp patients, of the author [21], Table 4, the measured pressure drop was uniformly found to be linearly and inversely proportional to carotid blood flow.

Among 14 patients of Crawford *et al.* [22] also with contralateral carotids patent the stump to systemic ratio measured at the time of carotid endarterectomy ranged from .39 to .76 and severe neurologic reactions only occurred in 3 patients when the contralateral carotid was occluded and stump pressures reached 12, 20 and 42 mmHg.

These figures demonstrate the wide range of collateral circulation available to support the intracranial blood pressure and flow in the circle of Willis upon sudden occlusion of the common carotid artery. The stump/systemic ratio is a direct measure of collateral available and is probably close to the values one would obtain with occlusion of the internal carotid artery alone. External carotid collaterals, though diagnostically helpful, probably are a minor contributor to pressure and flow support to the internal carotid territory.

Among 22 internal carotids, hemispheric brain vascular resistance calculated from pressure and flow measurements following endarterectomy, varied from 0.2 to 1 mm Hg/ml/min and averaged 0.6 [23]. The data to calculate collateral resistance was not available from this but measurements of stump pressure and Doppler evaluations of collateral circulation and circle of Willis pressure indicates that collateral resistance does not vary outside the limits of 0.1 and 1 mm Hg/ml/min and averages around 0.3.

If the equal resistance in the collateral channels equals that of the brain vasculature, hemispheric perfusion cannot diminish more than 50 percent of its normal value even when total occlusion of the internal carotid occurs and the additional effect of autoregulation will not allow brain perfusion to fall below a level to threaten cell metabolism when collaterals are this good. If collateral resistance is less than brain resistance, as often occurs, brain perfusion is not affected. Archie, et al. [24] have found in high grade internal carotid artery stenosis the ratio of collateral resistance to peripheral hemispheric resistance (R_c/R_p) is higher in TIA and stroke patients than in asymptomatic patients. Asymptomatic stenosis patients may well be so because they have adequate collateral to prevent ischemia. This hypothesis could explain why clinic patients with high

Table 4. Stump pressure studies in Selverstone clamp patients.

Patient	p/systemic	delta p_{max}	p/stump S/D	Stump/Systemic
FW	190	116	74/67	39
KP	142	66	76/65	54
EP	120	68	52/40	43
AK	104	69	36/33	35
JG	100	70	30/27	30

CAROTID   STENOSIS

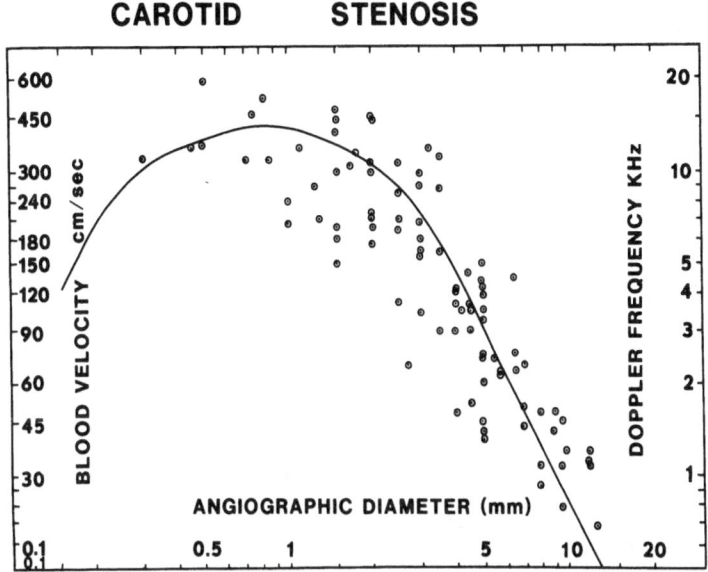

Figure 22. 1981 clinical experience in Seattle among 91 carotid arteries comparing angiographic micrometer measured diameter with the Doppler f_{max} and velocity based on assumption of a 60° angle of sound beam and stenosis jet. The log × log plot is made to demonstrate the power function of the relationship down to 2 mm.

grade obstructions often display strong collateral effects. It may also be that patients whom stroke without medical channels do so because of inadequate collaterals.

Transcranial Doppler offers a tool to separate the more vulnerable patients from the protected ones by mapping and grading the collateral pathways. See Chapter 15 for further details on transtemporal Doppler imaging.

Clinical experience

The foregoing concepts of Doppler frequency relationships to carotid stenosis severity were first tested in two Seattle vascular clinics in 1976. The highest Doppler frequency found at the origin of the internal carotid artery at the time of imaging was compared with the minimal internal carotid diameter measured on x-ray arteriography films. All patients during one calendar year were utilized if Doppler data and films were usable. If stenosis was not present on the x-ray film the internal diameter was measured 0.5 cm from the origin where Doppler frequencies are routinely recorded on magnetic tape.

Fig. 22 illustrates the relationship found between the maximum systolic frequency and the smallest diameter found on the available x-ray films. The ordinates used are logarithmic in order to spread out the points representing the

CAROTID STENOSIS

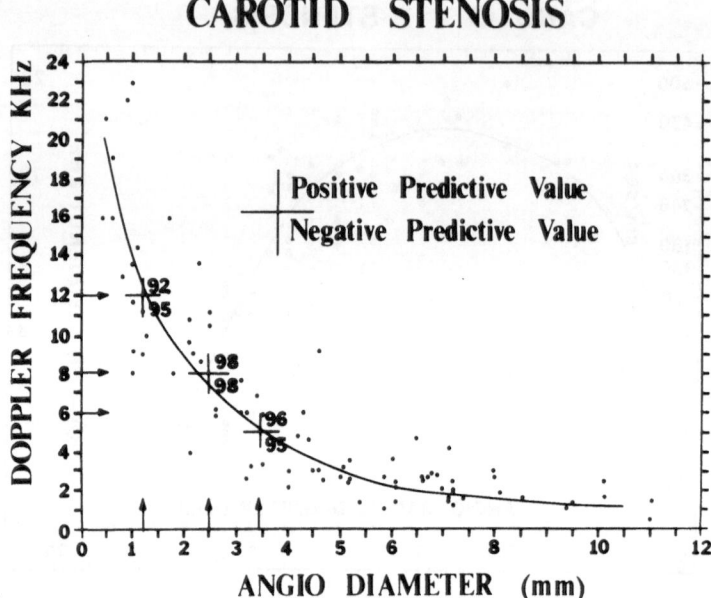

Figure 23. Seattle clinical experience with DOPSCAN (60° imaging with CW Doppler) of carotid bifurcations during year 1981–83. Predictive values are based on ± 1 mm error in diameter estimation. This appears to be the limit in the ability of Doppler frequency analysis in predicting morphological severity of carotid stenosis.

smallest diameter and to compress the frequency range. On such ordinates the theoretical relationship represented between frequency (velocity) and effective diameter approaches a straight line since the square of the diameter is proportional to the Doppler frequency. Fig. 23 represents a more recent comparison of 92 carotid arteries between Doppler frequency and angiographic measurements.

It is apparent that Doppler frequencies found in carotid stenosis do generally

Table 5. Predictive ability 5 MHz CW Doppler ultrasound.

Systolic Peak kHz	Internal carotid stenosis		
	%	Diameter mm	Range mm*
1–3	0	7.0	± 3.0
4–6	30	3.5	± 1.5
7–8	50	2.5	± 1.0
9–10	60	2.0	± 1.0
11–12	70	1.5	± 1.0
13–15	75	1.2	± 0.5
16–20	80	1.0	± 0.5
	90**	0.5	

* 90% confidence limits.
** special secondary signals necessary.

follow the experimental relationship [25], but scattering around a trend of the theoretical power function. The scatter in fig. 22 is due to problems of (1) the x-ray in identifying the true luminal diameter (2) unknown insonation angle and (3) collateral effects. Because of all of these limitations, the best then can currently be done by using Doppler to predict the morphologic severity of stenosis as presented in Table 5. The future of Doppler ultrasound lies more on its hemodynamic capability than its morphological accuracy.

References

1. Brown PM, Johnston WK: The Difficulty of Quantifying the severity of carotid stenosis, Surg, Sept, 468, 1982.
2. Gee W, Oller DW, Wylie EJ: Noninvasive diagnosis of carotid occlusion by ocular pneumo-plethysmography, STROKE 7: 18–21, 1976.
3. Brockenbrough EC, Lawrence C, Schwank WG: Ocular plethysmography: A new technique for the evaluation of carotid obstructive disease. Rev Surg 24: 299, 1967.
4. Brockenbrough EC: Screening for the prevention of Stroke: Use of a Doppler flowmeter. Information and Education Resource Support Unit Wash/Alaska Regional Medical Program, 1976.
5. Muller HR: The diagnosis of internal carotid artery occlusion by directional Doppler sonography of the ophthalmic artery. Neurology 22: 816, 1972.
6. Goldberg RE: Doppler physics and preliminary report of a test for carotid insufficiency. In: Goldberg and Sarin (eds) Ultrasonics in Ophthalmic diagnostic and therapeutic applications. Appendix I, 1976.
7. Hyman BN: Doppler sonography in a bedside noninvasive method for assessment of carotid artery disease. Am J Ophth 77 (2): 227, 1974.
8. Keneda H, Minami T, Taneda M, Irino T: The collateral flow via ophthalmic artery in internal carotid arterial occlusions – semiquantitative evaluation. No To Shinkei 29: 941, 1977.
9. Giddens DP, Mabon RF, Cassonova RA. Measurements of disordered flows distal to subtotal vascular stenoses in the thoracic aortas of dogs. Circ Res 39, 112–119, 1976.
10. Faye T: The cerebral vasculature. JAMA 84, 1717, 1925.
11. Holen J, Aaslid R, Landmark K, et al: Determination of pressure gradient in mitral stenosis with a noninvasive ultrasound Doppler technique. Acta Med Scand 199: 455–460, 1976.
12. Clark C: The fluid mechanics of aortic stenosis. I. Theory and steady flow experiments. J Biomechanics 9, 521–528, 1976.
13. Spencer MP, Arts T: Some hemodynamical aspects of large arteries. In: Reneman RS, Hoeks PG (eds) Doppler Ultrasound in the Diagnosis of Cerebrovascular Disease, Ch3: 59–75, Research Studies Press (A Division of John Wiley & Sons Ltd, England, 1982.
14. Reifel E, Tytus JS, Spencer MP: Monitoring internal carotid blood flow during graded occlusion for aneurysm. Bulletin of the Mason Clinic 20 (1): 29–35, 1966.
15. Faccenda F, Usui Yoshiyuki, Spencer MP: Doppler measurement of the pressure drop caused by arterial stenosis: An experimental study. In: Angiology, Westminster Publications, Inc, New York, Vol 36: 899, 1985.
16. West FW, Spencer MP, Clark SJ, Spencer MP: Noninvasive evaluation of severe carotid occlusive disease with continuous-wave (CW) Doppler ultrasound. Bruit 6: 46, 1982.
17. Waltz G, Sundt TM, Michenfelder JD: Cerebral blood flow during carotid endarterectomy. Circulation 45 (5): 1091–1096, May 1972.
18. Jarrett F: Noninvasive evaluation of the carotid circulation. Can J Surg 21 (4): 283–284, 1978.

146

19. Adams JE, Smith MC, Wylie J, Leake TB, Halliday B: Cerebral blood flow and hemodynamics in extracranial vascular disease: effect of endarterectomy. Surgery 53 (4): 449–455, April, 1963.
20. O'Brien MD, Veall N, Luck RJ, Irvine WT: Cerebral-cortex perfusion-rates in extracranial cerebrovascular disease and the effects of operation. The Lancet August 19, 1967: 392–395.
21. Spencer MP: Blood flow in the arteries. In: Cerebrovascular Evaluation with Doppler Ultrasound. 8: 97–112, (Spencer MP, Reid JM, eds), Martinus Nijhoff, Publishers, The Netherlands. 1981.
22. Crawford ES *et al.*: Hemodynamic alterations in patients with cerebral arterial insufficiency before and after operation. Surgery Vol 48, No 1, pp. 76–94, July 1960.
23. Spencer MP, unpublished data.
24. Archie JP, Feldtman RW: Collateral cerebral vascular resistance in patients with significant carotid stenosis. STROKE Vol 13, No 6, 1982.
25. Spencer MP, Reid JM: Quantitation of carotid stenosis with continuous-wave (CW) Doppler ultrasound. STROKE *10* (3): 326–330.

Vascular bruits

M.P. Spencer

According to recent studies (Sandok *et al.* [1], 1982; Wolf *et al.* [2], 1981) 4% of persons over 45 years of age have cervical bruits and in the age group 65–79 there is a 7% prevalence. In patients with TIA and carotid bruits 75% are associated with stenotic lesions of the carotid arteries (David *et al.* [3]. It is therefore important that the noninvasive examinations for cerebrovascular abnormalities begin with a careful auscultation of the head, neck, and chest in order to guide the examination to assure localization of the source.

Bruits or vascular murmurs are sounds generated in the arteries. They are distinguished from venous hums which arise from the veins. Bruits arise from vibrations of the walls of the larger vessels driven by turbulence in the underlying blood flow streams and transmitted to the body surface where they can be detected with a stethoscope or microphone. A bruit may also be produced by arterial venous fistulae. They usually have a random blowing quality but may in addition contain a superimposed resonant or harmonic quality. The most common morphology producing arterial bruits is a localized narrowing (stenosis) of the blood flow channel with widening of the channel downstream from the stenosis. Bruits may not be produced in the blood vessels by narrowing of the blood channel if a downstream widening is not present. Bruits may, however, be produced without narrowing in a large artery by higher than normal velocities (Fig. 1).

Turbulence is a condition which develops under special conditions usually associated in the arteries with velocities elevated above normal. Turbulence is a term to be distinguished from disturbed flow occurring in the normal carotid sinus as discussed in Chapter 5 on normal flow in the arteries. Turbulence is generally associated with highly unorganized flow velocities and flow streams but a special form called the 'von Karmen street' represents a special organization of vortices shed in a periodic fashion downstream of a stenosis and may explain the musical murmurs sometimes heard [4]. A non-dimensional parameter called the 'Reynolds number' (Re) is used to predict when turbulence will develop:

$$Re = v \, D/\eta$$

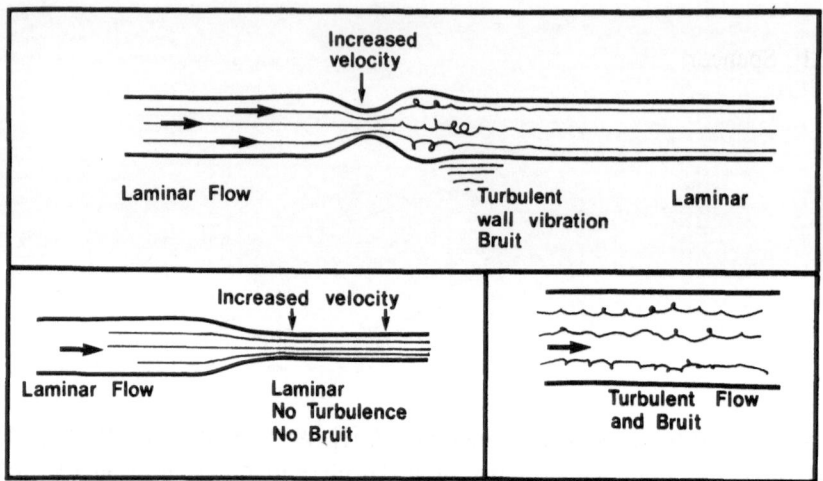

Figure 1. Three important arterial abnormalities which may or may not produce a bruit depending on the downstream channel widening.

where v is the spatial mean velocity downstream of the stenosis; D is the pipe diameter and η represents the kinematic viscosity of the blood. The Reynolds number concept explains how turbulence develops in large arteries without stenosis under high velocity conditions. Turbulence is usually present when the Reynolds number exceeds 2000. Fredberg [5] has shown in models how fluctuating wall pressure from turbulence develops at lower Reynolds numbers when stenosis is increasing in severity up to 90% area reduction. Bruit intensity appears to be independent of the Reynolds number when it exceeds 2000. Since even a moderate arterial stenosis produces Re>2000, we may record the bruit and analyse the frequency content to gain information about the severity of the stenosis. We shall see later how Lees *et al.* [6] has used spectral analysis of bruits to quantitate the severity of arterial stenosis. First we must learn more about auscultation and use of the stethoscope because it provides a key clinical sign of stenosis guiding the ultrasound examination to localize the source and severity of the pathology.

Stethoscopes possess two types of skin-contacting heads: the bell-type and the diaphragm-type. Both types utilize pneumatic tubes to transmit the skin vibrations to the ears. The bell-type contacts a small area of skin surface which acts as the sound transmitting diaphragm. The diaphragm-type stethoscope covers a broader area with a stiff membrane. The large stiff membrane transmits a louder sound but filters out the lower frequencies of the bruit. The frequencies transmitted by the bell-type may be modified by pressure against the skin. A lightly-applied bell better transmits the lower frequencies than the diaphragm-type, but pressure on the stethoscope will stretch the skin preferentially passing the higher frequency components. The bell is preferred for better localization of cervical bruits.

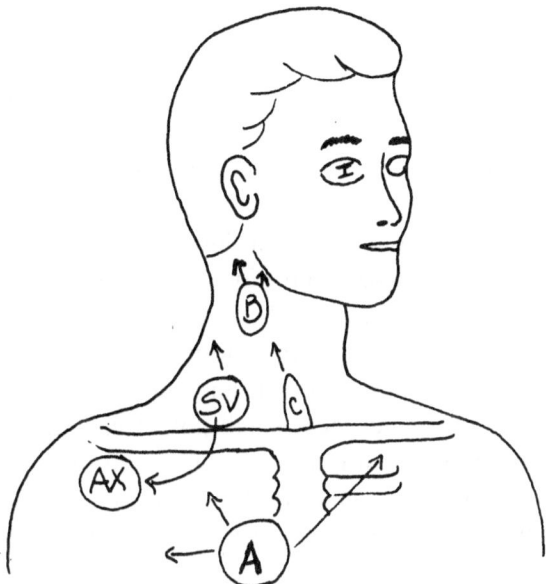

Figure 2. Shows locations where bruits are heard and, illustrates their transmission mode over bone and arterial channels. B = bifurcation; C = common carotid; V = vertebral; S = subclavian; AX = axillary; A = Aorta; I = internal 'siphon'.

Descriptive parameters

The observer should evaluate and describe the following four major characteristics of all bruits [7]: location and transmission, intensity and loudness, frequency content, and duration and timing.

Location

The location of loudest intensity should be identified. The surrounding area of transmission of the bruit representing its spread to secondary intensities should be determined. Vascular bruits tend to spread in the direction of blood flow particularly in an arterial channel and also are preferentially transmitted along the bones. For record-keeping, we recommend a diagram (Fig. 2) with an 'x' representing the position of loudest intensity and arrows representing the principal directions of spread over the skin surface.

Bruits arising from the internal carotid siphon generally are heard best over the closed eyelid. Transorbital pulsed Doppler however has shown that orbital bruits can arise from collateral effects in the anterior communicating and anterior cerebral arteries [8]. The bruit the patient can hear is usually high in the internal or vertebral artery near the temporal bone and middle ear. A useful technique for hearing the sounds the patient hears is to replace the bell or diaphragm of the stethoscope with a spare ear piece and place this into the external auditory meatus. By listening in this manner to sounds in the ear canal the sounds heard by the patient can be heard and the source from artery or vein proven by compressions on the cervical vessels.

Bruits at the bifurcation of the common carotid artery are best heard below the angle of the jaw in the upper neck and lateral to the larynx. If it, a 'carotid bruit' is well transmitted toward the mastoid bone or the lobe of the ear, it may indicate a high internal carotid source above the bifurcation. Sixty percent of carotid bruits (between the mid-neck and the angle of the jaw) arise from stenosis of the internal carotid artery and 20 percent from the external carotid [9], but 25–30% of the time a silent contralateral stenosis is present and can be detected by Doppler. The absence of bruit does not exclude the possibility of carotid artery stenosis and occluded common carotid arteries are never accompanied by a bruit [3]. The presence of bilateral carotid bruits indicates ICA stenosis in 71% of cases and 98% of patients with bilateral carotid bruits have ICA stenosis greater than 35% (Chambers) [9].

Sixty-five percent of bruits in the supraclavicular region at the medial end of the clavicle represent subclavian artery stenosis but may also represent vertebral artery stenosis. Subclavian bruits are transmitted along the axillary artery below the lateral end of the clavicle. Vertebral artery bruits tend to spread in a superior and posterior direction. Bruits in the innominate artery, at the origin of the left subclavian or in the aortic arch tend to be heard in the upper chest with a rumbling quality transmitting widely up both sides of the neck. Common carotid lesions near their origins in the chest have similar transmission modes into the lower neck.

Intensity

The loudness of a bruit may be clinically graded between I and IV with Grade I being the barely audible bruit and Grade IV being one that can be heard with a stethoscope close to but not touching the skin. In addition, Grade IV vibrations may be felt with the fingertips as a sensation called a 'thrill'. Most bruits detected of moderate loudness are designated Grade II or Grade III.

As stenosis of an artery progresses, the loudness of the bruit tends to increase up to approximately 70% reduction in the lumen area at which condition a maximum energy is released through turbulence and vessel wall vibration. This is because the volumetric flow through the stenosis is generally not greatly compromised by this degree of obstruction, but the momentum and dissipating energy in downstream turbulence has greatly increased. With further stenosis, volumetric blood flow is reduced and the bruit becomes softer until when the stenotic lumen is less than 1/2 mm in diameter, the turbulence produced is difficult to detect with

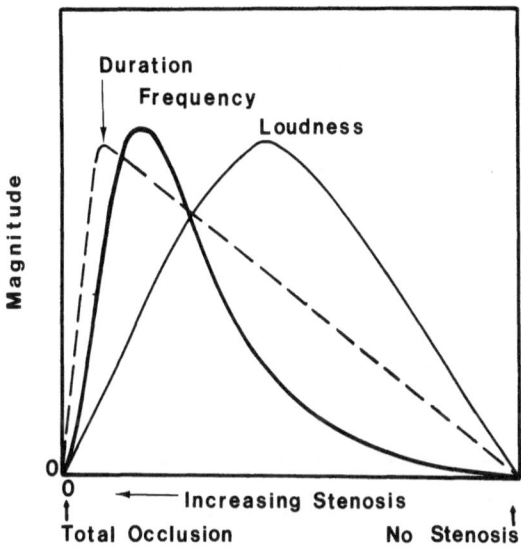

Figure 3. As stenosis increases, the magnitude of the bruit with respect to loudness, frequency, and duration also increases proportionally; however, seldom exceeds 500 Hz at which time it reverses until no bruit can be heard, even though the stenosis continues to increase.

a stethoscope. If there are many collateral channels available through which the blood flow is shunted to the vascular territory of the stenotic vessel, the bruit amplitude will decrease sooner and more rapidly. If there are no collateral channels, normal volumes of blood flow can pass through a 1 mm diameter lumen because of high blood velocity generated by a large pressure gradient.

Frequency content

All arterial bruits possess a blowing quality which means there is a random noisy audio spectrum. A superimposed harmonic, whining or musical quality indicates periodic vibration of a flexible arterial wall. It is possible a von Karmen street of vortices also produces the periodic vibrations but no special clinical significance has been indicated by the harmonic bruit. The upper frequencies of a bruit increase as the stenosis approaches the most severe degrees. The upper frequency content of the bruit spectrum is related to the blood velocity (Fig. 3). The upper detectable frequency generally does not exceed 1200 Hz, therefore, moderate hearing losses do not affect the observers ability to recognize bruits and analyze them. If a very faint, high frequency bruit of a tight stenosis is heard or suspected, the diaphragm stethoscope should be used to collect the maximum vibratory information.

The higher frequency components provide a sense of 'presence' to the sound usually at the point of maximum intensity and immediately over the bruit source.

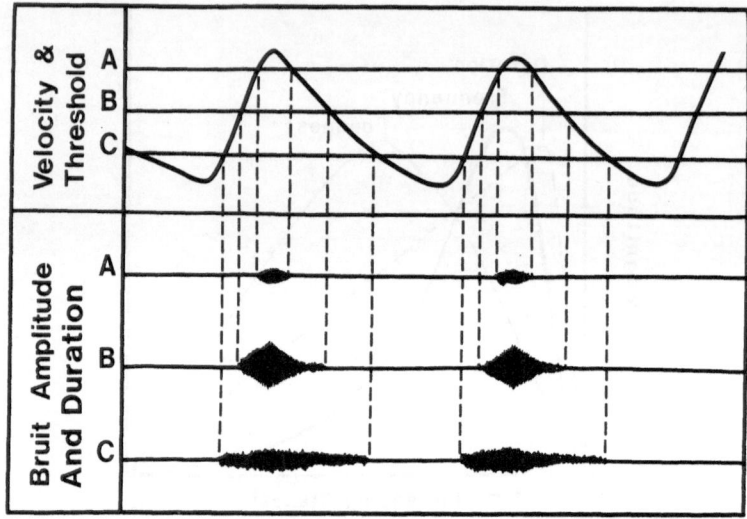

Figure 4. Diagramatic representation of how the blood turbulence threshold working on the arterial flow waveform changes the amplitude and duration of carotid bruits. 'A', 'B', and 'C' in the upper panel represent three stages of increasing stenosis with corresponding decrease in the turbulence threshold. 'A', 'B', and 'C' in the lower panel represent three bruits representing the three stages of stenosis selected in the upper panel. Note: the flow tracings are normalized to the same scale though 'A', 'B' and 'C' represent progressive increases in blood velocity.

The high frequencies are lost as the bruit spreads because the tissues tend to damp out the higher frequency components more than the low frequency components. The highest frequency qualities tend to be associated with bruits of longer duration within the cardiac cycle.

Duration and timing

With minor degrees of stenosis or irregularity in the arterial channel, the bruit will be of short duration in mid-systole (Fig. 4). As the stenosis increases, the duration of the bruit tends to expand to become pan-systolic. With the tighter degrees of stenosis down to 1mm diameter or with greater hemodynamic severity the duration spreads into diastole and may become continuous extending far into diastole (Fig. 5). Soft, long duration, high frequency bruits represent hemodynamically severe stenoses, a large pressure gradient throughout the cardiac cycle and indicating poor arterial collateral to the distal vascular bed.

Bruits caused by arterial-venous fistulae tend to be of long duration, very loud and transmit widely. Because of their loudness throughout the cardiac cycle, 'designated machinery bruit', they are generally not confused with a tight stenosis bruit. Through careful evaluation of the location, intensity, frequency and duration of vascular bruits, a good estimate can often be made concerning the severity and hemodynamic severity of arterial stenosis.

EXPERIMENTAL GRADED
COARCTATION

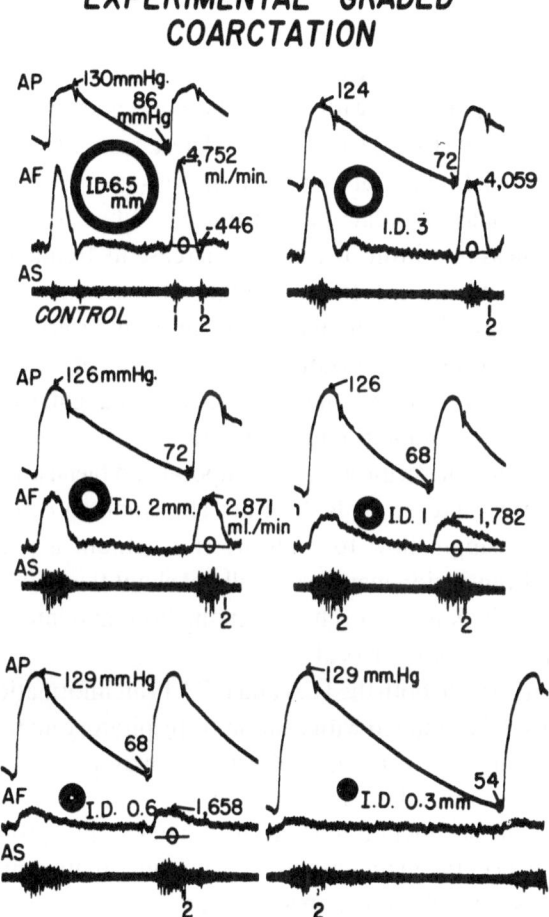

Figure 5. The sequence of events which takes place as a result of lumen reduction in experimental coarctation. The upper lefthand panel is the control, subsequent panels indicate the physiological changes which occur.

Table 1. Dynamic auscultation.

	ICAs	ECAs
Hyperventilation	*−	−0+
Breathholding	*+	−0+
5% CO_2	*++	0 or +
Compression temporal and facial arteries	0	*
Compression of contralateral common carotid	+	0 or +

* represents results which are most helpful.

Dynamic auscultation

Several simple maneuvers can be carried out, bedside, to diagnose internal carotid artery (ICA) stenosis with the stethoscope and to separate ICA from external carotid artery (ECA) stenosis [10]. These maneuvers include compression of the superficial temporal and facial arteries as well as hyperventilation, breathholding or pharmacologic administration. When a given maneuver increases the loudness of a bruit, it will also increase its frequency and duration. These three parameters also decrease together when a maneuver decreases one. Simultaneous compression of the temporal and facial arteries will diminish the loudness of an ECA bruit and will not change an ICA bruit (Table 1). Breathholding or administration of 5% carbon dioxide in air will augment an ICA bruit but have little, no effect, or diminish an ECA bruit.

These tests may not be reciprocal, i.e. temporal and facial artery compressions will not necessarily increase an ICA bruit. The common carotid artery is sufficiently large to supply flow to both arteries without a pressure drop and compression and ventilation maneuvers will not shunt flow from one bruit to the other. One should look for large changes in the bruit and interpret with caution changes that are weak or equivocal.

When bruits arise from both the ICA and ECA bruit information from dynamic auscultation must be evaluated with caution. If respiratory maneuvers or administration of CO_2 produce a marked effect, one may assume there is an ICA stenosis; but if temporal and facial artery compression decrease the bruit features one cannot rule out coincident ICA stenosis. When Doppler probes are placed on the site of turbulence, the maneuvers of dynamic auscultation may be used more effectively because Doppler function as a highly directional microphone to focus on either the external or internal carotid arteries.

Bruit spectral analysis

Quantitation of the relative spectral content of carotid bruits can be used to assess the severity of the stenosis [11]. The maximum energy of bruits lie between 100 and 600 Hz (Fig. 6). The position of the maximum intensity or 'break point' along the frequency amplitude plot increases with increasing degrees of stenosis. The 'break point' frequency can be used to estimate severity of stenosis according to the formula

$$d_1 = v_2/f_o$$

where d_1 = the stenosis lumen diameter in mm, and v_2 = the mean spatial velocity of blood upstream or downstream from the stenosis expressed in mm/sec and f_o = the break point frequency of the bruit in Hz. If v is assumed nominal at 500 mm/

sec then an f_o of 500 Hz represents a 1 mm diameter stenosis. v may also be estimated from this formula. The formula is an improved and quantitative expression of the observations reported previously [12], i.e., peak frequency is inversely proportional to diameter.

Duncan and Lees found a correlation coefficient of 0.64 between d_1 calculated and d_1 measured on x-ray contrast angiograms. There seemed to be a better ability to predict stenosis severities less than 3 mm. This method has difficulties in separating ECA stenosis from ICA stenosis and in diagnosing stenosis tighter than $d_1 = 1$ mm when bruits are not detectable. In a significant fraction of patients the signal-to-noise ratio is not adequate to produce the necessary spectral features. Further development of the concept using Doppler as a directional microphone and as a velocity detector, may prove useful.

Doppler detection of turbulence and bruits

Auscultation and phonography are closely akin to Doppler ultrasound in that Doppler detects both the turbulence and the wall motion, thus Doppler functions virtually as a directional microphone and can be used to study bruit phenomena. Bruits are represented on the directional Doppler spectrum as a symmetrical pattern shown above and below the zero frequency baseline. Please see Chapter 9. When the Doppler sample volume spans the artery wall the vibrations of the wall produce motion both towards and away from the transducer. Each velocity component of the wall motion produces a corresponding Doppler frequency component reproducing the bruit qualities. Hoeks [14] has demonstrated the reason why Doppler bruit qualities reproduce 'stethoscope' bruit qualities regardless of the ultrasound carrier frequency used. The excursion of the artery wall is apparently sufficiently small to fall within one ultrasound wavelength; i.e., much less than the 0.3 mm wavelength for 5 MHz ultrasound. Because of this a true Doppler effect does not occur, rather the phase of the ultrasound wave is modulated back and forth. This oscillating phase shift tracks the velocity of the artery wall producing in the Doppler demodulator a frequency spectrum reproducing the bruit spectrum. A true Doppler effect is produced only if the displacement is over more than one wavelength such as occurs as blood is translated along the axis of an artery across more than one wavelength. The fact that bruit frequencies are reproduced on the Doppler frequency spectrum with different carrier frequencies is, in fact, evidence that bruits are produced by small displacements in the artery walls and not directly by the underlying turbulence. The underlying turbulence moves through more than one wavelength and, of course, produces characteristic Doppler effects described in Chapter 9.

Doppler ultrasound probes function like a directional microphone and without the tissue attenuation effects imposed on stethoscopes applied to the body surface. Attention to the Doppler bruit qualities in the spectrum using the break point frequency relationship to blood velocity, both within the stenosis and downstream of the stenosis, may lead to improved Doppler diagnosis of hemodynamic and morphologic severity of stenosis.

References

1. Sandok MD, Whisnant JP, Furlan AJ, Mickell JL: Carotid artery bruits, prevalence survey and differential diagnosis. Mayo Clin Proc 57 *57:* 227–230, 1982.
2. Wolf PA, Kannel WB, Sorlie P, McNamara P: Asymptomatic carotid bruit and risk of stroke. The Framingham Study. JAMA *245,* No 14, April 10, 1981.
3. David TE, Humphries AW, Young JR, Beven EG: A correlation of neck bruits and arteriosclerotic carotid arteries. Arch Surg *107,* 729–731, 1973.
4. Aaslid R, Nornes H: Musical murmurs in human cerebral arteries after subarachnoid hemorrhage. J Neurosurg *60:* 32–36, 1984.
5. Fredberg JJ: Origin and character of vascular murmurs: Model studies. J Acoust Soc Am *61:* 1077, 1977.
6. Lees RS, Dewey CF, Jr.: Phonoangiography: A new noninvasive diagnostic method for studying arterial disease. Proc Ntl Acad Sciences *67,* 935, 1970.
7. Spencer MP, Reid JM: Cerebrovascular evaluation with Doppler Ultrasound, Martinus Nijhoff, 1981.
8. Spencer MP, Whisler DW: Transorbital Doppler diagnosis of intracranial arterial stenosis. To be published in STROKE, *17:* 6, November-December, 1986.
9. Chambers BR, Norris JW: Clinical significance of asymptomatic neck bruits. Neurology *35:* 742, 1985.
10. Kurtz KJ: Dynamic vascular auscultation: Am J Med *76:* 1066, 1984.
11. Duncan GW, Gruber JO, Dewey CF, Jr., Myers GS, Lees RS: Evaluation of carotid stenosis by phonoangiography. New Eng J Med 293: 1124, 1975.
12. Spencer MP, Fourney ME: Spectral analysis of murmurs produced in stenosis of large arteries. The Physiologist, *8:* (3) – August, 1965.
13. Spencer MP, Johnston FR, Meredith JH: The origin and interpretation of murmurs in coarctation of the aorta. Am Heart J *56:* 722, 1958.
14. Hoeks APG, Ruissen CJ, Hick P, Reneman RS: Methods to evaluate the sample volume of pulsed Doppler systems. Ultrasound in Med & Biol *10:* 427, 1984.

Free hand Doppler techniques for examination of the extracranial arteries with continuous wave Doppler

G.M. von Reutern

This chapter deals with only those aspects of Doppler-sonography, which refers specifically to the hand held techniques where a Doppler ultrasound probe is held in the fingers free to be moved in any position or angle on the body surface. These free-hand techniques are helpful in any laboratory regardless of additional equipment available. While the Doppler criteria for disease diagnosis are similar in all countries, the techniques of examination and equipment used for documentation purposes differ considerably. In European countries, from the beginning, Doppler devices received acceptance because when used as a hand held examination with audio output to speakers and analogue tracings of the mean audio frequency, they were efficient in time and economical in cost. The technician, generally under close supervision from a physician, performs all basic routines after which, if abnormalities are detected, the physician repeats certain parts of the examination to confirm or extend the observations. The hand held techniques have both advantages and disadvantages when compared to flow imaging. The main advantage of the imaging and spectral analysis is the standardized documentation and possibility of a post examination evaluation of data by the reviewing physician. The advantage of hand held techniques is the quick and free maneuverability of the probe and the easier feasibility of diagnostic compression tests. Both techniques yield excellent results if the examiner is careful and experienced. Which technique will be applied depends on how the ultrasonic laboratory is organized. In addition, the cost of the cerebrovascular Doppler evaluation in Europe is only a fraction of that in the United States thus producing less revenue for equipment purchase. For the demonstration of the essentials of the free hand technique it is irrelevant whether analog tracings are used or the spectrum analyzer.

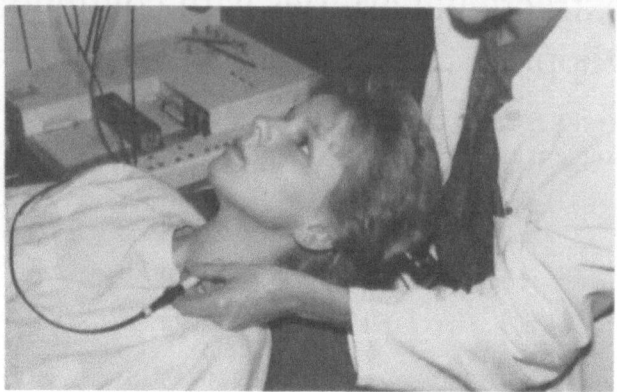

Figure 1. Convenient position of the examiner.

Patient examination

Position

The free hand Doppler examination should be performed with both the patient and the examiner in a comfortable position. The examiner should sit behind the patient's head as shown in Fig. 1. A reclining seat, similar to a dentist chair, with a head support gives free access to the head and neck from the side, front, or back. The head level should be such that both arms are in a relaxed working position, right angled in the elbow. The probe is held between the thumb and the rest of the fingers. The tip of the little finger should protrude slightly beyond the tip of the probe (Fig. 2). With this technique the artery underlying the skin can be felt and stabilized and the edge of the probe is not felt by the patient. In addition, interfering venous flow signals can be avoided by a gentle compression with the little finger.

Artery identification

Criteria for the Doppler-sonographic identification of arteries are based on a) probe position, b) shape of the pulse curve, and c) response to appropriate compression tests. The relative location of a velocity signal is a first preliminary criterion. The internal carotid artery, for example, is found only cranial to the carotid bifurcation and the thyroid artery only medial to the common carotid artery. Using the hand held technique the position of the probe has to be stored in the examiner's mind. Spatial resolution is possible by coordination of the hand, hearing and stepwise or continuous registration of Doppler signals while following arteries along their course by means of the continuity of the signals. (Figs. 3

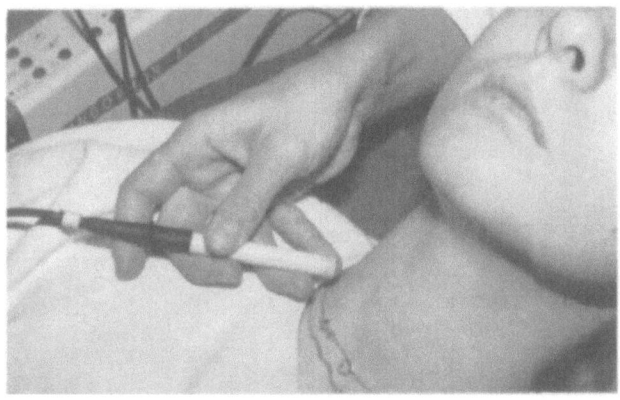

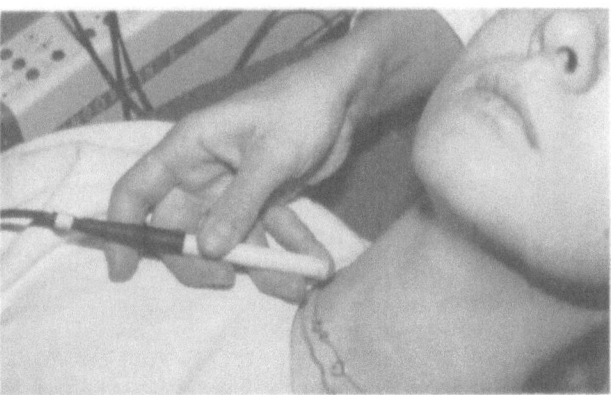

Figure 2. Touch of the probe providing a stable contact with the skin and freedom of movement. The protruding little finger (A) helps to stabilize the artery and can compress veins producing interfering signals (B).

and 9). The shape (waveform) of the recorded pulse curve or spectrum provides a 'signature' characteristic for each artery and flow condition. Normal and pathological waveforms of the cerebrovascular arteries are discussed in other chapters of this text.

Hand arterial compression maneuvers

Compression tests are helpful for correct identification under difficult conditions. They are especially useful in the differentiation of arteries with similar waveform characteristics such as the internal carotid, vertebral or thyroid arteries and do positively designate the source of pathologic Doppler signals. These compressions are always performed distally with respect to the insonated arterial segment.

160

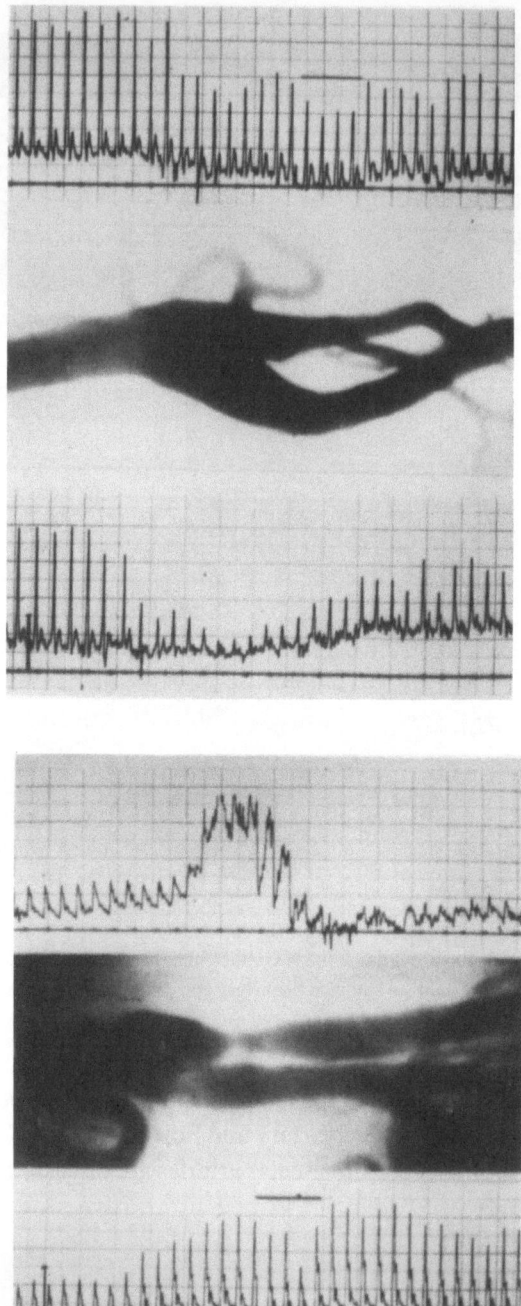

Figure 3A. Mapping of a normal bifurcation. External carotid artery above, internal carotid artery below. The relatively large carotid bulb causes a low Doppler frequency. Compression of the facial and temporal artery (—) identifies the external carotid artery.

Figure 3B. Mapping of a stenosis of the internal carotid artery (above). The examination of the stenotic segment of the internal carotid artery shows acceleration within the stenosis and disturbed flow pattern distal to the stenosis due to turbulence. Normal result of the external carotid artery.

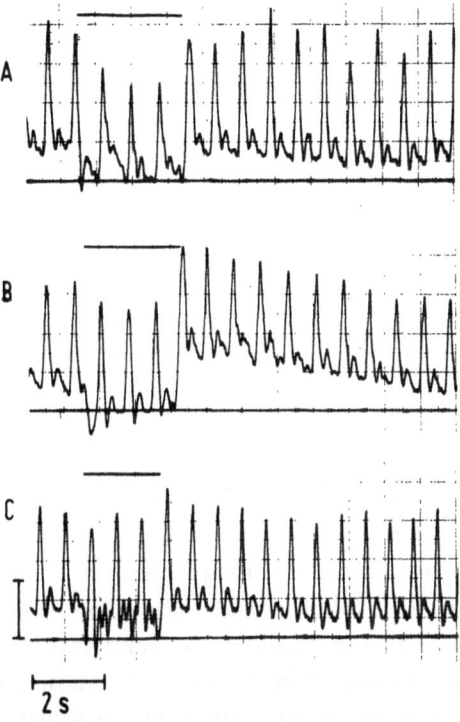

Figure 4. Three types of compression. Recording from the brachial artery. A: Occluding compression, B: peripheral arterial compression by means of isometrdic muscle contraction. The postischemic hyperemia is more pronounced than by simple occluding compression, C: Oscillating compression with little effect on flow volume. However, artery is identified by transmitted oscillations upstream.

Three types of compression are used:

1) A brief occluding compression for two or three pulse cycles. (Fig. 4).

After release of the compression the orginal flow is restored. Extracranial arteries, often occluded for diagnostic purposes, are the branches of the external carotid artery.

2) Prolonged ischemic compressions for several cycles to produce a strong reactive hyperemia.

Ischemia, however, is better induced by isometric muscle contraction than by passive occluding compression of an artery. Increase of flow velocity during postischemic hyperemia is often more prominent than the reduction of flow during the muscle contraction (Fig. 4).

3) Incomplete compression with rapid oscillations of the palpated artery.

Fast repetitive finger oscillations create modulations of the flow velocity waveform (Fig. 5) which are transmitted both upstream and downstream from the compression site. Artefacts can be caused by skin or head motion or by compression of nearby veins; they can be avoided if the finger is not tapping the skin but kept with continuous pressure against the artery while oscillating (Fig. 5).

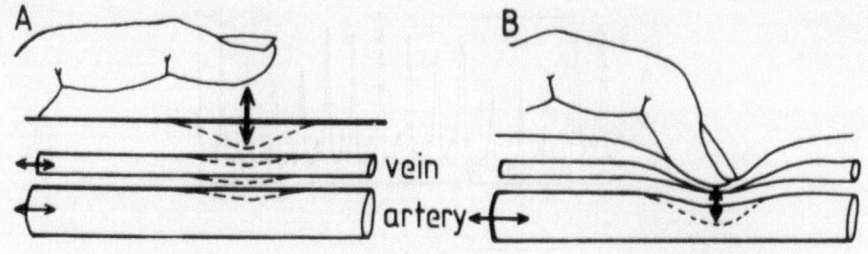

Figure 5. Correct compression technique. A: Tapping of the skin produces artefacts. B: Continuous pressure against the artery occludes veins. The finger approaches the artery. The strength of the pressure needed depends on how deeply the artery is lying. Then, oscillations can be applied creating modulations of the flow velocity signals downstream.

The external carotid artery and its branches

Every branch of the external carotid artery in the neck can be identified by means of compression maneuvers [3]. The parent artery can be identified by compression tests when doubt exists in the other two identification criteria. When occlusions or stenoses are suspected in the internal, external, or common carotid arteries, compression and oscillation tests are indispensible. In appropriate situations the examiner should not only occlude or oscillate the superficial temporal artery but also other branches of the external carotid artery. Of prime importance is separation of stenosis in the external carotid from stenosis of the internal carotid artery. When a signal of stenosis is found at the carotid bifurcation or at the origin of the external carotid, oscillation or occlusion of the homolateral temporal artery will modulate the stenosis signal. If the stenosis signal is arising from the internal carotid artery temporal artery manipulation will not alter the signal. Occasionally high velocity signals will be found from the superior thyroid artery which will not respond to temporal compressions but will respond to compression of the thyroid gland. Any eventually registered branch of the external carotid artery has to be recognized and differentiated from the internal carotid artery. Good results depend largely on the correct compression techniques (Fig. 5, 6).

For the examination of the origin of the *external carotid* artery, the superficial temporal artery can be compressed alone or together with the facial artery (Fig. 6). Sitting behind the patient and examining the left side, the probe is held with the left hand then the compression is done with the right hand. The right arm lies

$\longrightarrow$

Figure 6. Examination of the branches of the external carotid artery. A: Facial artery (compression test −−). B: Common trunk of the superficial temporal and the maxillary artery. Compression of the superficial temporal artery (left) and of the facial artery (right, without effect) C: Occipital artery. D: Thyroid artery. E: Lingual artery. Hyperemic reaction after pushing the tongue against the teeth.

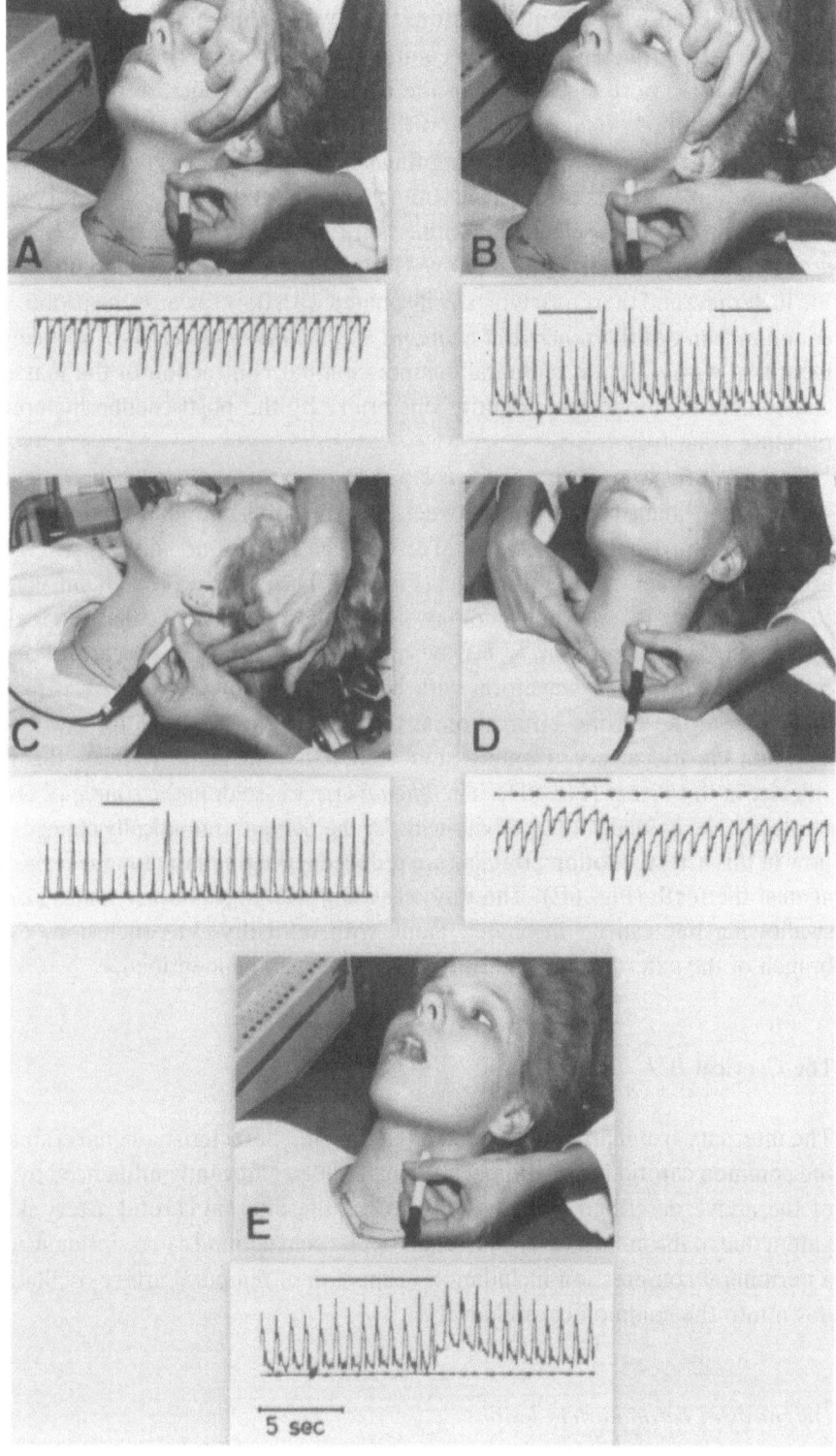

5 sec

on the forehead with a gentle pressure thereby avoiding head motion artefacts (Fig. 6). In general, the combined compression of the superficial temporal and facial artery is more effective than the compression of one artery alone. This combined compression is performed with the thumb just ventral to the antitragus and the aligned tips of the remaining fingers along the lower jaw.

Separation of signals from various branches of the external carotid artery distal to its origin requires selective compression of individual branches. *The facial artery* compression is described above (Fig. 6A). This artery is bending around the lower jaw and therefore typically insonated with flow towards the probe. The common trunk of the *superficial temporal* and the *maxillary artery* is sufficiently identified with only the temporal compression but contraction of the masseter and temporal muscle may identify this artery by the postischemic hyperemia response (Fig. 6B).

The identification of the *occiptal artery* is of great importance because this artery is the main connection between the vertebral and extracranial carotid system. Compression of the occipital artery is best performed distally where the artery crosses over the occipital bone (Fig. 6C). The probe position being ventral to the insertion of the sternocleidomastoid muscle or dorsal in the mastoid region.

The superior *thyroid artery* can be mistaken for the internal carotid artery because of the similar waveform with high diastolic flow. Its course is mainly medial from the carotid bifurcation at the origin of the external or end of the common carotid artery. Compression of the thyroid gland reduces the flow velocity in this artery (Fig. 6D). The *lingual artery* is seldom the source of errors because of its medial course. Swallowing by the patient dramatically changes the flow in this artery. Motion artefacts are reduced if the tip of the tongue is pushed against the teeth (Fig. 6E). The tiny *ascending pharyngeal artery* reacts also to swallowing but can be insonated alone with difficulty. In conclusion, every branch of the external carotid artery in the neck can be identified.

The Cervical ICA

The internal carotid artery is located by finding its characteristic signal cranial to the common carotid bifurcation. The signal is not significantly influenced by any of the above described compressions. When the internal carotid artery is not patent due to thrombosis every carotid Doppler signal found can be influenced by a peripheral compression including transmission of temporal artery oscillations down into the common carotid artery.

Diagnosis of carotid artery lesions

The freehand techniques offer advantages for the evaluation of both direct and indirect criteria of stenosis and occlusion. Direct criteria come from the signals directly recorded from the site of the arterial lesion. Indirect criteria are represented by differences of the velocity in arteries proximal or distal to a lesion. The full range of criteria to estimate the degree of stenoses are discussed extensively in the chapter on hemodynamics of arterial stenosis. We rely on the presence or absence of indirect criteria; side-to-side carotid differences, periorbital Doppler signs of collateral and on the spectral systolic peak frequencies and the quality of the spectrum directly recorded from the suspected artery. In our experience the systolic peak frequency is more closely correlated with the degree of stenoses than the quality of the spectrum; the latter depends more on the shape of the stenosis.

Indirect criteria

Side-to-side differences in the velocity signals from the carotid arteries are often found when stenosis or occlusion is present distal to the insonated arterial segment. This applies to obstructions either at the origin of the internal carotid or intracranial segments of the internal carotid artery or middle cerebral artery. Figure 7A and B illustrates an interesting case of stenosis of the supraclinoid segment of the left internal carotid artery. This 31-year old woman presented with aphasia and paresis of the right arm. Doppler sonography demonstrated greatly reduced velocities in the cervical left internal compared to the right but with normal responses in the supratrochlear artery to temporal artery compression. Selective catheterization of the carotid and vertebral arteries demonstrated severe stenosis of the siphon beyond the origin of the ophthalmic artery.

Tortuosities of the course of the common and internal carotid artery may lead to false positive results because of changes in the angle of insonation. When differences appear several different angles of insonation should be used from various levels to confirm true asymmetry. It is more reliable to compare the signals with the highest frequencies found from various probe positions using the lowest possible probe beam angle than to compare the signals of both sides in a standard probe angle. The reason for this that is the angle of insonation influences the recorded Doppler shift in a cosine function as explained in the chapter on physics. The lower the angle of insonation the less the influence of the unknown angle. A zero angle cannot be reached but one may reach angles of less than 30° keeping the side to side error less than 20 percent. The free hand technique makes this possible and represents an advantage of free hand over imaging techniques. Fig. 8 gives an example for the common carotid artery which is sometimes more tortuous on the right. Fig. 9 illustrates how to optimize the velocity signal of the internal carotid artery. In addition the drawing represents an example of how to document the examination. The speed of the motion of the probe along the artery depends on how easy it is to find and to follow the artery. Therefore, the

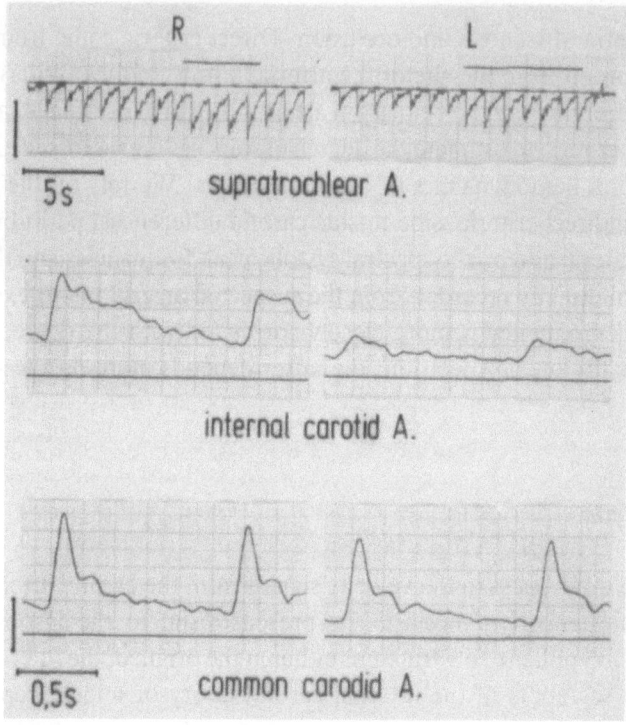

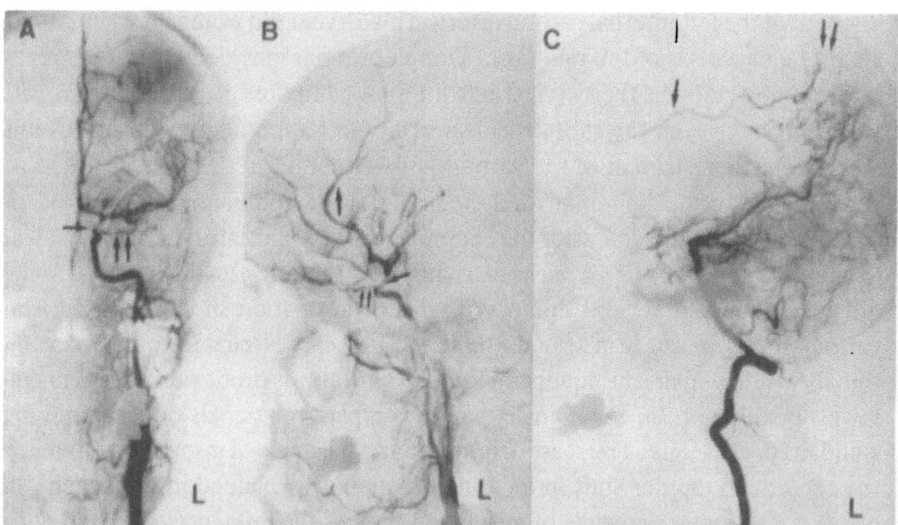

Figure 7A. Intracranial stenosis: 3 Doppler sonography: Supratrochlear artery with physiologic flow direction (flow towards the probe, increasing velocity with the temporal artery occlusion test. Reduced flow velocity of the left internal (in systole and diastole) and common carotid artery (mainly in diastole), indicating elevated resistance beyond the origin of the ophthalmic artery.

Figure 7B. Angiography of intracranial stenosis – same patient in 7A. Selective catheterization of the left carotid (A and B) and left vertebral artery (C). Stenosis of the distal carotid siphon shown (A) in the a.p. and (B) lateral projections indicated by the horizontal arrows (→) and (←). Normal filling of the ophthalmic artery is indicated by the double vertical arrows (↑ ↑). In addition occlusion of the callosomarginal artery is indicated in B by the single vertical arrow. In C retrograde filling is indicated by the single inverted arrow via cortical anastomeses indicated by the double inverted arrows (↑ ↑).

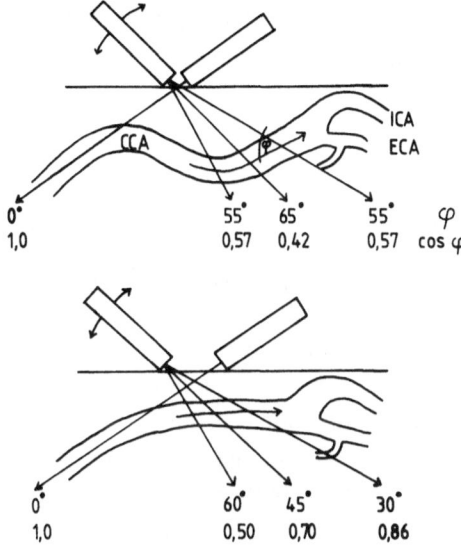

Figure 8. Influence of the course of the common carotid artery on the recorded Doppler shift. The error is higher with large angles between the ultrasonic beam and the vessel axis.

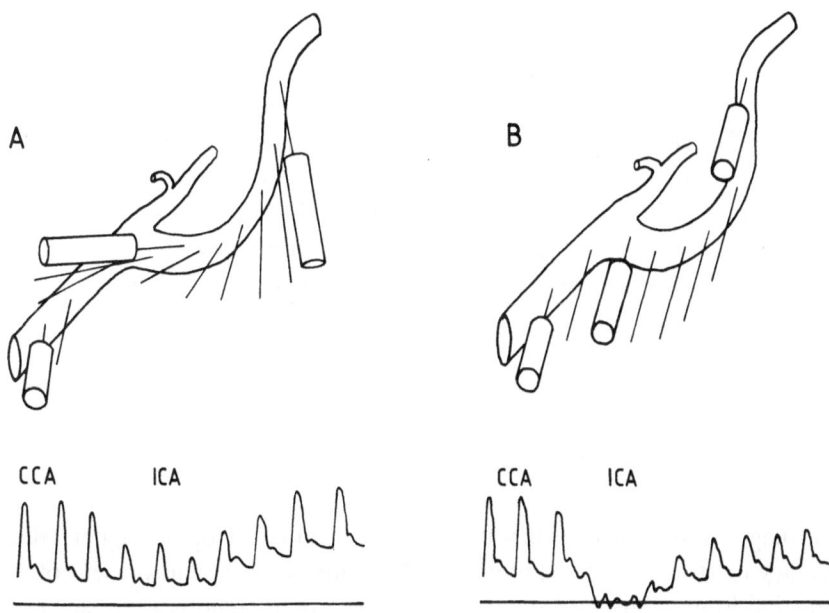

Figure 9. Scanning of the carotid bifurcation with free hand technique (A) and with a fixed angle of examination (B).

estimated distance between the insonated segment of the internal carotid artery and the bifurcation and the mandible should be noted on the records.

Direct criteria

The direct criterion for a vascular stenosis is based on the fact that diameter variations are reflected by local variations in blood velocity. The utilization of this principle for quantitation of artery diameter is subject to error if the probe angle is always fixed with respect to the body axis, because the exact course of the artery and the angle of insonation respectively is not known. The free hand method allows better estimation of the course of an artery. This is important in the interpretation of locally increased or decreased Doppler shifts. Fig. 10 shows pulse curves resulting from changes in the direction of an artery in the plane of the insonation compared with the results from a straight artery. From the situation in Fig. 10 a stenosis might be suspected, however, insonation from different angles makes a misdiagnosis of a stenosis unlikely. The same principle can be extended to the detection of arterial coiling.

In normal subjects the origin of the internal carotid artery is large compared to the distal segments. Therefore the Doppler-shift, which is normally recorded from the origin of the internal carotid artery, is relatively low and the spectrum often disturbed by flow separation. Plaques in this region of up to 50 percent local diameter reduction may only fill in the bulb. When this occurs the recorded Doppler frequency may be the same as recorded in the distal internal carotid artery and flow becomes laminar. Therefore the interpretation of a Doppler signal has to take into account the position of the probe beam in relation to the carotid bifurcation. The only sign of a low degree stenosis of the internal carotid artery at the origin may be the abrupt increase of the Doppler frequency as the probe is moved from the common to the internal carotid artery. The problem is the same for the hand-held technique as well as for flow imaging techniques. The carotid bifurcation, however, must be localized exactly using sometimes two or more scanning planes to separate the external and internal carotid arteries at their origins.

Criteria for diagnosis of arterial occlusion

The diagnosis of an occlusion is based on the fact that a Doppler signal indicating patency or stenosis is not found, yet there are indirect signs present of a flow reducing lesion. Special care must be taken when stenosis is so severe as to produce such a thin volume of blood in the stenotic segment that a very weak Doppler signal is produced. Sometimes it is not possible, in these cases, to follow the internal carotid artery cranialwards. The free hand technique may be helpful

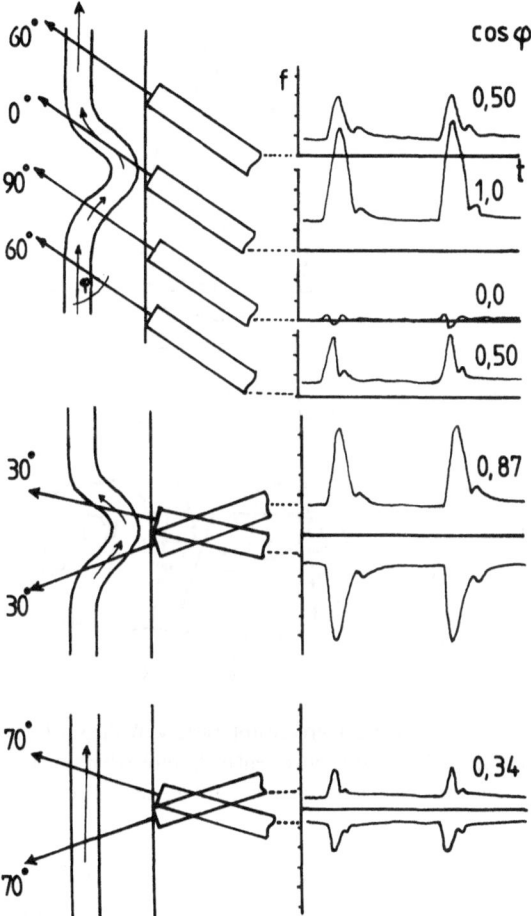

Figure 10. Interpretation of localized high Doppler frequencies due to a curved artery with a fixed probe position. A stenosis may be suspected because of locally elevated Doppler frequencies (above). If a small change in the angle of the probe induces reversal of flow direction, with both directions showing high Doppler shift, a curve in the vessel can be suspected.

in finding such weak signals because a lot of different positions and directions of the probe can be applied quickly moving around the bifurcation.

Avoidable pitfalls

The following are typical errors which occur for the beginner [10] but can be avoided by being alert to the special situation and diligence of the examining techniques.

1. Carotid occlusion
a) Prevention of false negative diagnosis.
   Mistaking vertebral artery for internal carotid artery. In a frontal view the

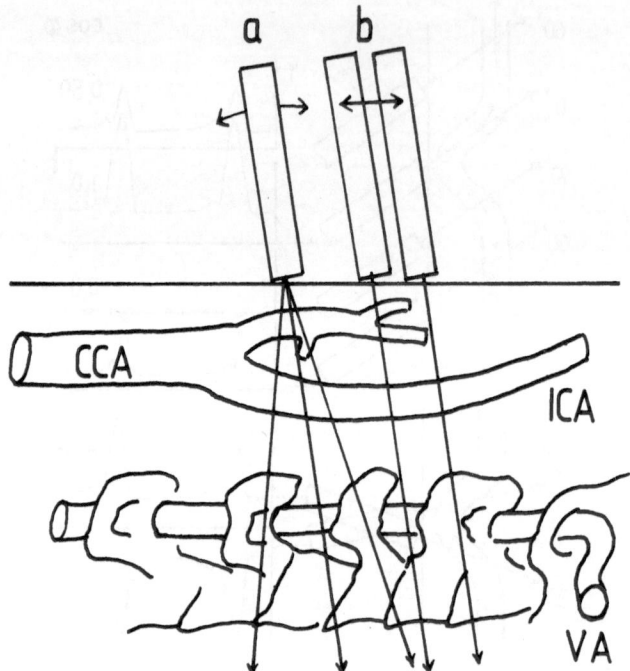

Figure 11. Mistaking vertebral artery for internal carotid artery. With a small change in the angle of the probe (a) or with a little up- or downwards movement of the probe (b) the signal of the vertebral artery is lost, whereas in general the signal of the internal carotid artery can continuously be followed.

vertebral artery lies, more or less, in line with the carotid artery. Therefore it is the vertebral artery that is frequently taken for the internal carotid which, in fact, is occluded. This mistake happens in patients with a slim neck and a large vertebral artery and is favored also by increased collateral flow in the vertebral artery. The finding of a Doppler signal like that from a normal internal carotid artery in the presence of indirect signs of obstruction makes it probable that the vertebral artery was insonated.

Several additional clues help recognize the vertebral artery (Fig. 11). Because of its depth in anterior-posterior direction, the angle of the probe is rather high when recording. Signals of the vertebral artery are lost when the angle of the probe is lowered. In addition, these signals disappear with little up or downward movement of the probe because the vertebral artery is partially covered by the transverse processes. On the other hand, only the internal carotid artery can be followed continuously downward until the bifurcation is reached.

In the presence of occlusion of the internal carotid collateral flow increases the blood velocity of the external carotid. This can produce Doppler signals which mimic the internal carotid. This error, that one branch of the external carotid artery is taken for the internal carotid artery, is easy to avoid by a systematic use of the compression tests (Fig. 6).

The diagnosis of an occluded common carotid artery can be made by careful palpation comparing the two sides of the neck. The need of palpation and auscultation should accompany the Doppler examination. On the other hand, Doppler sonographic diagnosis is sometimes difficult because one of the many collaterals can be taken for the common or internal carotid artery. This confusion is avoided because these collaterals can be easily obliterated by pressure with the probe (please refer to the chapter on vertebral subclavian artery abnormalities). When the common carotid is patent strong pressure of the probe is needed to occlude. The common carotid artery occlusion produces postocclusive flow effects in the branches of the external carotid artery. The differentiation against internal carotid flow is based on compression tests. Flow in the occipital artery is reversed in the segment from the anastamosis with the vertebral artery to the proximal external carotid artery serving as collateral artery. This is proven by compression of the facial and superficial temporal artery producing continuity effects.

In most cases of occlusion of the common carotid artery the internal carotid artery occluded as well. However, a patent bifurcation is possible when proximal disease is primary. Then, the occipital artery supplies the internal carotid artery. Here compressions of the occipital artery will modulate the internal carotid signal. This difficulty occurs rarely and is predictible from the context of the rest of the examination. Additional duplex scanning or angiography may be helpful to prove the patency of the internal carotid artery.

b) Prevention of false positive diagnosis

The possibility of overlooking a preocclusive situation with extremely tight stenosis was mentioned previously, but a second source of error is intracranial stenosis simulating an occlusion of the proximal internal carotid artery because flow in this segment is highly reduced and the Doppler result of the common carotid artery fits with the diagnosis of occlusion. Again, the identification of the internal carotid by negative compression maneuvers is mandatory.

2. Carotid stenoses

a) Prevention of a false negative diagnosis

The problem of how to enhance accuracy in low degree disease will not be discussed here. This belongs to the presentations of B-mode and spectrum analysis. Moderate and high graded stenoses of the carotid bifurcation, on the other hand, are demonstrated with a sensitivity close to 100%.

Stenoses of the proximal common carotid artery at its origin from the aorta will not be missed if the probe is also directed caudaly as a routine procedure in scanning the common carotid artery.

b) Prevention of false positive

The false positive diagnosis of an internal carotid artery stenosis may result from high flow in the superior thyroid artery. Especially high frequencies and turbulences may be related to the fact that the course of this artery is first upward and then turns downward (flow disturbance in arterial curve or kinking). Compression of the thyroid gland assigns these signals to the thyroid artery. In regions with endemic goitre this situation is frequent. High degree external carotid stenoses will not be taken for internal carotid stenoses if the appropriate compression tests are applied carefully. However, this error is the most common and can especially occur when the internal carotid and external carotid are reversed in their relative lateral projections.

3. Combined internal and external carotid lesions

In combined high degree lesion problems are encountered. It may be difficult to separate the Doppler signals of these stenoses lying close together and therefore the false diagnoses of an occlusion of one of both is possible. Spectrum analysis is in some cases helpful and demonstrates simultaneously the two stenotic signals with the influence of compression tests seen only on the signal of the external stenosis. But in this situation careful investigation of the region distal to the bifurcation is most helpful in analyzing all Doppler signals with the complete battery of compression tests. Compression tests are essential to separate internal and external carotid artery flow because the character of the postocclusive or poststenotic pulse curves of internal and external carotid arteries are similar.

Results

This section is provided as an example of what accuracy can be achieved by noninvasive diagnosis of extracranial carotid stenosis and occlusion of the carotid arteries using only noninvasive free hand Doppler criteria. We reported in 1976 on 76 carotid arteries examined with Doppler sonography and angiography [9], (Table 1).

The number of patients in this study was not large and the angiograms were not evaluated independently by a neuroradiologist. Our second correlation of Doppler-sonographic and angiographic data in 1978/1979 included 161 carotid arteries of 108 patients with cerebrovascular occlusive disease ranging in age from 39 to 77

Table 1.

Angiography Doppler- sonography	<50% or normal	>50% stenosis	Occlusion	Σ
normal	37	1		38
Stenosis >50%		19		19
Occlusion		1	18	19
Σ	37	21	18	76

years. Patients with tumors and other non-vascular disease were excluded. Indication for angiography was transient ischemic attacks in 55 patients, stroke with the possibility in view of surgical treatment in 33 patients and no symptoms but severe disease who were to be operated alone or in combination with aorto-coronary bypass procedures in 20 patients.

The angiographic evaluation of the degree of stenosis was made by measuring the diameter in relation to the region immediately upstream or downstream from the stenosis. In the most frequent cases of asymptomatic plaque formation this method of angiographic evaluation corresponds nearly to the cross-sectional area reduction [11]. Smooth plaques of less than 20% diameter reduction were not taken into consideration. Stenoses were divided into three groups: less than 50%, 50 to 70%, and greater than 70%. With regard to the intracranial arteries stenosis of the carotid siphon, the middle cerebral artery and occlusions of its major branches were noted. Angiograms were reviewed independently by Dr. A. Thron, radiologist. The results are shown in Table 2. We did not accept equivocal Doppler results as pathologic in order to reduce false positives. This was also the reason for our assumption that stenoses of less than 50% local diameter reduction (in the case of asymmetric plaques) or cross-sectional area reduction were undetectable. The sensitivity of the Doppler diagnosis in lesions of greater than 50% in the internal carotid artery near the bifurcation (stenosis or occlusion) was 98% and the specificity was 94%.

Differentiation of stenosis from occlusion

The greatest reliability of the Doppler-sonographic differentiation of stenosis and occlusion occurred when a stenosis was suspected. Only one false diagnosis of stenosis occurred despite no flow detection from the cervical carotid artery, due to misinterpretation of physiologic flow direction in the opthalmic artery resulting from an abnormal origin of the latter. Four errors in differentiation were noted

Table 2.

Angiography	'normal'	20–49	50–70	>70	Occlusion	Σ
Doppler-sonography						
'normal'	27	18	2			47
50–70			29	2		31
>70			2	54	1*	57
Occlusion	3***			1**	22	26
Σ	30	18	33	57	23	161

when the Doppler diagnosis was 'occlusion.' Review of these cases revealed reasons previously mentioned in the chapter of avoidable pitfalls. Once an intracranial stenosis was taken for an occlusion. A severe stenosis of the internal carotid artery was taken for an occlusion in presence of a similar severe stenosis of the external carotid artery. One occlusion of the common carotid artery and one occlusion of the inominate artery was the source of error.

The sensitivity of the Doppler test for occlusions of the internal carotid artery was 96%. However, in practice the question is not if Doppler-sonography is suitable to select patients with total occlusions of the internal carotid artery among all examinations; the real problem is the differentiation between complete occlusions and severe stenoses. This is essential for the clinician because the impact of these two findings on management and treatment decision differ considerably. Therefore, the positive predictive value of each of these two Doppler-sonographic findings is of primary interest. The predictive value of the sonographic diagnosis was higher for stenoses (98%) than for occlusions (84%). The reason being the fact that the diagnosis of occlusion relies mainly on the absence of a Doppler signal whereas a stenosis can be proven positively. The limited reliability of the Doppler-sonographic differentiation between stenosis and occlusion of the internal carotid artery, in patients with additional severe stenoses of the external carotid artery and occlusions of the common carotid artery can be recognized during the examination and given consideration. The predicitive value of the remaining 'uncomplicated' diagnoses of occlusion was 96% (occlusions correctly identified 22, intracranial stenosis taken for occlusion 1). The high percentage of severe stenoses in this series compared with occlusions was a result of selection. Angiography was only indicated for occlusion if the diagnosis was uncertain for the above mentioned reasons or if this occlusion was contralateral to a stenosis. No patient of this study underwent extra- intracranial bypass surgery because this indication was limited to repeated ischemic attacks in known occlusions of the internal carotid artery. In conclusion we believe that the Doppler-sonographic diagnosis of an occlusion of the internal carotid artery is more reliable than shown in Table 2.

As completely different methods have to be compared both with inherent limitations, we only noted discrepancies between the categories of 50–70% and more than 70% stenosis with less than 50% being considered as Doppler negative. Two overestimations by Doppler were due to tortuosity and kinking of the internal carotid artery with registration of localized high frequencies and turbulence. For the good differentiation between stenoses of more or less than 50% degree also a factor of selection was probably responsible, angiography being more indicated in 60–70% stenoses than in borderline cases of 50% stenoses. In addition, the good correlation of the Doppler and angiographically determined degree of stenosis was due to a long-standing, close communication between the neuroradiology and the Doppler laboratories, which brought a common terminology. However, documents of this study were evaluated independently.

External carotid artery

The diagnosis of 12 stenotic lesions greater than 70% and 5 occlusions of the external carotid artery were confirmed by angiography.

Intracranial stenosis

Less reliability was found for those stenoses situated intracranially or in the region of the base of the skull. Among 11 high degree (over 70%) stenoses of such localization, 5 could be demonstrated by Doppler-sonography (4 out of 6 isolated and 1 out of 5 combined proximal and intracranial stenoses).

Comparison of the free hand examination with flow imaging

It has also been shown by others that the free hand Doppler sonography yields reliable diagnoses in carotid artery disease [5, 6, 7]. Neuerburg-Heusler e.g. found a sensitivity of 93% for >50% stenoses and occlusions of the internal carotid artery. Sensitivity for occlusions was 97%. Among 30 occlusions and 34>50% stenoses only 2 errors of differentiation occurred. Comparable results were found by Trockel *et al.* [12], Reimer *et al.* [8] and Fischer *et al.* [4]. All these figures compare favorably with the findings of others using flow imaging procedures. In the series of White [13] for instance, the differentiation of severe stenosis and occlusion of the internal carotid artery by Doppler was correct in only 82%. Bloch *et al.* [2] found a sensitivity of 83% for hemodynamically significant internal carotid artery stenosis with a specificity of 96%. The Doppler results of Blackwell *et al.* [1], also using flow imaging, were in total agreement with angiography in 12 occlusions of the internal carotid artery but the Doppler correlated only 70% to 85% with angiography in stenoses.

We carried out a comparative study between our free hand method with the flow mapping technique of the Institute of Applied Physiology and Medicine, Seattle, WA. During a three-month period in 1982, 50 patients with cerebrovascular disease and/or carotid lesions were selected and examinations were carried out by separate technicians blinded to one anothers results. One nearly occluded internal carotid artery was correctly identified with the free hand method, whereas, an occlusion was suspected by flow imaging. One occlusion was overlooked by flow imaging because a branch of the external carotid artery was taken for the internal carotid artery. No additional significant differences were noted comparing the reliability of both methods.

Conclusions

Doppler-sonography with the free hand techniques, as used routinely in European countries, yields reliable diagnostic information. The free hand technique provides freedom of movement with the probe and is advantageous especially in tracing and evaluating signals originating from tortuous or abnormally situated vessels. The equipment is less expensive than that of imaging. Accuracy is as good or better than use of imaging. Flow imaging, on the other hand, is a well standardized method and allows documentation and division of labor between the physician and a vascular technician. The routine use of the compression test, as described in this chapter, is of great importance regardless of documentation technique.

Doppler is not very accurate in diagnosing stenosis <50%. This diagnostic gap can be bridged by the use of B-mode duplex scanners which seem to detect the low degree lesions better than those of high degree. Duplex-scanning is also helpful in common carotid occlusions and may improve the positive predictive value of the diagnosis of internal carotid occlusion.

References

1. Blackwell E, Merory J, Toole JF, McKinney W: Doppler ultrasound scanning of the carotid bifurcation. Archives of Neurology 34: 145, 1977.
2. Bloch S, Baltaxe HA, Shoumaker RD. Reliability of Doppler scanning of the carotid bifurcation: Angiographic correlation. Radiology 132: 687, 1979.
3. Büdingen HJ, Reutern von G-M, Freund HJ: Doppler-Sonographie der extrakraniellen Hirnarterien. Thieme, Stuttgart, 1982.
4. Fischer M, Wiehler S, Vogelsang H, Alexander K: Zum Stellenwert direkter und indirekter Methoden der nichtinvasiven Diagnostik von Karotisobstruktionen. In: Mahler F, Nachbur B, (eds) Zerebrale Ischämie, Huber, Bern, Stuttgart, Wien, 1984.
5. Keller HM, Schubiger O, Krayenbühl C, Zumstein B: Cerebrovascular Doppler examination and cerebral angiography – alternative or complementary? Neuroradiology 16: 140, 1978.
6. Neuerburg-Heusler D: Dopplersonographische Diagnostik der extrakraniellen Verschluß-krankheit. VASA Suppl. 12: 59, 1984.
7. Pourcelot L: Indications de l'ultrasonographie Doppler dans l'etudes des vaisseaux périphéres. L'Année du Practicien 25: 4671, 1975.
8. Reimer F, Wernheimer D, Lange J, Friedrich B, Maurer PC, Becker HM: Die Ultraschall-Doppler-(USD)-Sonographie der A. carotis. Ein klinischer Erfahrungsbericht. Verhandlungen der deutschen Gesellschaft für innere Medizin, Vol. 86., J.F. Bergmann Verlag, München, 1980.
9. Reutern von G-M, Büdingen HJ, Hennerici M, Freund H-J: Diagnose und Differenzierung von Stenosen und Verschlüssen der Arteria carotis mit der Doppler-Sonographie. Archiv für Psychiatrie und Nervenkrankheiten 222: 191, 1976.
10. Reutern von G-M, Thron A: Dopplersonographie des artères carotides. Résultats et causes d'erreurs. Actualités d'Angéiologie 5: 9, 1980.
11. Spencer MP, Reid JM: Quantitation of carotid stenosis with continuous-wave (C-W) Doppler ultrasound. Stroke 10: 326, 1979.

12. Trockel U, Hennerici M, Aulich A, Sandmann W: The superiority of combined continuous wave Doppler examination over periorbital Doppler for the detection of extracranial carotid disease. Journal of Neurology, Neurosurgery and Psychiatry 47: 43, 1984.
13. White DN, Curry GR: A comparison of 424 carotid bifurcations examined by angiography and the Doppler echoflow. In: White D, Lyons EA, (eds) Ultrasound in Medicine and Biology Vol. 4, pp. 363–376, Plenum Press, New York, London, 1978.

Quantification of carotid stenosis using continuous wave Doppler and spectral analysis

Ph. Arbeille, F. Lapierre, F. Patat, M. Berson, D. Besse and L. Pourcelot

Continuous wave (CW) Doppler examinations have been performed for more than 10 years for peripheral circulation to assess atherosclerosis patients. By means of the audio signal and velocity curve (analogue tracing) it is possible to detect stenoses >60% by area [1, 8, 13, 15, 20]. Real time 2-D echography provides good visualization of the vessel walls and shows most of the atheromatous buildup; however, using this technique, it is sometimes difficult to estimate the extent of stenosis. This is especially the case of the hypoechogenic plaque, where limits are not well defined, or of calcified plaque, behind which the lumen and the vessel wall is masked by acoustic shadow [2, 9, 10, 14, 15, 16].

Spectral analysis of the Doppler audio signal, more recently developed, has considerably increased the performance accuracy of the Doppler examination. This new display mode of the Doppler signal provides information on the velocities within the vessel. It is possible to detect hemodynamic disturbances caused by stenosis of 15% by area and to quantify higher degrees of stenosis according to the amplitude of the spectrum disturbance [2, 3, 4, 5, 6, 7, 11, 12, 17, 18, 19, 21, 22].

Since 1981, a real time spectrum analyser and a 4 MHz CW Doppler have been used. The Doppler includes a dephasing module to separate positive and negative Doppler audio signals. This direction capability makes possible display of arterial and venous spectra separately or negative frequency shifts due to whirling phenomena. To date more than 1500 patients with cerebrovascular symptomathology (TIA – Transient Ischemic Attack) and carotid atheromatous disease have been investigated in our laboratory with this device.

The purpose of this chapter is to describe and extend the possibilities and the limitations of the CW Doppler spectrum analysis for the quantification of carotid disease. The degree of stenosis has been evaluated in accordance with a classification in five grades of spectrum disturbances and with the help of a stenosis (STI) calculated from the most disturbed spectrum recorded immediately downstream from a stenosis. The results obtained through spectrum analysis have been compared to those obtained from physical study of endarterectomy specimens and angiography data.

Materials and methods

Equipment

The system used consists of a 4MHz CW Doppler unit (Angio-Dop 482 DMS) connected to a real time FFT frequency analyser (Angioscan I Unigon Industry Inc.).

Patient examination

At the bifurcation of the common carotid artery the internal and external carotid branches can be identified both by listening to the audio signal and viewing the Doppler spectrum. Diastolic flow can be observed on the internal carotid spectrum but is less prominent on the external carotid spectrum. The internal carotid is then explored from its origin and followed up the patient's neck as far as possible.

The technician subjectively evaluates the spectrum disturbances according to a group of parameters which will be defined later and records the most disturbed spectrum. Generally, atheromatous lesions are located at the origin of the internal carotid and it is quite important to be sure this area has been well investigated. For that reason the examination is repeated by placing the probe in the submaxillary area and exploring the internal carotid in reverse down to its origin.

Spectral analysis of the Doppler signal

Frequency analysis of the audio signal gives the partition of the red cells among the different velocities present in the velocity profile of the explored vessel section. By 'partition' we mean the distribution of frequencies according to the distribution of velocity flow streams. (Please see Chapter 2 for further details on spectral representation.) The frequency spectrum is displayed on a videomonitor with frequencies on the vertical axis, time on the horizontal axis and amplitude of each frequency as the intensity of a gray scale (Fig. 1). On the normal spectrum we observe an homogeneous partition of the brightness on the high and middle frequency domain and a well defined limitation of the upper border of the spectrum (Fig. 1).

Modifications of the spectrum are due to modifications of the velocity profile and certain features can be directly related to the degree of stenosis. In Chapter 9 we see how the increase in velocities and Doppler frequencies are used to quantitate degrees of stenosis. In this chapter we will explore how the use of spectral disturbances can also provide quantitative information. In the case of a

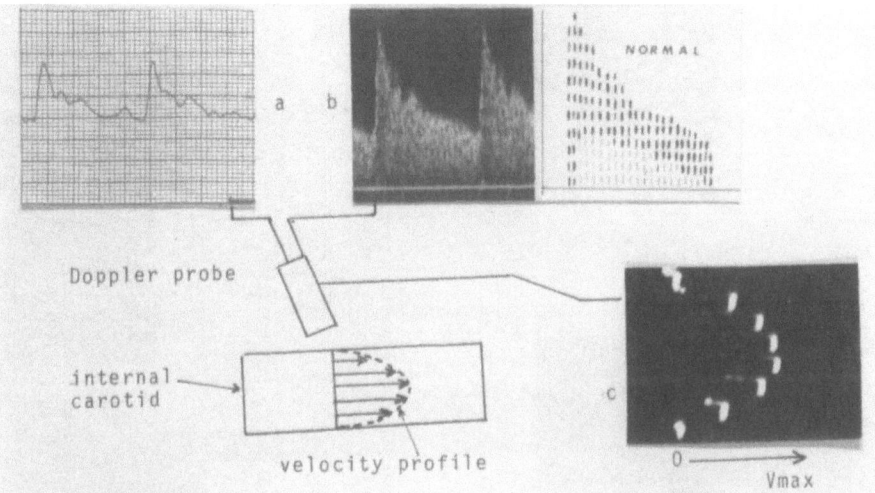

Figure 1. Doppler exploration of a normal internal carotid. a) velocity curve (CW Doppler + zero crossing system). b) frequency spectrum (CW Doppler + spectral analyser). c) velocity profile (multigate pulsed Doppler).

very low grade stenosis the increase of the velocities of the central (axial) stream and the decrease of the velocities on the edges just following the stenosis, does not affect the Doppler analog velocity curve but can be easily detected on the frequency spectrum. This method is much more powerful than the conventional Doppler analogue tracings for the detection of the low hemodynamic disturbances. In case of great flow disturbances when the velocity curve from zero crossing techniques gives information on mean velocities, the spectrum disturbances show different grades of disorder.
– Doppler spectrum will be characterized qualitatively with three parameters (Figs. 1 & 2).
– the upper border of the spectrum in systole and diastole. This is well defined in a normal spectrum (Fig. 1) but not in the case of a disturbed spectrum.
– the brightness distribution on the spectrum. On the normal spectrum the most intense brightness occurs on the high and middle frequencies but moves toward the low frequencies (disturbed spectrum) as the degree of stenosis increases (Fig. 2).
– the presence of negative frequency shifts. In systole this phenomenon is related to whirling phenomena of downstream flow disturbances.

Criteria for degrees of stenosis with spectral classification in five grades

Different types of abnormal spectrum have been observed on 1500 atheromatous patients explored; they have been classified in five grades according to the spectral amplitude of the disturbances (Figs. 2 & 3).

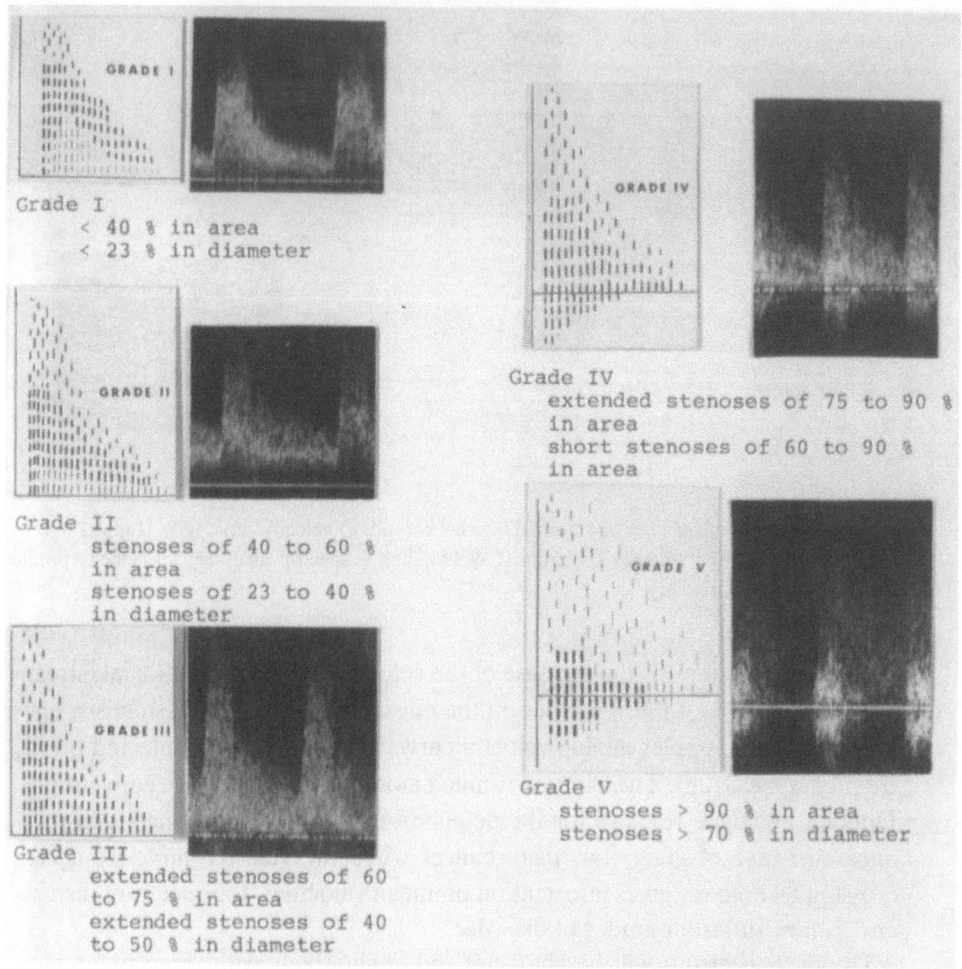

Figure 2. Different grades of carotid spectral disturbances. Note that the most intense brightness move toward the low frequencies domain as the degree of stenosis increases.

Grade I is characterized by a mild spectral broadening in higher frequencies, essentially in systole, with loss of energy density in this part of the spectrum. *Grade II* shows the same kind of modifications but occurs both in systole and diastole. *Grade III* is characterized by a more noticeable expansion of the spectrum to higher frequencies with the majority of the brightness on the lower frequency domain. *Grade IV* shows a strong spectral broadening causing an increase of the brightness of the lower frequencies, and negative frequency shifts in systole due to vortices. *Grade V* is characterized by severe disturbances during all of the cardiac cycle, with brightness of very strong intensity both on the positive and negative low frequencies and a very low brightness intensity on the upper frequencies of the spectrum. This aspect corresponds to a turbulent flow (unsteady flow). As the degree of stenosis increases the maximum systolic

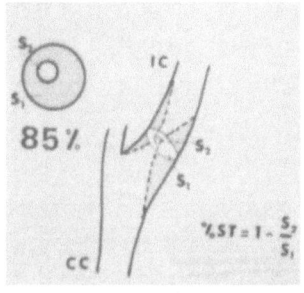 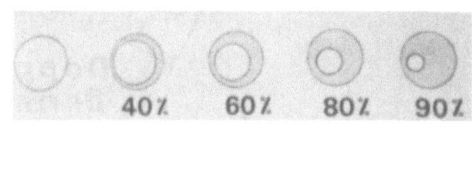

Figure 3. Degree of stenosis expressed in percentage of the lumen reduction.

frequency increases and the brightness moves toward the low frequencies domain.

All of the abnormal spectra described have been reproduced on an experimental plastic tube device, with different values of stenosis, and with flows ranging between 300 and 500 ml/min. Grade I corresponds to stenosis of less than 40%; grade II occurs for stenosis of 40 to 60%; grade III is obtained for elongated stenosis of 60 to 75%, grade IV corresponds to short stenosis of 60 to 90% and elongated stenosis of 75 to 90%, grade V concerns very tight stenosis, higher than 90%.

For the *in vivo* evaluation of the degree of stenosis with the CW Doppler spectrum analysis, the same classification has been used. Each grade is related to an interval of possible values for the degree of stenosis. This degree of stenosis is expressed as the percentage of the arterial area occupied by the atheroma (Figs. 2 & 3).

For stenoses whose degree ranges between 60 and 90%, the modifications of the spectrum representation of the velocity profile depends on the *shape* of stenosis. Short stenoses of 60 to 90% degree, with an abrupt downstream slope, produce vortices and provide spectrum disturbances of grade IV with negative frequency shift. With elongated stenoses the shape of the downstream outlet slope is generally not abrupt, for stenosis between 60 and 75% whirling phenomena do not occur and these lesions provide spectrum disturbances of grade III. For stenosis more than 75%, however, their outlet slope is not abrupt, vortices exist and the spectrum shows negative frequency shift (grade IV).

In summary: All the stenosis between 60 to 90% provide spectrum disturbances of grade III or IV, but grade III concerns only elongated stenosis of 60 to 75%.

Criteria of the stenosis index (STI)

On the classification in five grades one can note that, as the degree of stenosis

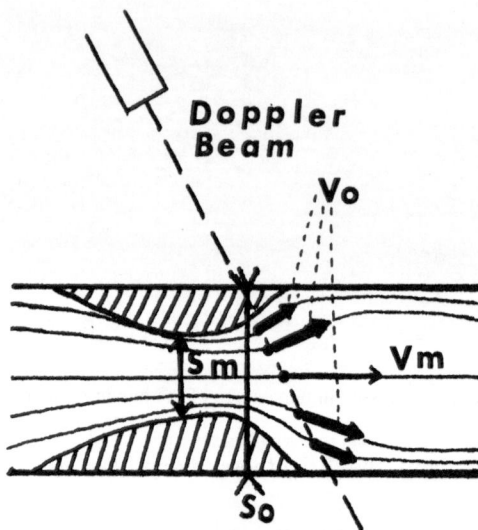

Figure 4. Principle for quantitating stenosis severity using Doppler spectral features. Vm represents the maximum velocity or frequency within the stenosis and in the outlet. Vo represents the velocities and the frequencies within the major intensity domain of the spectrum. Sm represents the minimal cross-section within the stenosis and So the normal, non-stenotic, cross-section.

increases, the maximum sytolic frequency increases and the most intense bright-ness moves toward the low frequency domain. In order to quantify the spectral disturbance and therefore the degree of stenosis, a stenosis index STI has been proposed (Fig. 4):

$$STI = 0.9 \left(1 - \frac{Vo}{Vm}\right)$$

With Vm representing maximum velocity in the central stream of the stenosis. Vo represents the mean velocity in the post stenotic outflow (i.e., the mean velocity represented within the major intensity brightness) (Fig. 5). 0.9 is a constant. If we consider that the Vm in the downstream section of the artery is the same as within the stenosis, we can record both Vo and Vm at a point 2–3 mn after the stenosis. From Figure 4 we see that the ratio Vo/Vm is proportional to Sm/So:Sm and So are respectively the cross-section of the residual lumen and the cross-section of the normal artery at the level of the stenosis. Then (1 – Vo/Vm is proportional to the degree of the stenosis. Finally since Vo/Vm is proportional to Fo/Fm the stenosis index becomes: STI = 0.9 (1 – Fo/Fm with Fm the maximum systolic frequency and the Fo the mean frequency on the most intense brightness area during the systole (Fig. 5). The index of stenosis is calculated only on disturbed spectra. Also, because of the expression we use, this index applies only for stenosis greater than 25 to 30% by area. For all the stenoses of more than 90% the index remains constant equal to 0.9 because Fo is equal to zéro.

$$STI = 0,9(1 - \frac{Fo}{Fm})$$

$$STI = 0,53$$

stenosis degree = 53 %

Fm

Fo

0

Comparison of Doppler degree of stenosis with endarterectomy data

Carotid endarterectomy pieces are cut out in transversal cross-sections of 2 mm thickness from the common carotid up to the limit of the internal carotid. The diameters D1 of the whole artery and D2 of the residual lumen are measured under a microscope on the narrowest section of the artery. When the arterial lumen is not circular, D2 is obtained by averaging the extreme values of this parameter. As for the other methods, the degree of stenosis is expressed as the percentage of the lumen occupied by the Atheroma:

$$\% St = (1 - \frac{D2^2}{D1^2})$$

Comparison of the Degree of Stenosis with Angiography

Radiographic evaluation is performed on biplane x-ray incidence. The degree of stenosis is calculated as follows: $\% St = (1 - D2^2/D1^2$ with D2 the diameter of the lumen at the narrowest part of the artery, and D1 the extrapolated diameter of the artery at the same level. The advantage of this mode of calculation is that the degree of stenosis is expressed from the same parameters for the three methods (angiography, spectrum analysis, anatomopathology).

Results

Every patient examined for this study came from the Neurosurgical Department of the hospital. Their age ranged between 50 and 85. Fifty eight patients were explored on both sides by ultrasound and angiographic methods: 20 of them had bilateral lesions, 38 unilateral lesions. Fifty patients already had a TIA during the 5 previous years; 8 patients were asymptomatic.

We consider that we have a perfect correlation between the results of the

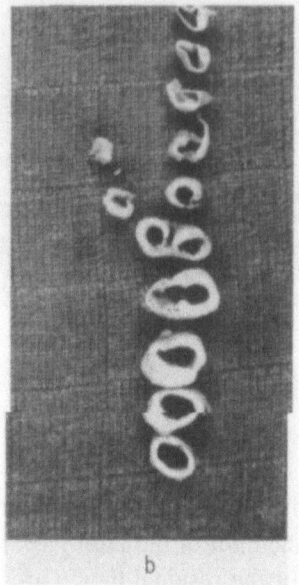
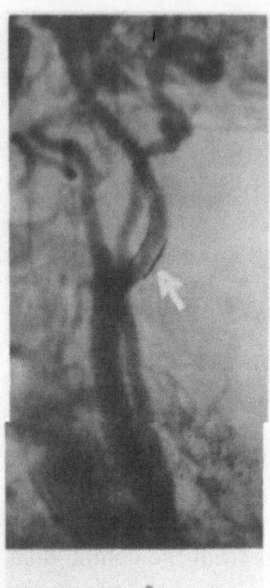

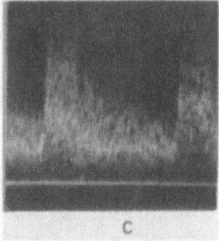

Figure 6. degree of stenosis evaluated by the three methods: a) angiography 50%. b) anatomic study 54%. c) spectrum analysis. – grade II (40–60%). – STI 0,53 (53%).

different methods when the degree of stenosis measured on the pieces of endarterectomy or on the angiography is in accordance with the classification of the spectrum disturbances in 5 grades and with the stenosis index value (STI).

Comparison between the results of spectrum analysis and those of the physical study of the endarterectomies (Table 1, Figs. 6, 7, 8, 9).

The comparative study concerns 72 endarterectomies. We obtained a perfect concordance between the results of the spectral method (classification in grades) and the physical study on 68 out of the bifurcations, that is to say on 94% of the cases (Fig. 7, 8, 9), Table 1.

In three cases, the Doppler spectrum method underestimates the lesions. In

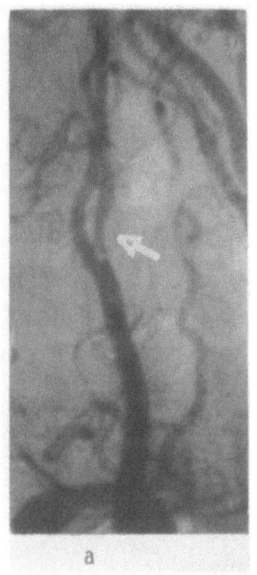

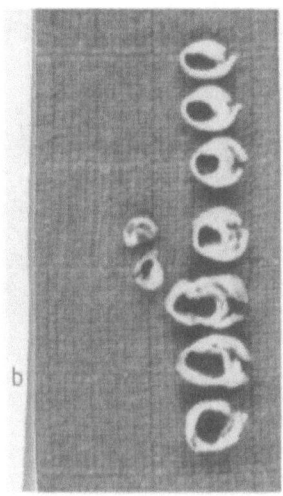

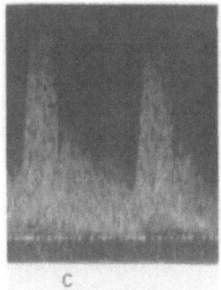

Figure 7. a) angiography 70%. b) anatomic study 73%. c) spectrum analysis. – grade III (60–75%). – STI = 0.71 (71%).

Table 1. Comparison of spectrum analysis and anatomic data.

Anat-Path Grade	<40%	40%–60%	60%–90% 60%–75%	>90%	Stenosis Index ST. I
V				27	= 0.9
IV			22	1	0.6–0.9
III			10		
II		7	2		0.4–0.6
I	2				<0.4

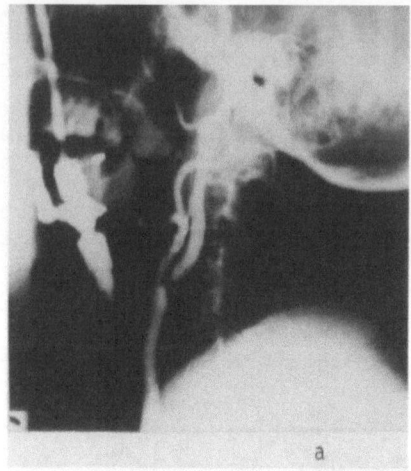
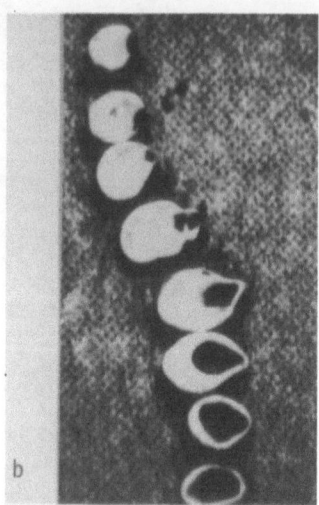
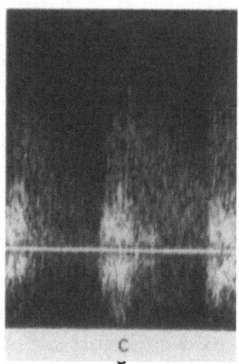

Figure 8. Degree of stenosis evaluated by the three methods: a) angiography 97%. b) anatomic study 96%. c) spectrum analysis. – grade V (>90%). – STI = 1 (>90%).

one case, Doppler examination does not detect any internal carotid signal. The physical study of the endarterectomy showed a very tight stenosis. The sensitivity of the method is of 95%, the specificity of 98%.

The comparison between the stenosis degree measured on the pieces of endarterectomy and the values of STI showed that the values of STI expressed in percentage are quite equal to the stenosis degree expressed in percentage of the lumen reduction (Fig. 9). Moreover the values of STI are in agreement with the classification in five grades (Table 1).

Comparison of spectrum analysis and angiographic data (Table 2, Figs. 6, 7, 8)

Seventy eight bifurcations were investigated. The quality of the x-ray incidences

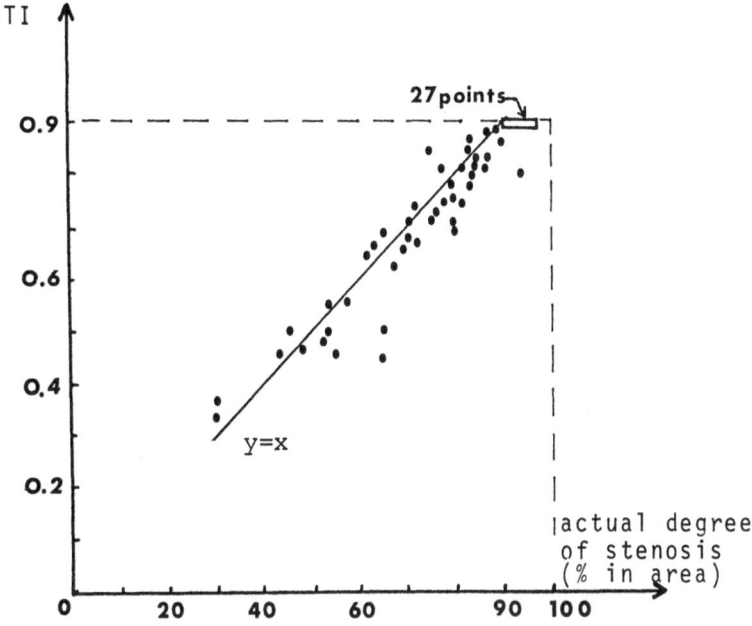

Figure 9. Relationship between the stenosis index measured on the spectrum and the actual value of the degree of stenosis measured on the piece of endarterectomy.

was not good enough in eight cases to perform objective measurements of the degree of stenosis. These eight cases were not taken into account in this study. In 12 cases, angiography could not be considered as a reference method because it did not show any abnormality whereas echography showed atheromatous defects and spectrum analysis detected hemodynamic disturbances. In these 12 cases, one patient with TIA was operated only on the basis of ultrasound findings (grade IV) the stenosis was of 80%. On the last 58 cases the results were in agreement in 54 cases, that is to say in 93% of the cases. In two cases, the lesion was evaluated more severely on the angiography than on the spectrum, in one case it was the contrary. In one case, Doppler examination does not detect any signal but the

Table 2. Comparison of spectrum analysis and angiographic data.

Grade	Angio N	<40%	40%–60%	60%–90% 60%–75%	>90%	Stenosis Index ST. I
V					14	= 0.9
IV	1			10		0.6–0.9
III				6 1		
II	5	1	16	1		0.4–0.6
I	6	4				<0.4
N	4					

angiography showed a very tight stenosis. The probable reasons of these mistakes will be developed in the discussion.

Discussion

The results of this study show that it is possible to appreciate the degree of the carotid stenosis by a simple subjective (5 grades) or semi-quantitative (STI) evaluation of the spectrum disturbances. The accuracy of these ultrasound methods is better than those of the angiography for the bifurcation assessment. Moreover the stenosis index expressed in percentage gives directly the value of the stenosis degree (Figs. 6, 7, 8).

The information provided by this method on the bifurcation could be very helpful for the surgeon and contribute to the decision and the choice of a therapy. For several patients the endarterectomy was decided on the clinical data, the Doppler spectrum, and an electroencephalogram with compression only. It is sure that spectrum analysis does not give any information on the distal circulation and an angiography by venous punction will be discussed.

1. Several remarks have to be mentioned about the advantages and the drawbacks of this method. The exploration of the bifurcation with this method has always been possible whatever the patient morphology.

2. The use of a CW Dopler (and not a pulsed one) seems to be better for the detection of hemodynamic disturbances. This system is able to explore the entire arterial section, and the absence of a precise location of the Doppler sample volume eliminates the problems due to the movement of the vessel during each cardiac cycle, and the relative position of sample volume and plaque surface, especially in low grade stenosis.

3. The dephasing system which separates the positive and negative Doppler audio signals is necessary to display separately arterial and venous spectrum and to detect possible negative frequency shifts due to whirling phenomena.

4. The classification in five grades enables us to evaluate the degree of stenosis without the help of a computer. This system is very easy to use because first of all there is no numeric processing of the spectrum; second, the difference between the five grades is simple and precise enough to obtain from different examiners the same diagnostics on the same patient. Third, the hemodynamic disturbance (degree of stenosis) can be quantified with the stenosis index and this parameter is very useful in comparing the evolution of the disturbance from one examination to another.

5. The exploration of the internal carotid by spectrum analysis of the Doppler signal must be performed from the origin of the vessel, which is not always easy to localize, and to continue as far as possible. Atheromatous defects and the hemodynamic disturbances they induce are generally located at the bifurcation. Spectrum disturbances progressively decrease when we move the

probe far from the stenosis consequently, if the internal carotid origin is not well located, we are not sure the maximum disturbed spectrum has been recorded and the lesion may be underestimated, whatever the system being used 3, 19.

6. This method is simple to use and is very accurate for the stenosis degree evaluation, but must be performed by skilled Doppler operators.

Summary

Conventional Doppler examination (zero crossing system) allows the detection of important hemodynamic disturbances due to severe stenoses (>60% by area). Spectral analysis of the Doppler audio signal allows the detection and the quantification of all the hemodynamic disturbances caused by stenoses superior to 15% by area. Two methods are proposed for the evaluation of the carotid stenosis extend with the help of the spectral analysis of the CW Doppler audio signal.

The first method is based on a classification in five grades of the spectral disturbances according to three parameters: the upper limit of the spectrum, the repartition of the brightness, the existence of negative frequency shifts in systole. Each of these grades have been related to an interval of possible values for the degree of stenosis.

Grade I, stenosis <40% by area (dia-23%); grade II, 40–60%; Grade III, 60–75% (elongated plaque); grade IV, 75–90% (elongated plaque) and 60–90% short stenosis; grade V >90%.

The second method consists of the evaluation of a stenosis index (STI) which is proportional to the degree of stenosis. For this calculation, maximum and mean systolic frequencies are measured on the spectrum. The value of the STI, appears to be equal to the stenosis value expressed in percentages of lumen reduction.

The values of the degree of stenosis provided by these two methods have been compared to actual degree of stenosis measured on the carotid surgical specimens (pieces of endarterectomy); the physical study of the piece of endarterectomy is considered as the gold standard method of confirmation for the Doppler spectral analysis. We also compare the Doppler data with angiographic measurements.

The comparison between spectral grades, STI, and physical findings covers 72 specimens. The results were in agreement in 94% of the cases (sensibility 95%, specificity 98%). The comparison between spectral and angiographic findings covers 78 specimens. In eight cases angiography did not allow to evaluate the degree of stenosis. In 12 cases it was normal, whereas echography showed atheromateous plaques and spectral analysis showed hemodynamic disturbances. Of the remaining 58 cases, the results of spectral analysis and angiography were in agreement 54 times. Spectral analysis and CW Doppler are very simple to use and very accurate for the evaluation of carotid stenosis but they must be performed by skilled Doppler operators.

192

References

1. Ackerman RH: A perspective on noninvasive diagnosis of carotid disease. Neurology, 29, 615–622, 1979.
2. Arbeille Ph, Pejot Cl, Berson M, Fleury G, Besse D, Patat F, Pourcelot L: Intérêt de l'association échotomographie-analyse spectrale du signal Doppler dans l'exploration du système carotidien. Rev Europ Biotech Med, Vol 4, n° 6, 473–478, 1982.
3. Arbeille Ph, Lapierre F, Patat F, Benhamou A-E, Alison D, Dusorbier Ch, Pourcelot L: Evaluation du degré des sténoses carotidiennes par l'analyse spectrale du signal Doppler. Arch Mal Coeur, n° 10, 1097–1107, 1984.
4. Barnes RW, Russel HE, Bone AE, Slaymaker EE: Doppler cerebrovascular examination: improved results with refinements in technique. Stroke, 8. 489. 1977.
5. Barnes RW, Bone GE, Reinestson J, Slaymaker EE, Hokanson DE, Strandness DE Jr: Noninvasive ultrasonic carotid angiography: prospective validation by contrast arteriography. Surgery, 80, 328–335, 1976.
6. Barnes RW, Rittgers SE, Putney WW: Real time Doppler spectrum analysis: predictive value in defining operable carotid artery disease. Arch Surg, 117, 52–57, 1981.
7. Blackshear WM, Phillips DJ, Chikos PM, Harley JD, Thiele BL, Strandness DE Jr: Carotid artery velocity patterns in normal and stenotic vessels. Stroke 11, 67–71, 1980.
8. Coghlin BA, Taylor MG, King DH: Cardiovascular applications of ultrasound In Reneman R (ed) Ch 5, North Holland, Amsterdam 1974.
9. Comerato AJ, Cranley JJ, Cook SE: Real time B-mode carotid imaging in diagnosis of cerebrovascular disease. Surgery, 89, 718–729, 1981.
10. Evans TC, Taenzer JF: Ultrasound imaging of atherosclerosis in carotid arteries. Appl Rad J 8, 106–115, 1979.
11. Gosling RG: Extraction of physiological information from spectrum analysed Doppler shifted continuous wave ultrasound signals obtained noninvasively from the arterial system. In: Hill DW, Watson WB (eds) IEEE Medical Electronics Monographs. London, pp 13–22, 1976.
12. Lewis RR, Basley MG, Hyams DG, Gosling RG: Imaging the carotid bifurcation using continuous wave Doppler shift ultrasound and spectral analysis. Stroke, 9, 465–471, 1978.
13. Miyazaki M, Kato K: Measurement of cerebral blood flow by ultrasonic Doppler technique: hemodynamic comparison of right and left carotid artery in patients with hemiplegia. Jap Circ J, 29, 383–386, 1965.
14. Nigam AK, Olinger CP: A large aperture real time equipment for vascular imaging. Acoustical Holography, 7, 65–77, 1977.
15. Planiol Th, Pourcelot L: Ultrasonics in medicine . In: de Vlieger M, White DN, McCready VR (eds) Excerpta Medica, Amsterdam, pp 104–111, 1975.
16. Pourcelot L: Vascular imaging. In: Wagai R, Omoto R, (eds) Proceedings of the 2nd Meeting of the World Federation for Ultrasound in Medicine and Biology. Miyazaki, Japan, 22–27, July 1979. Excerpta Medica, pp 1–10, 1980.
17. Reneman RS, Spencer MP: Local Doppler audio spectra in normal and stenosed carotid arteries in man. Ultrasound Med Biol, 5, 1–11, 1979.
18. Rittgers SE, Putney WW, Barnes RW: Real time spectrum analysis and display of directional Doppler ultrasound blood velocity signals. IEEE Trans Biomed Engr, BME-27, 723–728, 1980.
19. Rittgers SE, Thornhill BM, Barnes RW: Quantitative analysis of carotid artery Doppler spectral waveforms – diagnostic value of parameters. Ultrasound in Med and Biol, 9, 3, 255–264, 1983.
20. Rutherford RB, Hiatt WR, Kreutzer GW: The use of velocity waveform analysis in the diagnosis of carotid artery occlusive disease. Surgery, 82, 695–702, 1977.
21. Smallwood RH, Brown BH, Rodgers AW: A real time frequency analyser for ultrasonic Doppler signals. J of Med Engr and Tech, 1, 221–222, 1977.
22. Smallwood RH, Brown BH: A measure of blood flow from a frequency analysed ultrasonic Doppler signal. J of Med Engr and Tech, 2, 73–74, 1978.

Vertebrobasilar arterial abnormalities

G.M. von Reutern

Introduction

The investigation of the posterior circulation (subclavian vertebral and basilar arteries) differ from that of the carotid arteries in several aspects.

1. The positioning of the probe is more difficult for the vertebral artery and special training is necessary.

2. Criteria which are useful for the detection of carotid obstructions, such as side-to-side differences of the Doppler signals, are not reliable because of frequent anatomical variations.

3. The impact of pathologic Doppler findings on the management of patients is not as evident as for the carotid arteries.

Examination of the carotids alone does not seem to be advisable. To achieve more accuracy both the vertebrals as well as the carotids ought to be examined, also yielding information about the collateral compensation resulting from obstructions. Even though the vertebral arteries are not often objects for surgery, the detection of stenoses and occlusions may help to understand the underlying pathopysiology of cerebrovascular symptoms. Also the examination of the vertebral arteries allows to suspect basilar artery occlusion and with the advent of transcranial pulse Doppler the diagnosis of basilar artery stenoses is possible which may lead to therapeutic decisions.

Techniques of examinations

The examination of the vertebral artery was first performed at the level of the atlas loop [5, 6, 9]. Here the vertebral artery has to be differentiated from the internal carotid and occipital artery only. Close to the origin of the vertebral artery the network of important arteries is much more dense. Between these two regions the insonation of the vertebral arteries is hindered by the lateral processes of the vertebra. Sometimes with large vertebral arteries, flow signals may be

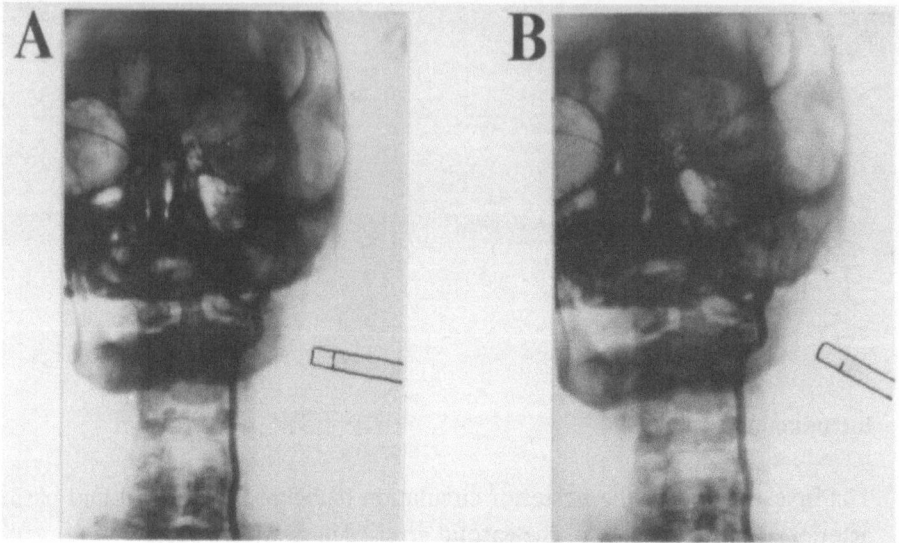

Figure 1. Two positions of the probe to examine the vertebral artery in the atlas region. If the ultrasonic beam is directed slightly inferiorly or horizontally (A) flow towards the probe can be registered with generally higher Doppler frequencies than when the probe is directed slightly superiorly and to the opposite eye or ear (B) resulting in a flow direction away from the probe.

recorded stepwise in each intravertebral space. Because this approach is not always successful the examination along the course between the transverse foramina, is not a routine procedure.

Vertebral arteries

Atlas loop. The probe is positioned behind the tip of the mastoid process and directed slightly anterior and superior aiming somewhere between the contralateral eye and ear (Fig. 1). The more the vertebral artery is elongated the more the loop courses posterior and anterior. This probe position records flow away from the probe and does not exclude confusion with the internal carotid artery which sometimes runs in the submandibular region quite close to the vertebral artery. This mistake especially occurs if the signal of the vertebral artery is weak and difficult to find due to hypoplasia. A second probe position for the investigation of the vertebral artery avoids this misinterpretation. The probe is placed a few millimeters more anterior and inferior and directed horizontally or slightly posterior inferior. Flow is now towards the probe. The recorded frequencies are often higher than those of the first probe position. The occipital artery can be found about 0.5 to 1.0 cm superior to the vertebral artery. In the normal subject the characteristics of the pulse curve is like that of a branch of the external carotid

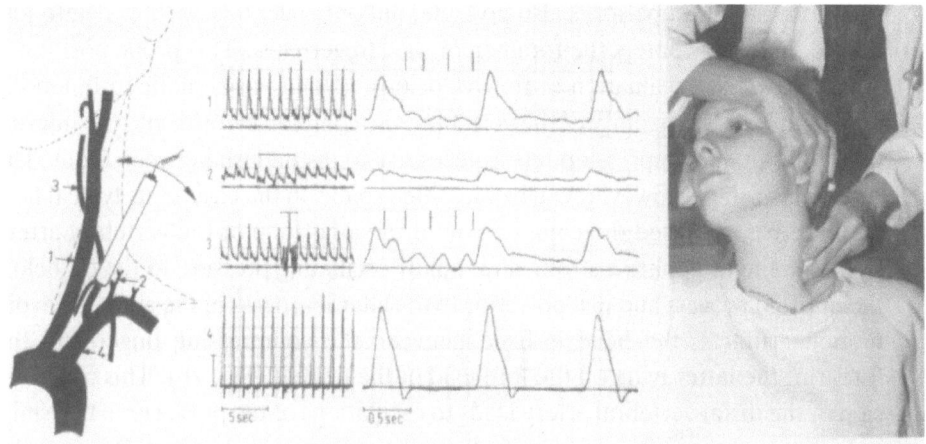

Figure 2. Examination of the proximal vertebral artery: By changing the angle of insonation, the following arteries can be identified: 1. Common carotid artery. The distal vertebral artery oscillating compression has only a weak effect (‖‖‖), probably by simultaneous compression of the occipital artery. 2. Inferior thyroid artery. Low amplitude modulation. Flow direction can be towards or away from the probe, compression of the thyroid gland (——) identifies this artery. The distal vertebral artery compression has no effect. 3. Vertebral artery. Clear cut effect of the oscillating compression at the atlas loop (‖‖‖). 4. Subclavian artery. During the compression tests motion artefacts have to be avoided (see text). (Modified after (12))

artery whereas the pulse curve of the vertebral artery is similar to that of the internal carotid artery. Therefore, under normal conditions, there is no reason for a misinterpretation. Under pathologic conditions however, the peripheral compression of the occipital artery as described in the previous chapter, allows to differentiate between the occipital and the vertebral artery. Also pressure with the probe itself will occlude an occipital artery but in most cases not the vertebral artery. However this criterion is not reliable.

Proximal vertebral artery. The vertebral artery can be examined from the ostium up to the entrance of the transverse foramen of the fifth vertebra. Doppler signals can be obtained from most of this segment if the probe points inferior posterior by being placed laterally to the common carotid artery. Tracing the vertebral artery is facilitated by the following procedure (Fig. 2). First, flow velocity from the common carotid artery is recorded, then that of the proximal part of the subclavian artery. For this only a change in the direction of the probe is required. The vertebral artery is found between these two arteries, directing the probe slightly more posterior. Once the typical signal of the vertebral artery is found, the signal is followed while the probe is moved down along the vertebral artery as far as possible until only signals of the common carotid artery or the subclavian artery can be heard. This guarantees that the vertebral artery has been followed as close to it's origin as possible. The investigation of the proximal vertebral artery with the probe aiming superior is also possible, but only over a very short length just before this artery enters the foramen of the 5th vertebra. This probe position is advisable for the evaluation of flow velocities beyond poststenotic turbulences. Due to the close proximity of the vertebral, the common carotid, and the inferior thyroid artery a compression test is necessary to distinguish between them. The subclavian artery, however, can be identified solely on the basis of its typical flow pattern. We proposed the compression of the atlas loop of the vertebral artery [11]. One finger applies a strong and rapidly oscillating pressure to the pit below the mastoid process and just posterior to the lateral process of the atlas. To avoid motion artifacts, the head is fixed between the compressing finger and the forearm, the latter lying on the forehead of the patient (Fig. 2b). This compression of the distal vertebral artery leads to oscillations of the pulse curve transmitted upstream to positively identify the proximal vertebral artery. Because the same compression has a weak effect on the common carotid artery (via occipital artery) the response is considered positive only if clearcut oscillations appear (Figs. 3 and 7). This test presents certain advantages compared to occlusive compression of the common carotid artery recommended by others [3, 5, 6]. A common carotid artery occlusive compression induces an increase of the flow velocity in the vertebral arteries because of intracranial collateral flow through the posterior communicating artery. In the case of anatomical abnormalities (hypoplastic vertebral artery ending in the PICA) or occlusions, this test will be falsely negative. On the other hand, the distal vertebral artery compression is positive also under these conditions. In addition, compression of the carotid arteries may be avoided. Another advantage is that flow volume is not reduced by an oscillating compression test. We have never observed negative side effects from oscillating compression of the vertebral artery.

Subclavian artery

The subclavian artery is easy to investigate. The probe is placed in the supraclavicular region and directed laterally towards the distal segment or medially towards the aorta (proximal segment). The signal is usually strong and the pulse curve characterized by the resonant wave form with a steep systolic increase in frequency and a reverse component in early diastole (Fig. 2).

Cervical branches of the subclavian artery

Anatomy and pathophysiology. The vertebral artery is the first branch of the subclavian artery, followed by the thyrocervical and costocervical trunks (Fig. 3). The inferior thyroid artery originates from the thyrocervical trunk. This artery is important with respect to the Doppler investigation because it can be mistaken as

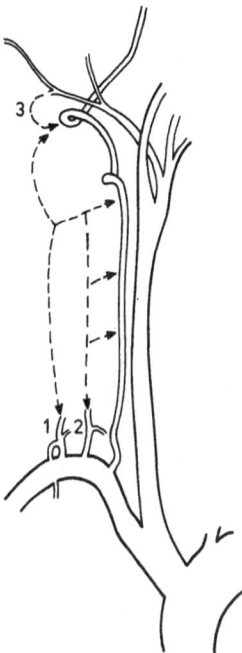

Figure 3. Schematic representation of the cervical collateral arteries. 1) Costocervical trunk. 2) Thyriocervical trunk. 3) Muscular branches of the vertebral and occipital artery. With subclavian artery obstructions, the flow in the cervical arteries is towards the arm; with vertebral artery obstructions, the flow is directed towards the distal vertebral artery.

the vertebral artery, both lying close together and showing similar pulse curve characteristics. The other cervical branches of the thyro- and costocervical trunk supply the skin and muscles of the neck and normally show a different pulse curve shape. They also serve as a collateral network between the subclavian, the vertebral, and the external carotid artery (especially the occipital artery). The vertebral artery is connected in every intervertebral space by small segmental branches with the ascending cervical artery and at the level of the atlas loop with the occipital artery via several small muscular branches. If an occlusion occurs at the origin of the subclavian, the vertebral, or the common and external carotid arteries, these collaterals become functional, enlarging in diameter so that they are visible on angiograms. These collaterals are, however, of secondary import-ance and in cases of vertebral artery occlusions they are less developed if the blood supply to the basilar artery is mainly supported by the collateral vertebral artery. In cases of subclavian steal flow towards the lower pressure arm is provided by both vertebral arteries. If these main channels are occluded or not developed, flow through the cervical collateral arteries is always high and may be detected with continuous wave Doppler. The direction of blood flow through these collaterals depends on the localization of the occlusion. In the case of an occlusion of the subclavian artery, flow is directed towards the arm, while with vertebral artery occlusion flow is directed cranially.

Cervical collaterals should be taken into consideration during a Doppler examination because they can be mistaken for a normal vertebral or common carotid artery, thereby leading to a false negative diagnosis. On the other hand, the presence or absence of such collaterals is a reliable diagnostic criterion.

Technique of examination. Cervical branches of the thyro- and costocervical trunks cannot be detected in normal subjects using conventional Doppler equipment with an emission frequency of 4.0 to 5.0 MHz because they are too small. If by chance a small branch is detected rather low frequencies are recorded. The pulse curve is similar to that of a branch of the external carotid artery without flow during diastole. In the case of collateral flow, flow volume and flow velocity is increased. The characteristic of the pulse curve is somewhere between that of an external and that of an internal carotid artery. These collateral arteries with increased flow, can be detected with conventional CW Doppler equipment and are found over the total length of the neck. However, three regions can be distinguished: the supraclavicular, the mid neck and the mastoid region.

An unequivocal differentiation between these collaterals and the vertebral artery is only possible in the mid neck region, where the vertebral artery runs through the transverse foramina and is therefore covered by bone. The cervical collaterals however, which are found mostly adjacent to the lateral edge of the sternocleidomastoid muscle or posterior in the neck, run more superficially. Therefore they can be compressed by a finger or by the Doppler probe. By producing a total occlusion with the probe no flow can be recorded (Fig. 4). The same compression does not influence the flow velocity in the vertebral artery if recorded between the transverse processes of the vertebra.

In the supraclavicular region, the differentiation between collaterals and the vertebral artery by means of a compression with a probe is not possible. These collaterals react as well as the vertebral artery to the distal vertebral oscillating compression. A large mid neck compression with the index placed lateral to the sternocleidomastoid muscle reduces flow in the collaterals of the supraclavicular region but not in the vertebral artery. Therefore as a result of both compressions, the compression at the atlas level and in the mid neck region it is theoretically possible to differentiate between the proximal vertebral artery and collaterals in the supraclavicular region. However, the compression in the mid-neck region is not easy to perform without creating motion artefacts because the probe is close to the compression finger and the compression has to be rather strong.

In the mastoid region one may have the impression of multiple different vessels (collaterals and vertebral artery). The Doppler signals show different amplitudes and flow directions. Within this 'network' those signals with the lowest frequency modulation are most likely to belong to the vertebral artery (postocclusive flow in a relative large artery). A direct compression with the probe does not differentiate reliably between collaterals and the vertebral artery in this region.

Only during a careful investigation of the neck region one may discover the

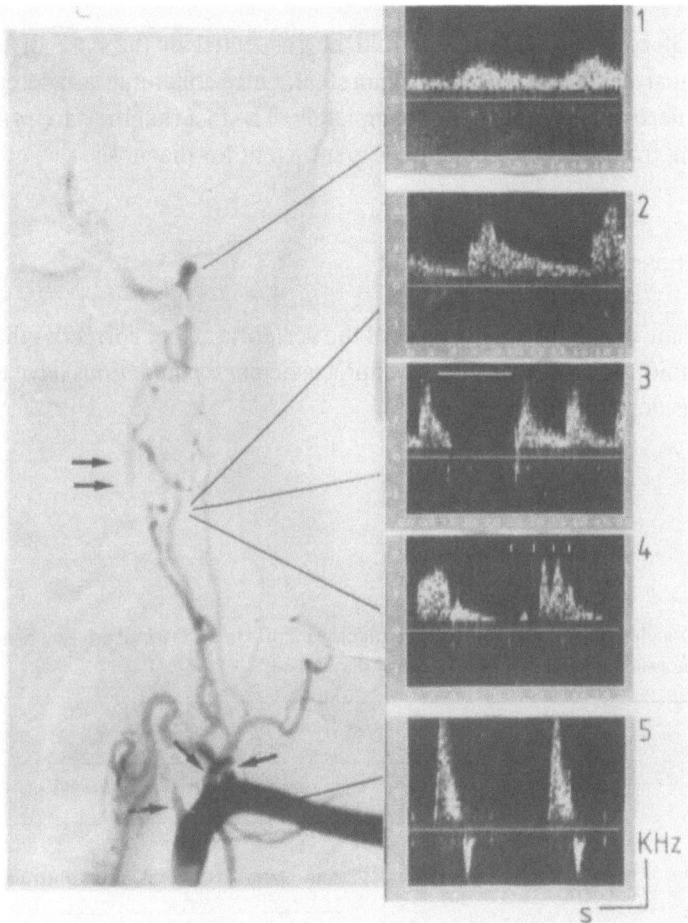

Figure 4. Occlusion of the proximal vertebral artery: ♂ 57 y, repeated TIA of the left hemisphere with occlusion of the left internal and severe stenosis of the right internal carotid artery. In addition, proximal occlusion of the left vertebral artery. On the left: Selective catheterization of the left subclavian artery showing the stump of the occluded vertebral artery (→), filled up distally (⇥) from cervical arteries, branches of the thyrocervical (↘) and costocervical trunk (←). Right hand panels: 1) Peak systolic frequency of the left vertebral artery at the atlas loop 1 KHz with low amplitude modulation ('soft audio signal'), 2) multiple cervical collateral arteries with higher frequency modulation compared with the vertebral artery. 3) they can be obliterated by compression with the probe, 4) reacting to distal oscillating compression of the vertebral artery, and 5) normal result of the subclavian artery.

collaterals as described above. Such a time consuming investigation is not necessary in the case of a normal distal and proximal vertebral artery. The additional search of collaterals is recommended if it is difficult to find signals from the vertebral artery either proximal or distal, or if the signals supposed to belong to the vertebral artery differ with respect to the amplitude modulation proximal and distal. Of course, collaterals should be suspected in the case of a proximal vertebral artery stenosis or subclavian steal. Once collaterals are detected, again it is not necessary to track them completely. The fact that they are present and a recording from a few selected areas is sufficient for diagnosis.

Obstructions of the vertebral artery

To evaluate proximal obstructions of the vertebral artery correctly, the results of the mastoid, the mid neck and the supraclavicular examinations have to be taken into consideration (Table I).

Table I. Doppler-sonographic findings in patients with proximal vertebral artery stenoses and occlusions. ↕ normal, ↓ diminished, ↓ severely diminished.

		Type of lesion of the proximal vertebral artery				
		stenosis			occlusion	
		moderate	severe			
			contralateral vertebral artery obstruction			
			not present	present	not present	present
distal vertebral artery (atlas loop)	f-peak	↑ ↓	↓	↑ ↓	↓ ↓	↑ ↓
	frequency modulation	↑ ↓	↓	↓	↓ ↓	↓
mid neck region (collaterals)		0	+	+ +	+	+ + +
proximal vertebral artery (supraclavicular region)		elevated peak frequencies and moderate turbulences	elevated peak frequencies and severe turbulences		no stenotic signal from the vertebral artery perceived	

+ = Few collateral present, relative low diastolic frequencies.
+ + = Some collaterals with relative high systolic and diastolic frequencies.
+ + + = Multiple collaterals, high frequencies, signals similar to the normal vertebral artery or even to a stenosis.

Vertebral artery stenoses

The diagnosis of a vertebral artery stenosis relies mostly on direct criteria, just as for the carotid arteries. The insonation of the proximal vertebral artery, where most stenoses occur, therefore, is essential. The Doppler spectra are similar to that recorded from an internal carotid artery stenosis (see chapter 9), characterized by elevated frequencies and spectral broadening. However, it is more difficult to predict the degree of vertebral artery stenoses on the basis of Doppler results than it is for carotid stenoses, for the following reasons:

1. Doppler frequencies within a stenosis: The range of frequencies recorded in normal vertebral arteries is wider than in carotids, due to remarkable side-to-side differences in diameter and flow volume. In addition peripheral resistance and eventually collateral flow effect the recorded frequencies of a stenosis. In consequence it is advisable to compare Doppler frequencies recorded from the proximal vertebral artery with those recorded from the atlas loop (including both flow directions towards and away from the probe) for confirming the diagnosis of a stenosis. Poststenotic turbulences are a useful additional parameter.

2. Tortuosity of the normal proximal vertebral artery is frequently found. In addition this artery originates from the subclavian artery more or less inferior and posterior. An inferior origin mostly results in an S-shaped course of the proximal vertebral artery (Fig. 5). Therefore, the downward movement with the probe along the vertebral artery should be continued as far as possible. Nevertheless, in some patients it is not possible to reach the origin of the vertebral artery or the site of the stenosis. This is the reason why the diagnosis of a moderate stenosis can fail. However, a severe stenosis will be detected because of marked turbulences extending distally.

3. Severe turbulences are a reliable criterion for a stenosis. This is not true for low degree turbulences (spectral broadening and small irregularities in the maximum envelop curve) Please see chapters 6 and 8. These changes may also occur in large tortuous vertebral arteries with a high flow volume. In these cases an examination at the level of the atlas loop gives a similar result making the diagnosis of a stenosis unlikely. Stenoses in the subclavian artery proximal to the origin of the vertebral artery, eventually create turbulences extending in the proximal vertebral artery. But this condition can be differentiated because these turbulences are not severe and the signal of the subclavian artery is pathologic.

Proximal vertebral artery occlusions

The fact that no signal can be recorded from the vertebral artery either proximally or distally is not a sign of an occlusion but of hypoplasia or aplasia [11, 12]. An occlusion can only be stated if the postocclusive segment is filled up by collaterals (Fig. 4). This results in a Doppler signal of the vertebral artery which is recorded

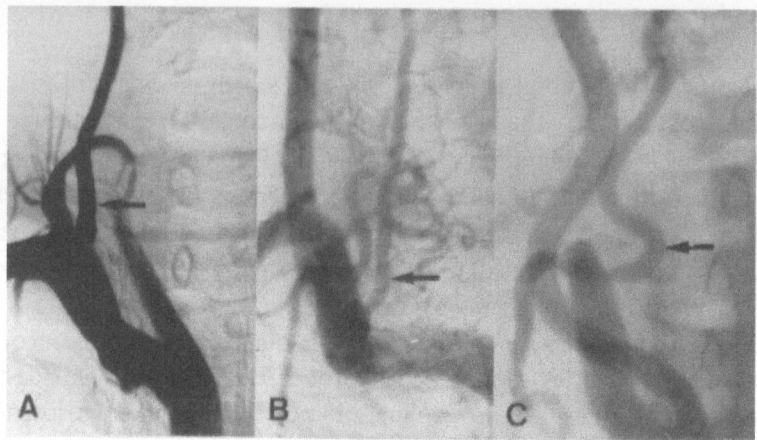

Figure 5. Anatomical variations of the origin of the vertebral artery. Three examples showing the right vertebral artery: A) Origin from the top of the subclavian arch close to the thyrocervical trunk. B) Origin of the vertebral artery located more proximal with elongated subclavian artery which runs first nearly parallel to the vertebral artery. C) S-shaped proximal vertebral artery (in addition distal occlusion of the subclavian artery) from (12) with permission of the authors.

at the atlas loop. In most instances this signal is of low frequency and reduced frequency modulation (pulsatility). The audio signal is 'soft'. This pathologic signal should prompt the examiner to search for collaterals. If they are present, the next question is whether a stenosis or an occlusion is responsible for these abnormalities. The answer can be found by direct examination of the proximal vertebral artery where stenosis and occlusions are localized.

The criterion for a stenosis is a positive one, which means that the already described signs of accelerated and turbulent flow can be shown. The criterion for an occlusion is a negative one. No signal will be detected, which can be attributed to a high degree vertebral artery stenosis. Only severe stenosis with considerable poststenotic pressure drop can cause the development of enhanced flow through cervical collateral arteries (Table I). However, it may be more difficult to spot the signal of the stenosis of a nearly totally occluded vertebral artery than that of a carotid stenosis of similar degree.

Enhanced flow in the thyrocervical and costocervical trunk can imitate a moderate (seldom a severe) vertebral stenosis. This is complicated further by the fact that both, the vertebral artery and the collaterals react positively to an oscellating compression of the atlas loop (Fig. 4). If the collateral flow is very high the mid neck compression differentiates between a collateral and a vertebral artery. On the other hand, if flow is not so high a relative high frequency modulation characterizes the collaterals.

Distal vertebral artery obstructions

An occlusion of the vertebral artery beyond the atlas loop occurs rarely and is associated with infarctions of the dorsolateral oblongata (Wallenberg syndrome). It is difficult to differentiate distal occlusion against marked hypoplasia, because the pulse curve of the vertebral artery is similar in both conditions characterized by a high resistance index. The proximal vertebral artery may remain perfused in distal occlusions because an outflow is possible through small segmental branches and muscular branches at the atlas loop.

The following criteria suggest a distal occlusion:

1. Absent or nearly absent flow in diastole. Vertebral arteries with hypoplasia generally show low systolic and diastolic frequencies but flow is still detectable during diastole, at least by ear analysis of the signal. Because the energy of the signal in a hypoplastic vertebral artery is low, the recording with a zero crossing Doppler device is often not possible or the true wave form is not displayed. Therefore one has to rely more on the examiner's ear and, if available, on a spectrum analyzer. Fig. 6 shows the Doppler recording and angiogram of a right sided distal vertebral occlusion.

2. To differentiate low flow conditions as distal vertebral artery occlusion against hypoplasia information is needed concerning the diameter of the vertebral artery. Duplex-scanning is therefore helpful. On the other hand if Duplex-scanning is not available a strong Doppler signal of the proximal vertebral artery with the above mentioned wave form indicates a normal vertebral artery diameter with a distal occlusion. In cases of hypoplasia the proximal vertebral artery is difficult to find and the Doppler signal is of low energy. Of course this criterion is not very reliable and therefore the differentiation between hypoplasia and distal vertebral artery occlusion remains difficult without B-mode-imaging.

A stenosis of the vertebral artery byond the atlas loop can only be suspected by means of extracranial Doppler examination if this stenosis is clearly flow reducing. With the recently developed transcranial Doppler sonography it is possible to demonstrate this lesions directly and to prove even moderate ones. For this the probe is placed in the midline of the nape aiming through the occipital foramen. The gate can be moved along the vertebral artery to the origin of the basilar artery (pulsed Doppler). However the differentiation between hypoplasia and distal occlusion of the vertebral artery is not possible.

Basilar artery occlusions

A unilateral vertebral artery occlusion is compensated by high flow velocities on the contralateral side. If both vertebral arteries have pulse curves indicating a high peripheral resistance, a diagnosis of basilar artery occlusion must be considered [13]. The reduction of flow velocity in both vertebral arteries is especially

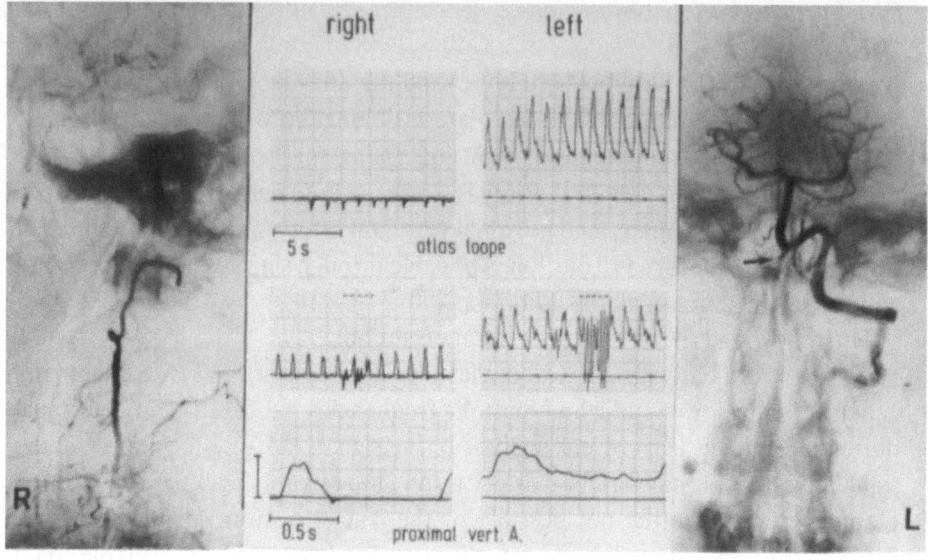

Figure 6. Occlusion of the distal vertebral artery: ♂ 53 y, right side lower brainstem infarction 2 days after a myocardial infarction. Doppler-sonography: (Analogue tracings) upper 2 panels show tracings from the atlas loops. High flow velocity in the left vertebral artery and diminished velocity in the right vertebral artery; Lower 4 panels show on both sides, the proximal vertebral identified by distal oscillating compression (– – – –). Demonstrating the side-to-side differences (the two outside panels) bilateral retrograde brachial artery injection demonstrates the right vertebral artery is slightly hypoplastic and slow contrast filling which ends at the level of the atlas loop. This late exposure does not show filling of cerebellar arteries or of the basilar artery. The left side angiogram shows a normal vertebral and basilar artery wall as well as a stump of the distal right vertebral artery.

pronounced in proximal basilar artery occlusions and less pronounced if the distal basilar artery is occluded (top of the basilar artery occlusion). A unilateral distal vertebral artery occlusion can be seen in patients with infarction of the dorsolateral oblongata (Wallenberg syndrome).

The findings of a basilar artery occlusion is especially valuable if a 'lockes-in-syndrome' is present or for the evaluation of fluctuating brain stem deficits. The early non-invasive diagnosis is very important because anticoagulation may be indicated and recently local fibrinolyzis was proposed for basilar artery occlusions [13].

Stealing from the vertebral artery

The subclavian steal effect is characterized by reversed flow in the vertebral artery on the side of a subclavian artery stenosis or an occlusion localized proximal to the origin of the vertebral artery. The blood supply usually comes from the contralateral vertebral artery, whose flow volume and flow velocity

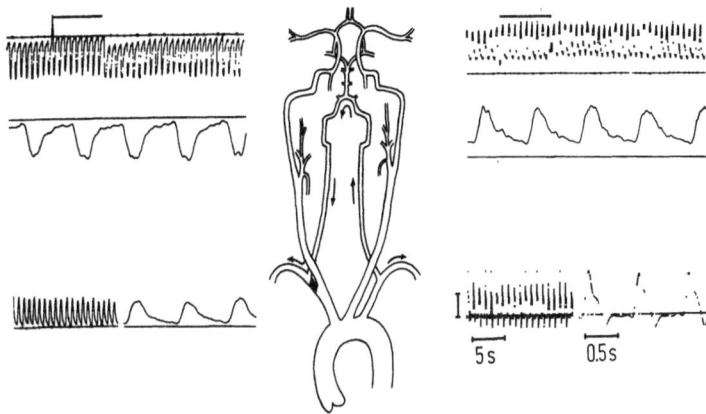

Figure 7. Subclavian steal with occlusion of the right subclavian artery: Above pulse curves of the vertebral artery recorded at the atlas loop, below pulse curves of the subclavian artery. Flow in the right vertebral artery is reversed. This is proved by manual compression of the right upperarm (———). The same compression has a weaker effect on the left vertebral artery which proves flow from left to right.

increases to maintain normal flow direction and flow volume in the basilar artery as well as to 'feed' the steal. This common condition is called a 'vertebro-vertebral' steal [4]. Other types of steal may also exist, sometimes combined. The reason for the development of other than vertebro-vertebral steal types, is a vertebral artery insufficiency, either homo- or contralateral to the subclavian artery occlusion. If the contralateral vertebral artery is hypo- or aplastic, the anastomosis between the occipital artery and the homolateral vertebral artery at the level of the atlas loop becomes functional. This situation may be referred to as 'externo-vertebral' artery steal. In addition the occipital artery can fill the cervical collaterals of the thyro-cervical and costocervical trunk which now show reverse flow, indicating flow towards the arm ('externo-subclavian' steal). This proximal collateral pathway is also important in hypo- or aplasia of the homolateral vertebral artery.

Vertebro-vertebral-steal. A typical recording of subclavian steal is shown in Fig. 7. The systolic peak frequency of the subclavian artery on the side of the occlusion is reduced and there is no reverse flow in early diastole. The signal of the vertebral artery showing reverse flow is always very similar to that of the subclavian artery. Flow velocity during diastole is lower than on the side with physiologic flow direction. Brachial artery compression and release proves the flow reversal of the vertebral artery: During the compression flow velocity in the vertebral artery is reduced, while after the compression flow velocity increases due to postischemic hyperemia. It is preferable to compress the arm of the patient manually instead of inflating a cuff, because the effect is more rapid and correlates therefore better with the beginning and the end of the compression. Postischemic hyperemia is

206

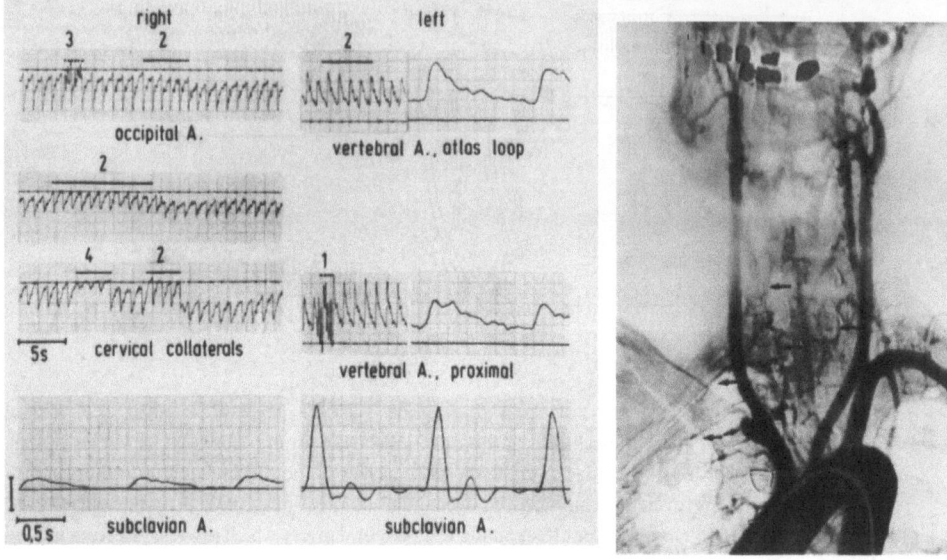

Figure 8. Externo-subclavian steal: ♂ 31 y, traumatic occlusion with aneurysm of the right subclavian artery 7 years before. At the time of the examination the patient had no complaints. Doppler-sonography: Normal findings from the left subclavian and vertebral artery (investigation of the atlas loop and proximal). Oscillating compression of the distal vertebral artery (1) identifies the vertebral artery. Compression of the right arm and clenching of the fist (2) has no effect on the left vertebral artery. On the right side severely diminished amplitude of the subclavian artery. The vertebral artery is not found. The occipital artery, identified by peripheral oscillating compression (3), shows a hyperemic reaction after compression of the right arm (2). The same is true for multiple cervical collaterals identified by compression with the probe (4). Angiography: Aortic arch injection. Short stump of the right subclavian artery (→), collateral network (←) supplied by intercostal, inferior thyroid and cervical arteries.

more pronounced if in addition to the compression the patient stretches his arm and clenches his fist as hard as possible.

External-subclavian steal. In this type blood mainly derives from the occipital artery which anastomoses with the vertebral artery as well as with cervical branches of the thyrocervical and costocervical trunk. In the mastoid region both pathways are used in the case of contralateral vertebral artery hypoplasia or occlusion. Usually only cervical branches are used in cases with homolateral vertebral artery insufficiency (Fig. 8). These collaterals are identical with those described for proximal vertebral artery occlusions, but flow is directed armwards and the pulse curve is similar to that of a reversed vertebral artery. The identification of the collaterals is only possible by compression with the probe (see vertebral artery occlusion). It is useful to prove such 'atypical steal' phenomena before performing angiography, because special selective injections have to be applied to find out the exact pathology.

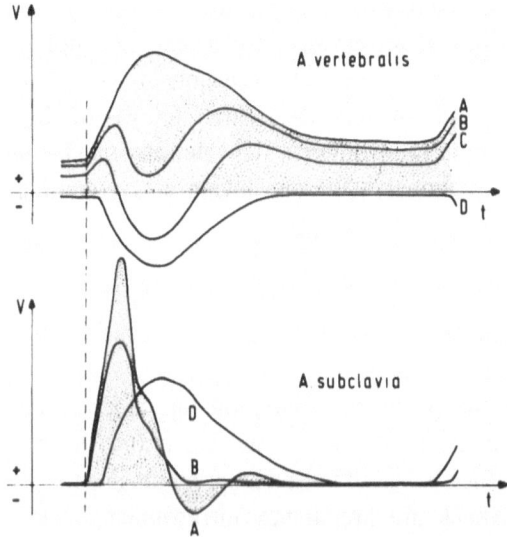

Figure 9. The transmission from physiologic to reversed flow in the vertebral artery. Semischematic representation of results obtained by EKG triggering. A: Normal waveforms of the subclavian and vertebral artery. B: Stenosis of the subclavian artery (poststenotic recording). The reverse flow phase early in diastole of the subclavian artery disappears. Flow direction of the vertebral artery is still physiologic but a dip appears during peak systole. C: Intermittent steal with alternating flow direction. Flow reversal in the vertebral artery occurs only during systole. The arise point of systole is not shifted. D: Complete subclavian steal with occlusion of the subclavian artery. Increased latency of the arise points of the vertebral and subclavian artery on the side of the occlusion.

Intermittent steal. During the transition from physiologic flow in the vertebral artery to reverse flow intermediate stages without effective blood transport exist. However, occlusion is prevented presumably because the blood is always in alternating motion. The development of steal phenomenon is characterized by the following characteristic stages [7, 8, 10].

1. A dip appears during middle systole, which signifies a reduction of the peak flow (Fig. 9).

2. With increasing degree of the subclavian artery stenosis, a flow reversal occurs but first during systole only (alternating flow direction). Early in systole, flow accelarates in the normal physiologic direction but decelerates shortly afterwards. In diastole the flow direction is again normal with slightly diminished flow velocity.

3. Complete reversal appears after further reduction of the normally directed systolic and diastolic flow.

Severe stenoses at the origin of the vertebral artery may also lead to a small mid-systolic dip. Vertebral stenosis can be identified by the direct recording from the stenosis. Alternating flow direction in the vertebral artery is a reliable sign of subclavian artery stenosis. It occurs with subclavian artery occlusion only in patients with additional aortic valve insufficiency. Complete reversal of flow, on the other hand, occurs either with occlusion or with stenosis of the proximal subclavian artery [10]. In most cases, the stenosis of the subclavian artery is indicated by turbulent flow, but very tight stenoses can be mistaken as occlusion, most of the flow volume in the subclavian artery coming from the vertebral artery.

Transcranial Doppler

Examination of the posterior circulation has recently been extended to the intracranial segments of the vertebral artery and the basilar artery.® These arteries are examined by use of pulsed Doppler placing the probe near the midline at the back of the neck and directing the ultrasound beam towards the level of the eyes. The intracranial vertebrals are easily found at 5–7 cm depth. The conjunction of the vertebral arteries is found at approximately 7.5 cm in depth. The basilar artery may be traced to 10 cm in some subjects. Doppler examination of the intracranial vertebral and the basilar arteries allows detection of intracranial stenoses and of effects of extracranial obstructions such as vertebro-vertebral steal. Of special interest are the effects of subclavian steal on the basilar artery flow velocities. The posterior cerebral artery can also be examined with transtemporal Doppler. Please see Chapter 16 for further information and references on transcranial Doppler diagnosis.

Conclusion

Doppler-sonography proves to be superior to angiography for the functional evaluation of the posterior circulation. Depending on the clinical background angiography can sometimes not be replaced because it demonstrates many important morphological details. Most problems for the interpretation of Doppler results occur with physiologic variations of the diameter of the vertebral arteries. A side-to-side comparison of the Doppler peak frequencies is therefore not a valuable criterion for obstructions. Improved accuracy in diagnosing severe obstructions of the proximal vertebral or subclavian artery is reached with the demonstration of cervical collateral arteries.

   Careful application of compression tests is the key for a correct diagnosis in the posterior circulation. The extracranial vertebral arteries should be evaluated by examination close to the origin and additionally at the atlas loop. Intracranial examinations with pulsed Doppler sonography will be of value to evaluate intracranial aspects of the posterior circulation.

References

1. Aaslid R, Markwalder T-M, Nornes H: Noninvasive transcranial Doppler ultrasound recording of flow velocity in basal cerebral arteries. Journal of neurosurgery 57: 769, 1982.
2. Arnolds BJ, Reutern von G-M: Transcranial Dopplersonography. Examination technique and normal reference values. Ultrasound in Medicine and Biology, (in print).
3. Franceschi C: Investigation vasculaire par ultrasonographie Doppler. Collection de médicine ultrasonore Masson, Paris, 1977.
4. Gänshirt H: Der Hirnkreislauf. Georg Thieme Verlag, Stuttgart, 1972.
5. Keller H, Müller A, Meier W, Schönbeck M: Transorale Doppler-Sonographie unter Schleim- hautanaesthesie zur Beurteilung der Strömungsverhältnisse in den Aa. vertebrales (Vertebralis- Doppler). Deutsche Medizinische Wochenschrift 100: 943, 1975.
6. Keller HM, Meier WE, Kumpe DA: Noninvasive angiography for the diagnosis of vertebral artery disease using Doppler-ultrasound (vertebral artery Doppler). Stroke 7: 364, 1976.
7. Marcadé JP: Techniques d'enrégistrement de la vélocité vertébrale par effet Doppler. Actualités d'Angéiologie III, 4: 5, 1978.
8. Pourcelot L, Ribadeau-Dumas JL, Fagret D, Planiol Th: Apport de l'examen Doppler dans le diagnostic du vol sousclavier. Revue Neurologique 133: 309, 1977.
9. Reutern von G-M, Büdingen HJ, Freund H-J: Dopplersonographische Diagnostik von Stenosen und Verschlüssen der Vertebralarterien und des Subclavian-Steal-Syndroms. Archiv für Psychia- trie und Nervenkrankheiten 222: 209, 1976.
10. Reutern von G-M, Pourcelot L: Cardiac cycle dependent alternating flow in vertebral arteries with subclavian artery stenosis. Stroke 9: 2229, 1978.
11. Reutern von G-M, Clarenbach P: Value of Doppler examinations of the cervical collateral arteries and the vertebral ostium in the diagnosis of stenoses and occlusions of the vertebral artery. Ultrason 1: 153, 1980.
12. Reutern von G-M: Doppler-Sonographie der hirnversorgenden Arterien mit besonderer Berück- sichtigung der direkten Kriterien. Kriessmann A, Bollinger A, Keller H (ed.) Praxis der Doppler- sonographie, pp. 183–211, Georg Thieme, Stuttgart, New York, 1982.
13. Ringelstein EB, Zeumer H: The role of continuous-wave Doppler sonography in the diagnosis and management of basilar and vertebral artery occlusions, with special reference to its appli- cation during local fibrinolysis. Journal of Neurology 228: 161, 1982.

Doppler imaging

M.P. Spencer

For the purposes of this chapter 'imaging' is defined as a two-dimensional projection of the relative position of remote three dimensional structures or phenomena [1]. X-ray imaging has been a field of medicine since Roentgen's great discovery. More recently ultrasound imaging has developed because of the noninvasive aspects of ultrasound as compared to those of ionizing radiation. Ultrasound, however, is limited by its longer wavelength and provides less resolution than x-rays. 'Mapping' may be a more appropriate term for the first Doppler imaging devices because like a road map their primary use has been to separate the sources of the main information of Doppler shifted frequencies providing little morphological detail.

Both pulsed wave Doppler (PWD) [2], and continuous wave Doppler (CWD) [3], may be used in generating images in blood flow channels. For the superficial vessels CWD has a great advantage because like a flashlight beam finding an object in a dark room sweeping searches rapidly locate the region of interest. It is usually not clinically important to know exactly how far away the object is, only that it is present in approximately its expected location and, in the case of a blood flow channel, to quickly display the blood velocity profile characteristics and diagnostic characteristics. Overlapping or superimposed vessels sometimes present a problem with CWD imaging but are usually dealt with by their inherent separate flow characteristics seen on a frequency spectral display. CWD imaging combined with spectral analysis remains an excellent cost-effective instrumentation.

CWD imaging was first introduced for the carotid arteries whose superficial position minimized the need for range resolution and where the importance of diagnosis of surgically accessible stroke-producing lesions was important. A 5 MHz probe (chosen as a compromise on minimum beam diameter and audibility of stenosis jet frequencies) was mounted on a mechanical arm suspended over the supine subject. Two potentiometers mounted in the arm sensed the probe position producing x-y coordinates in two dimensions in a plane parallel to the body axis, (Fig. 1A and B). A cursor always represented on the viewing screen

CAROTID DOPPLER IMAGING

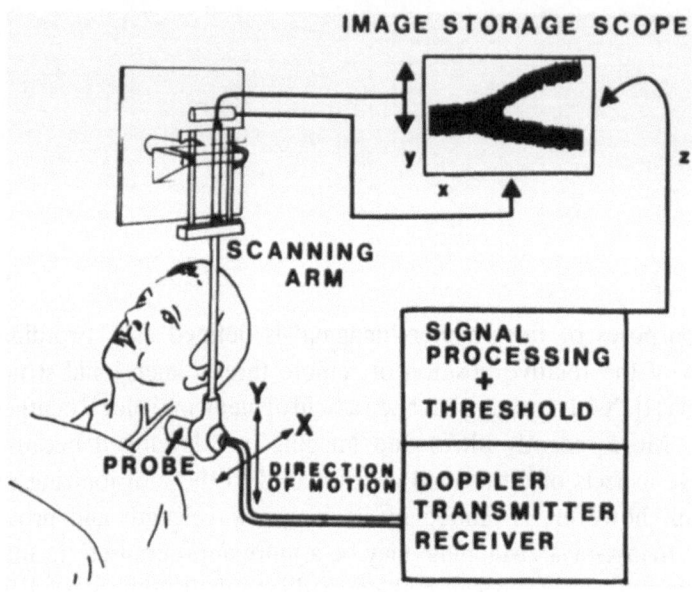

Figure 1A. Principle of CW Doppler imaging. The brightness of the oscilloscope beam (Z) is increased when the ultrasound beam passes through the flowing blood. The artery image is projected in one plane only (x-y). See text for further explanation.

provided the operator with constant information on the position of the probe moving over the skin surface.

When the probe is moved by the operator to pass the sound beam through a carotid artery the Doppler shifted signal stores a spot on the viewing screen while a display of the real-time spectrum of Doppler frequencies is displayed. Continuous motion of the probe beam back and forth across the arteries while following the common carotid to its branches paints an image of the carotid bifurcation. This method's principle advantage is to facilitate a careful search of the regions of maximum interest which, with the carotids, is at the end of the common carotid and the origin of both the internal and external carotid branches. If abnormal signals are found the vessel source can be identified by the relative position on the projection plane and by the Doppler spectral characteristics. By providing a constant angle of the soundbeam, usually 60° with the body axis, repeated examinations can follow the progress of a stenotic lesion [4]. The primary spectral feature of stenosis being the elevated frequency providing the means for diagnosis and quantitation of the lesion.

Color coding of the direction of Doppler signals was first provided by Brandestini [5] using a TM-mode of superimposed structural image and Doppler

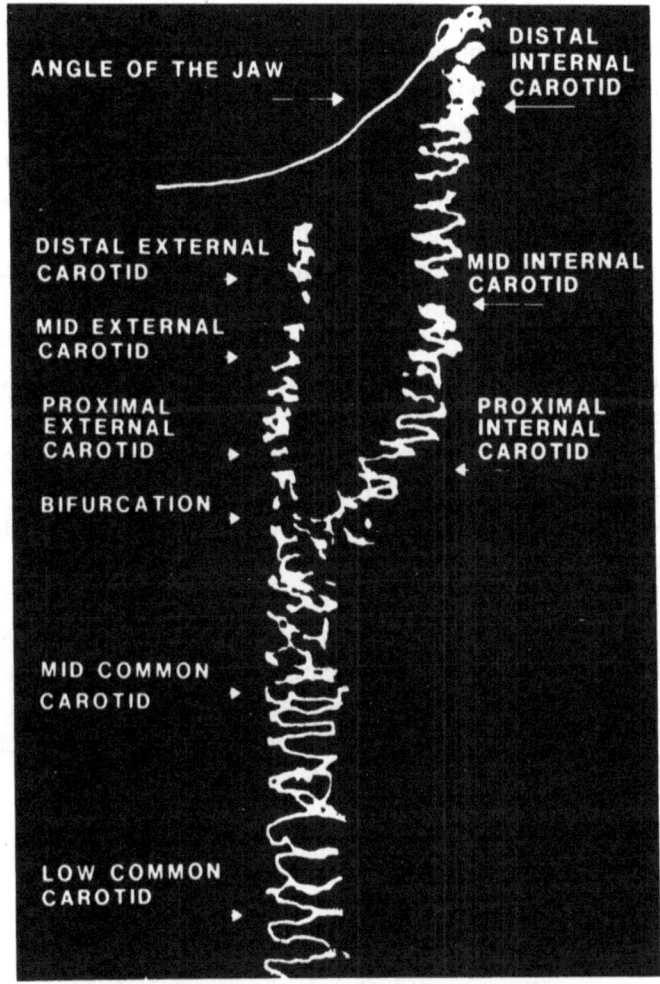

Figure 1B. CW Doppler image of the common carotid artery bifurcation as developed by the equipment in Fig. 1A. The labeled sites represent routine recording positions when searching for arterial stenosis signals.

signals. This system found principle use in pediatric cardiology by Stevenson [6]. Color coding of carotid CW frequencies and direction was proposed by Reid and Spencer [7] and first used clinically by Curry and White [8]. A color is assigned to different frequency ranges so that the site of stenosis represented by elevated frequencies stand out against the adjacent color representing lower frequencies. Morphological representations of the artery dimensions are poor with continuous wave systems due to limitations of lateral resolution and lack of depth resolution.

The single gate PWD imaging system of Hokanson [2] provides greater spatial resolution and has been used clinically by Sumner [9]. This system uses a mechanical arm, similar to CW imaging equipment, senses the position of the probe in two dimensions parallel to the body axis, while the third dimension (depth in the body) is sensed and controlled by range gating of the pulse echo receiver. Sumner used both the Doppler audio signal and the morphological representation of the flow channel to diagnose carotid stenosis. The technician must first locate the common carotid by operating both the arm position and the range depth gate. The equipment then provides an automatic gate movement which repeats a sequence through the artery while the arm is moved to follow the artery direction. The range resolution of PWD approaches one wavelength of ultrasound in practicality and is better than the lateral resolution and does provide an improved anatomical resolution over CWD imaging. The improved morphological resolution is gained at the cost of increased complexity of the equipment and scanning techniques and foregoing the high frequency resolution of CWD.

A highly refined multigate PWD imaging system by MAVIS® was developed to improve the ease of operation and speed of carotid artery imaging [10]. This cleverly designed equipment uses an onboard computer to calculate volumetric blood flow (Fig. 2). Unfortunately, the diagnostic potential of this sytem was not improved by the blood flow capability because of its primary limitation to the common carotid and poor correlation between volume flow in the internal carotid and cerebral symptoms. It is, however, of great interest for research and physiological studies. Determination of flow in a stenotic internal carotid is hampered by the short segment of usable artery and the presence of turbulence. High cost and low clinical relevance of current blood flow measurement in the carotid reduced its popularity.

The multigate imaging system of Brandestini [5] was color coded for direction of blood flow and operated in a TM-mode. This equipment was particularly advantageous in pediatric cardiac Doppler imaging [6] where anatomy, motion and blood flow patterns are most complex. Nowicki and Reid [11] conceived of an infinite gate pulsed Doppler (IGPD), using a moving target indicator technique from radar technology. The analog and digital techniques used operate on the A-mode echo to remove stationary signals and allow the echo shifted in phase by the Doppler effect to pass through. The Doppler effect is thereby distributed along the line of the ultrasound beam.

The 'ideal' equipment for ultrasonic and Doppler examination, which present technology can provide, includes a 2-D B-Mode image superimposed with a 2-D color Doppler image coded for direction and frequency with an option to focus either a PWD or CWD on any region of special interest. A single gate PWD simultaneous with B-mode and color Doppler is needed as well as a CWD for quantitating high velocities. All modes should be available separately when maximum resolution is required. This ideal equipment should provide the following capabilities:

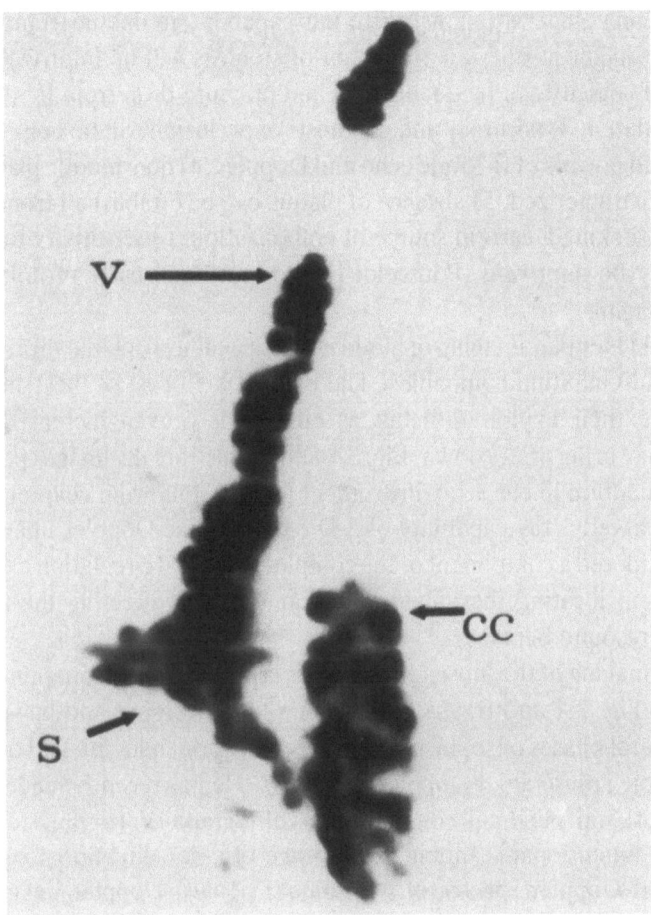

Figure 2. PW Doppler image of the subclavian (S), vertebral (V) and common carotid (CC) arteries achieved with MAVIS pulsed Doppler imaging equipment. Notches and gaps along the vertebral artery represent overlying bone of the vertebral canals. Cross-sectional views made with the depth capability separate the overlying carotid from the deeper subclavian artery.

Mode	Application
B-Mode Tissue Echo	– Nonstenotic Plaque and Occlusion Diagnosis
B-Mode Color Doppler	– Abnormal Flow Patterns
Pulse Doppler	– Vessel Identification
CW Doppler	– Jet Velocity Quantification

The availability of 2-D Doppler is helpful to rapidly lead the examiner to regions of special interest for guiding the focus of PW or CW Doppler single line beams and in reducing angle problems. With this capability in one instrument: 1) The accuracy of diagnosis and quantification of stenosis will be improved, 2) maximum blood velocity can be quantitated and pressure drop from by the stenosis can be calculated, 3) accuracy and diagnosis of occlusion will be helped by using the combined powers of B-Mode echo and Doppler, 4) nonstenotic plaque can be found and characterized, 5) absence of plaque can be established from consideration when seeking a carotid source of embolization, 6) sensitivity to ulcerated plaques may be improved. Pourcelot [12] proposed an early prototype of 2D Doppler imaging.

In 1985 2-D Doppler imaging of blood vessels became available through Aloka, Toshiba, and Quantum companies. The present high cost of these instruments may impede their exploitation but as efficacy is proven increased numbers produced may bring prices down. Fig. 3A and B illustrate the images produced by the U.S. Quantum linear array instrument and the following chapter illustrates the Aloka curved array capability of 2-D color cardiac Doppler imaging which may be considered a component of the complete cerebral circulation examination and helpful in locating the valves and chambers for directing the single line Doppler ultrasound beam.

Doppler imaging of the intracranial vessels is presently in the mapping phase of technology, Fig. 3A and B. Aaslid has been the developer and has proceeded through several phases of sophistication. His basic principles are laid down in the Chapter 16 on Transcranial Doppler Diagnosis. He has recently made extensive use of the desk top 'personal' computer and color graphics programs to introduce anatomic 3-dimensional scanning and storage of color directional coded maps with selected Doppler spectra of intracranial signals. Doppler imaging of the intracranial vessels is important to identify the various components of the branches of the circle of Willis. The only alternative to spatial orientation assistance is 2-D B-Mode imaging which is presently limited by the need to use 2–3 MHz for skull pentration problems. Doppler imaging of other regions of the body is a needed technology. Future possibilities include the retina and the abdominal vasculature. The advantages in these new regions as in cardiac, cervical and intracranial imaging, will be to speed the examination process and give assurances regarding vessel identification before quantitative Doppler beams are applied. Doppler imaging capabilities will also assist in the determination of patency or occlusion of coronary bypass grafts.

References

1. Spencer MP, Reid JM *et al.:* Doppler imaging. In: Hegyeli RJ (ed) Atherosclerotic Reviews, Vol. 10. Raven Press, New York, 1983.
2. Hokanson DE, Mozersky DJ, Sumner DS *et al:* Ultrasonic arteriography: a new approach to arterial visualization. J of Biom Engrng, Vol 6, 420, 1971.

3. Reid JM, Spencer MP. Ultrasonic Doppler technique for imaging blood vessels. Science, 176, 1235, 1972.

4. Chambers BR, Norris JW: The case against surgery for asymptomatic carotid stenosis. STROKE 15: 964, 1984.

5. Brandestini MA, Eyer MK, Stevenson JG. M/Q-mode echocardiography: The synthesis of conventional echo with digital multigate Doppler. In: Lancee CT (ed) Developments in Cardio-vascular Medicine, Echocardiology, Vol 1, pp 441–446. Martinus Nijhoff. The Hague, The Netherlands, 1979.

6. Stevenson JG, et al. Pulsed Doppler echocardiography applications in pediatric cardiology. In: Lance CT (ed) Echo Cardiology, Vol I. Martinus Nijhoff Publisher, The Hague, 1979.

7. Reid JM, Spencer MP. Apparatus for ultrasonic arteriography. U.S. Patent 4, 109, 642, 1974.

8. Curry GR, White DN. Color-coded ultrasonic differential velocity arterial scanner. J of Ult in Med & Biol. Vol 4, 27, 1978.

9. Sumner DS, Moore DJ, Miles RD. Doppler ultrasonic arteriography and flow velocity analysis in carotid artery disease. In: Bernstein EF (ed) Noninvasive Diagnostic Techniques in Vascular Disease, Ch 34, 3rd Edition. C.V. Mosby Publisher, 1985.

10. Fish PJ. Multichannel resolving Doppler ultrasonography. Ult in Med, Amsterdam Excerpts Medica, 153, (Kazner, deDlieger, Muller, eds). 1975.

11. Pourcelot LG. Real time blood flow imaging. In: Lance CT (ed) Echocardiology. Martinus Nijhoff, Publishers, 1979.

→

Figure 3A. On the right: color Doppler image of the normal carotid bifurcation in the neck overlying a B-mode image achieved with a linear array. Tic marks represents centimeters. On the left: diagram representing major features of the image. The diagonal line represents the skin surface separated from the array by a diagonal wedge which provides an angle sufficient to produce a Doppler effect. Red color represents blood flow away from the transducer, white mosaic represents higher velocities, and bright blue represents reversed flow in an eddy at the origin of the internal carotid artery (I). (E) = external and (C) = common carotid arteries.

Figure 3B. On the right: color Doppler image of stenosis in a carotid stenotic artery. On the left: solid line represents artery wall and plaque outline, dashed line = gradient where blood velocities increase sufficiently to produce a color image. R & W represent red and white color representation of flow away from transducer, light blue (B) represents aliasing produced by high velocities through the stenosing plaque.

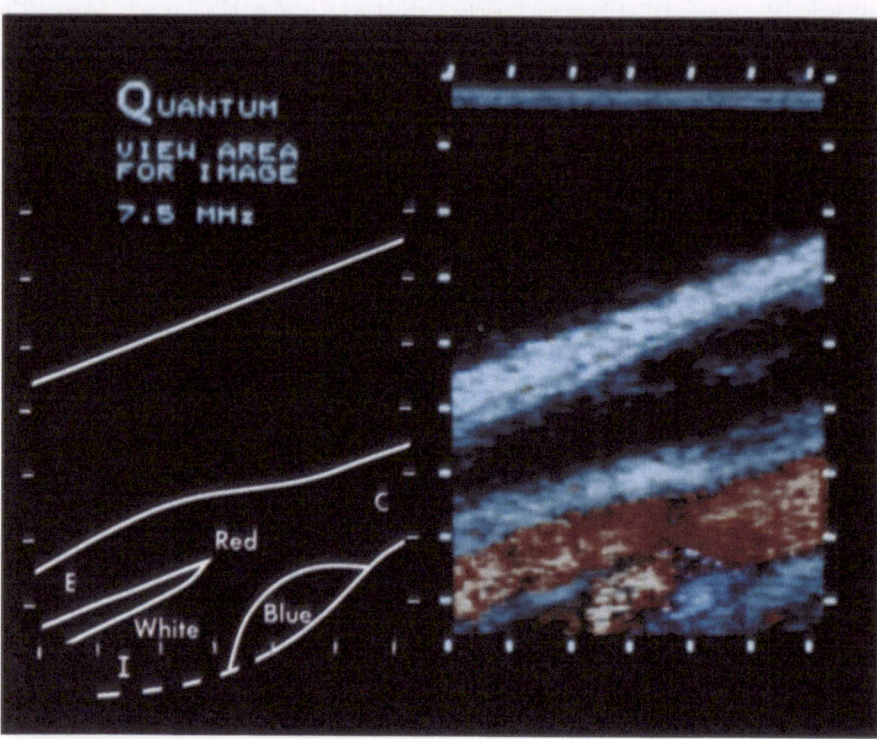

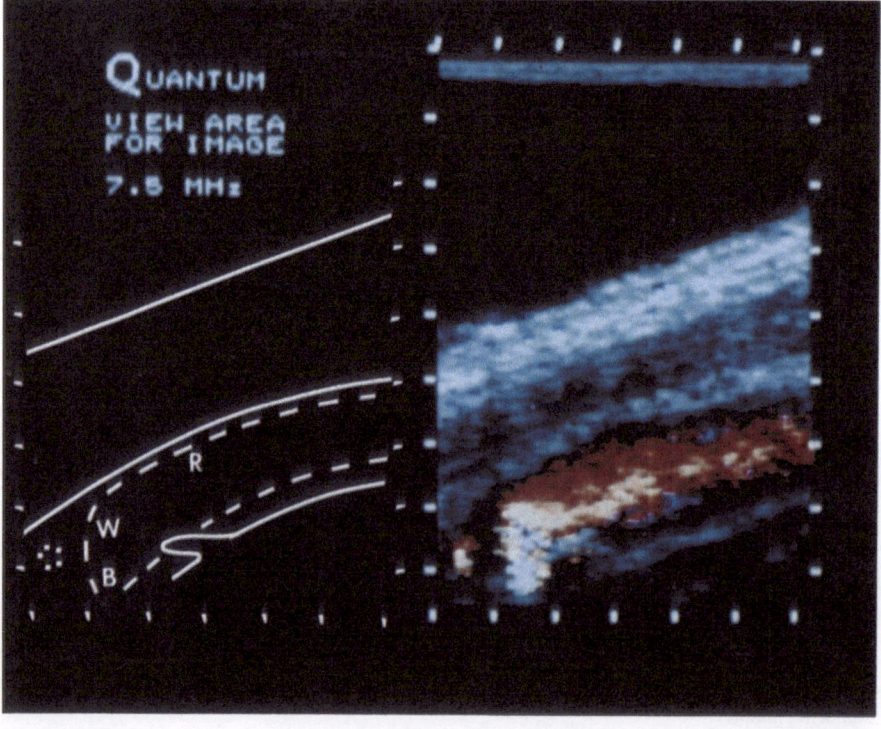

Clinical application of real-time Doppler color flow mapping of the carotid artery

S. Takamoto and R. Omoto

Non-invasive blood flow visualization of the carotid artery using the Doppler method was first introduced by Hokanson et al. [1]. Soon after Spencer and Reid [2] also obtained the carotid artery flow imaging by using the continuous-wave Doppler, Curry and White [4] developed color-coded flow imaging using the continuous-wave mode. Eyer, Brandestini et al. [3] also obtained color-coded carotid flow image with the aide of the multi-gated pulsed Doppler and the microprocessor system. However, these carotid flow imagings were not performed in real-time.

In 1983 Namekawa [5], Omoto and associates [6, 7] developed real-time color flow mapping two-dimensional Doppler echocardiography (2-D Doppler) mainly for the purpose of real-time visualization of the intra-cardiac and intra-aortic flow. 2-D Doppler displays real-time blood flow images non-invasively in color superimposed on the B-mode gray scale image (2-D echo). Direction, velocity and variance of the velocity of the flow were displayed in color. However, its application to the peripheral arteries was not fully carried out due to an insufficient color flow display of a slow flow at the superficial site by the original sector transducer (3.5 MHz). Recently the new 2-D Doppler system with a curved linear array transducer (5 MHz) has been developed for the examination of the peripheral vessels. The authors have first reported clinical application of this 2-D Doppler to the examination of the carotid and the lower limb arteries [8].

This chapter introduces clinical application of this real-time color flow mapping to the carotid artery using this new 2-D Doppler system.

Instrumentation

The new 2-D Doppler system is the ALOKA XA-340, a linear array system which has 2 and 4 KHz pulse repetition frequencies. The transducer is a convex type (curved linear array), 27(W) ⋆ 15(D) ⋆ 57(L) mm size, with 5 MHz frequency (Fig. 1). The minimal velocity detected in color is 2 cm/sec at 2 KHz and the

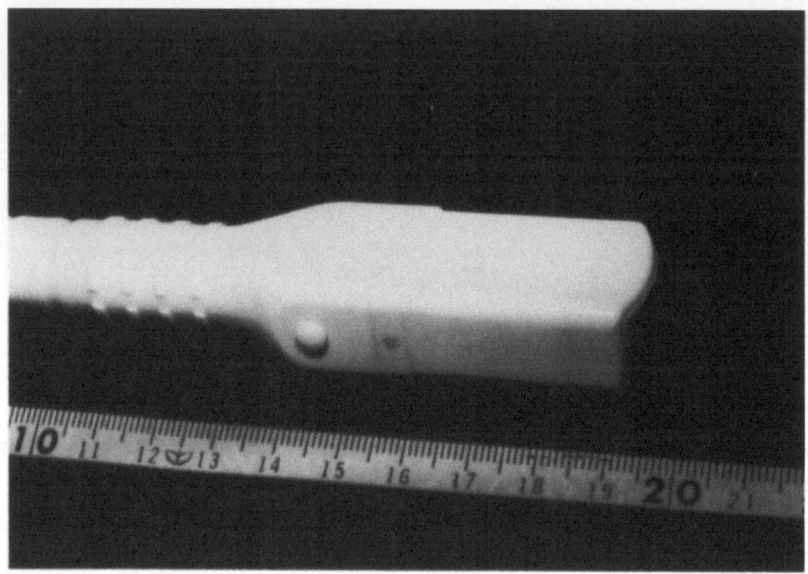

Figure 1. A curved linear array transducer (5 MHz) of Aloka XA-340.

maximal velocity detected in color without aliasing is approximately 30 cm/sec at 4 KHz. Flow towards the transducer is displayed in red and flow away from the transducer is displayed in blue. Velocity of the flow is displayed in one of eight steps which is proportional to the brightness of the color. Variance of the velocity is displayed in mixture of the green color: red color turns to be yellow and blue color to blue-green, cyan blue.

Normal carotid artery

This small-sized convex type transducer facilitates scanning of the carotid artery from its root to the distal branches percutaneously in color. Flow in the axial zone of the carotid artery is displayed with brighter color than in the peripheral zone near to the arterial wall. Due to the curved array display flow at the proximal carotid artery is displayed in red color which means flow towards the transducer (Fig. 2-f); the middle of the carotid artery which is perpendicular to the Doppler beam was displayed with both red color at the proximal, blue color at the distal segment with black color between them (Fig. 2-e). Black color or non color means that Doppler beam cannot detect a small vector of the flow to the transducer due to perpendicular Doppler beam projection to the flow. The distal carotid artery is displayed in blue (Fig. 2-d). Since the jugular vein is displayed in the different color from the carotid artery due to the opposite direction of the flow, it is easy to differentiate them even if both vessels are overlying each other.

On the external carotid artery side of the internal carotid artery and just distal to the bifurcation a yellow-colored representation of disturbed swirling flow is frequently seen (Fig. 2-d). This phenomenon of boundary layer flow separation by multigate pulsed Doppler was also observed in the velocity pattern of the human carotid artery [9] and in model experiments [10].
It was thought to be caused by artherosclerosis of the carotid bifurcation. With further study, this real time two-dimensional color display of the swirling flow at the carotid bifurcation may lead to further precise studies of physiology and genesis of atherosclerosis of the carotid bifurcation.

Differentiation of the internal and external carotid artery is sometimes difficult even by Duplex scanning, since position of both arteries are variant and velocity wave forms are changed by the various lesions. However, 2-D Doppler can detect color flow in 2 mm size arteries and if 2-D Doppler displays a small arterial branch, its main stem is the external carotid artery.

Plaque or ulcer of the carotid artery

This 2-D Doppler can detect even a small disturbed flow at the site of a plaque or ulcer on the carotid arterial wall. Since this small disturbed flow is displayed with the opposite color to the neighboring normal flow, it is very easy to detect it. Fig. 3 shows the small red disturbed flow at the site of the plaque and ulcer, while the normal flow is displayed in blue color. Spectral analysis of the velocity of the flow at such a mild lesion is reported to show spectral broadening at the peak systolic frequency [11]. This small disturbed flow observed by 2-D Doppler might cause spectral broadening of the carotid flow spectral analysis. However, spectral broadening of the velocity pattern has some limitations of accuracy to evaluate such a mild lesion. This 2-D Doppler can detect and evaluate such a lesion by a small disturbed flow very easily, even if B-mode image and spectral analysis fail to detect a small lesion of the plaque or ulcer on the carotid arterial wall.

Stenosis of the carotid artery

When the carotid bifurcation is affected by atherosclerosis the velocity of blood becomes accelerated. Through the stenotic portion with pulsed Doppler and aliasing when a low pulse repetition rate is used spectral analysis shows a bi-directional wide-band signal. 2-D Doppler expresses such a high velocity flow as a mosaic pattern with yellow and blue dots.

Fig. 4 shows a severe stenotic lesion of the external carotid artery at the bifurcation. 2-D echo shows the irregular wall and double stenoses at the bifurcation. 2-D Doppler shows a jet flow ejected from the stenotic lesion, which was expressed as a mosaic pattern with blue and yellow dots. Real-time spacial and

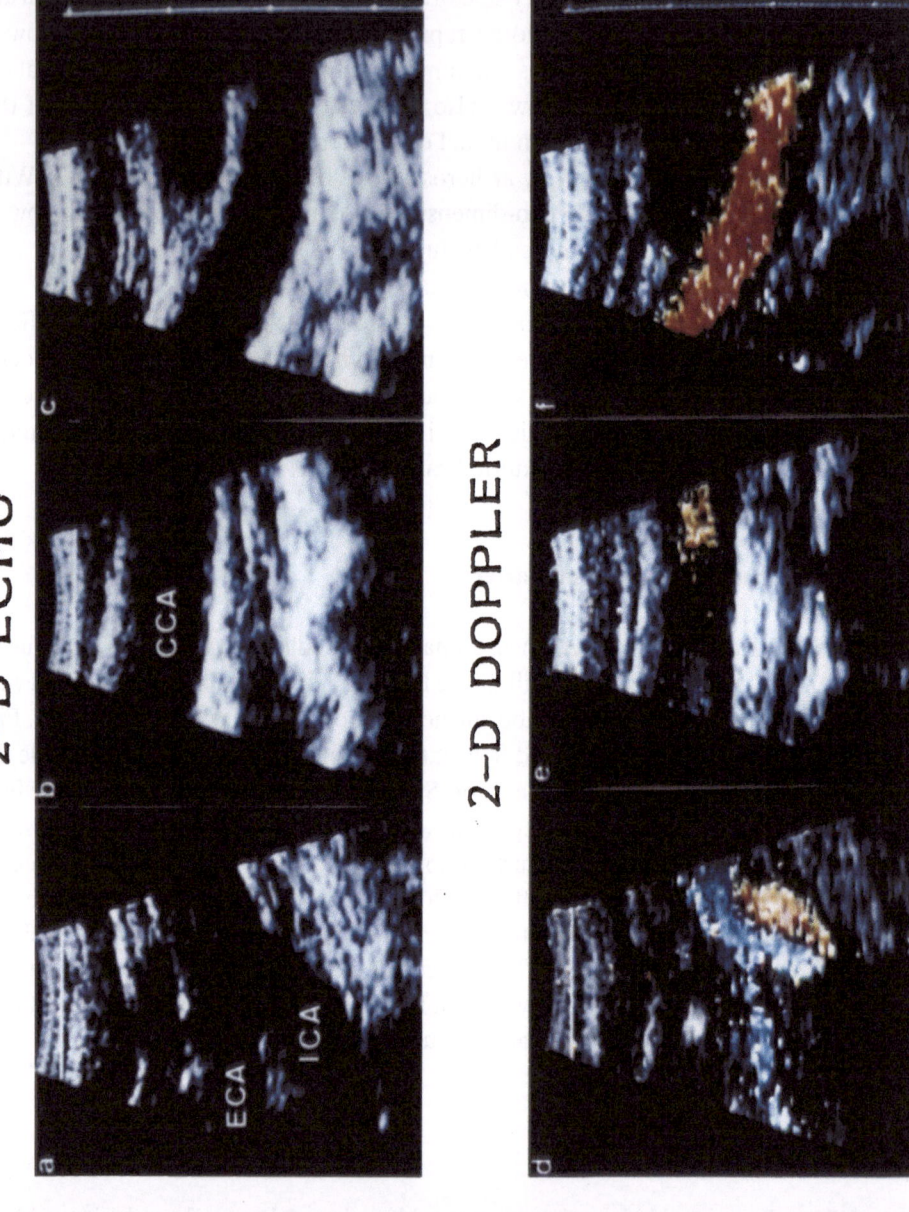

Figure 2. The normal carotid artery. The upper panel shows 2-D echogram of the normal carotid artery. The lower panel shows color flow mapping 2-D Doppler images of the normal carotid artery. The right (f) is the proximal common carotid artery which is displayed in red color. The center (e) is the middle portion of the common carotid artery. Note that flow directs from the right (yellow) to the left (blue). The left (d) is the bifurcation of the carotid artery. Note that a yellow-colored swirling flow is shown at the root of the internal carotid artery. CCA: common carotid artery, ICA: internal carotid artery, ECA: external carotid artery.

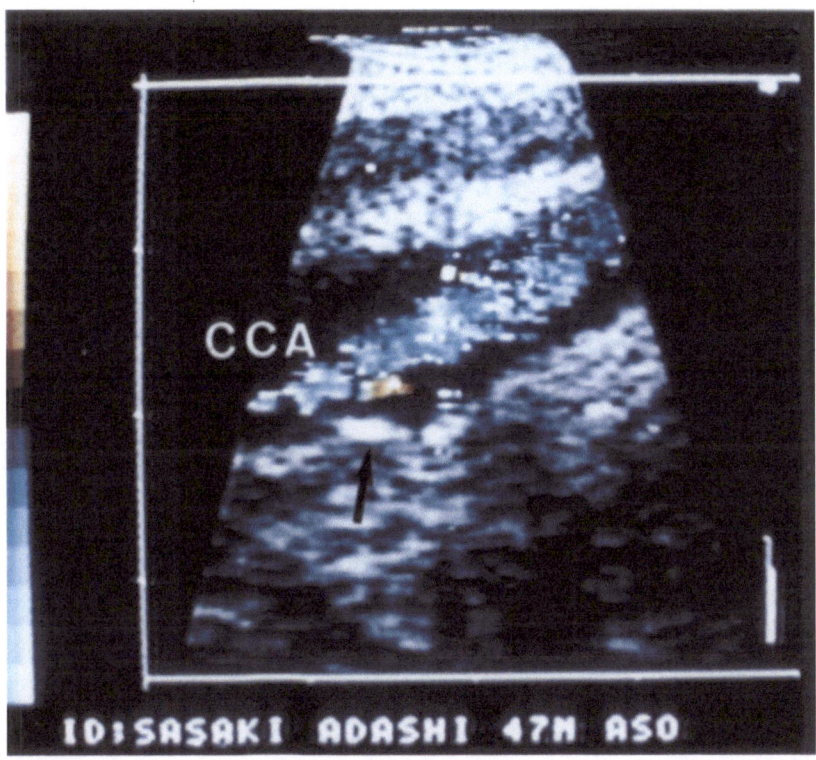

Figure 3. Plaque and ulcer at the wall of the carotid artery. At the posterior wall of the common carotid artery (CCA) a small plaque (AQ) with ulcer formation exists. At the lesion a yellow-colored small disturbed flow is displayed in a normal blue-colored flow.

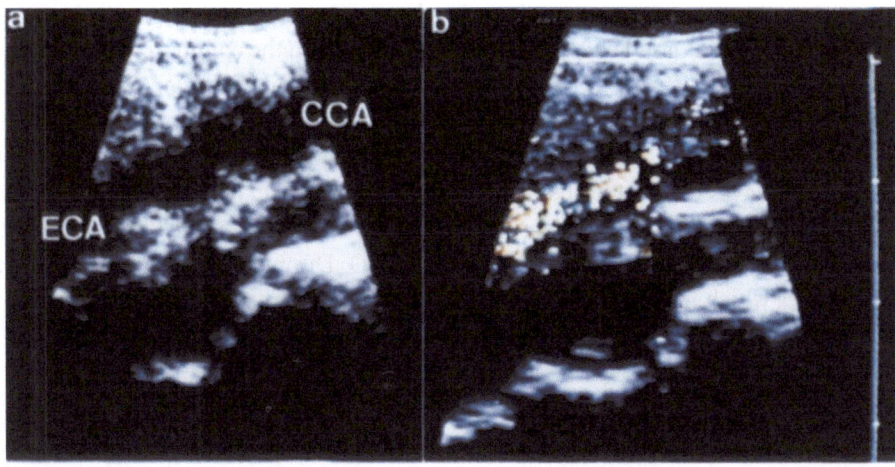

Figure 4. Severe stenosis of the carotid artery. 2-D echogram (a) shows irregular wall and stenosis of the common (CCA) and external (ECA) carotid artery. 2-D Doppler (b) shows a jet flow through the stenotic lesion as a mosaic pattern with blue and yellow dots which means high velocity flow. The internal carotid artery was displayed as a mosaic pattern also in the other view.

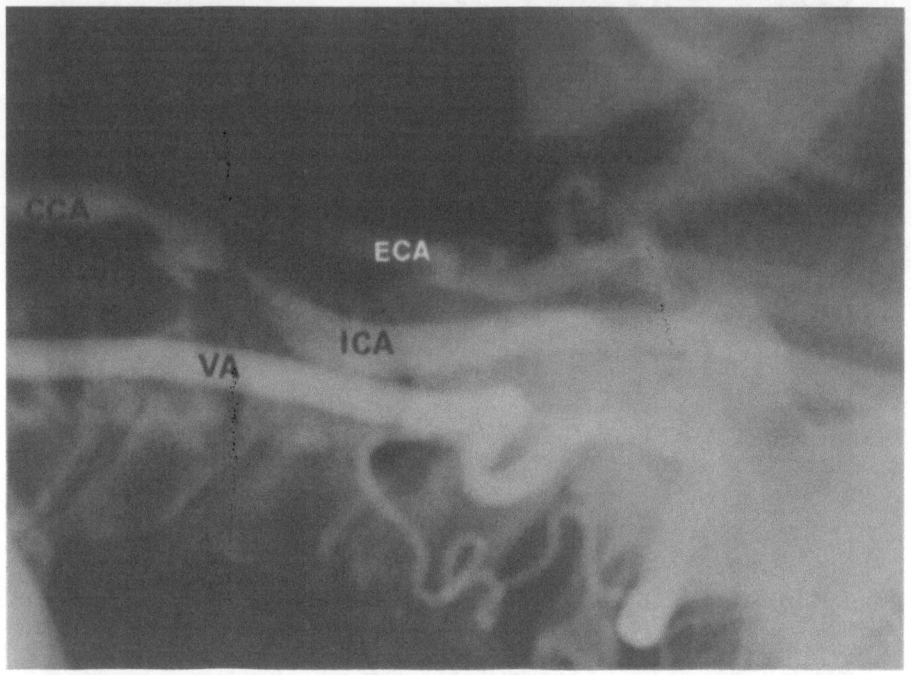

Figure 5. An angiogram of the carotid artery of the same patient as Fig. 4. Both the internal and external carotid artery are severely stenotic. CCA: common carotid artery, ICA: internal carotid artery, ECA: external carotid artery, VA: vertebral artery.

characteristic display of this flow dynamics of stenosis will lead to more accurate diagnosis than conventional noninvasive diagnostic tools. In this case the internal carotid artery was not displayed in the same plane with the common carotid artery and it was very difficult to identify it only by 2-D echo. However, 2-D Doppler showed a mosaic pattern in the internal carotid artery indicating a severely stenotic lesion. Fig. 5 is an angiogram of the carotid artery of the same patient which displays severe stenotis of both the internal and external carotid arteries. Therefore, even if 2-D echo cannot display the total image of the bifurcation due to elongation or tortuosity of the artery, 2-D Doppler can display the flow dynamics which are useful in diagnosing the severity of stenosis.

Discussion

Alhough several instruments have been developed for the carotid flow imaging, they do not offer a real-time flow image nor two-dimensional information of the flow dynamics. This 2-D Doppler supplies real-time 2-D image not only of the anatomical structure but also of the flow dynamics of the carotid artery simultaneously. By this 2-D Doppler physiology of the carotid flow and hemodynamic changes after some intervention can be easily observed. Even a small change of the flow state such as the small disturbed swirling flow at the plaque of the arterial wall and at the root of the internal carotid artery can be observed easily. Real-time non-invasive imaging of the flow may offer advantages of time-saving, repeatability and easy handling of the carotid examination.

With the small-sized convex type transducer the Doppler ultrasound beam can be projected with various angles to the peripheral arteries even if parallel to the skin, minimum detectable velocity is 2 cm/sec at 2 KHz at Doppler beam vector, the 5 MHz transducer provides high resolution as to display flow in a 2 mm diameter artery. This leads to a vivid color flow display of a slower flow at the peripheral arteries. By color flow imaging it is easy to scan the entire carotid system separating the artery from the vein. Even if the non-stenotic artery becomes tortuous and 2-D echo suggests a stenotic image, 2-D color Doppler can image a normal flow pattern at both the distal and the proximal sites to differentiate between changes in artery direction and true stenotic lesions. 2-D Doppler can supply three dimensional informations of the carotid artery by scanning longitudinally and cross-sectionally. Thus, 2-D Doppler is very useful in obtaining the total image of the carotid artery with not only the anatomical structure but also flow dynamics.

This easy-handling and easy-interpreting 2-D Doppler can be used intra-operatively to evaluate the effects of the surgery. 2-D Doppler can also be applied to evaluate the other peripheral vascular diseases such as obstructive lower limb arterial diseases and the peripheral artery aneurysm. 2-D Doppler might replace the angiography for the carotid artery disease and the peripheral vascular diseases.

In conclusion, real-time color flow mapping two-dimensional Doppler echography using a curved linear array transducer (5 MHz) is useful to display a real-time image of the flow dynamics and the structure of the carotid artery simultaneously. It can be a useful noninvasive diagnostic tool for the carotid artery disease.

References

1. Hokanson DE, Mozersky DJ, Sumner DS, Strandness De, Jr.: Ultrasonic arteriography, a new approach to arterial visualization. Biomed. Eng. 6: 420, 1971.
2. Reid JM, Spencer MP: Ultrasonic Doppler technique for imaging blood vessels. Science 176: 1235, 1972.
3. Curry GR, White DN: Color coded ultrasonic differential velocity arterial scanner (Echoflow). Ultrasound Med Biol 4: 27, 1978.
4. Eyer MK, Brandestini A, Phillips DJ, Baker DW: Color digital Echo/Doppler image presentation. Ultrasound Med Biol. 7; 21, 1981.
5. Namekawa K, Kasai C, Tsukamoto M, Koyano A: Real-time blood flow imaging system utilizing auto-correlation techniques. In Lerski RA, Morley P (eds), Ultrasound '82. Pergamon Press, Oxford, p 203, 1982.

6. Omoto R, Yokote Y, Takamoto S, Tamura F, Asano H, Namekawa K, Kasai C, Tsukamoto M, Koyano A: Clinical significance of newly developed real-time intracardiac two-dimensional blood flow imaging system (2-D Doppler). Jpn Circ J 47: 974, 1983.

7. Omoto R, ed.: Color atlas of real-time two-dimensional Doppler echocardiography. Shindan-to Chiryosha, Tokyo, 1984.

8. Takamoto S, Umaki K, Otani S, Irie T, Kasai C, Koyano A, Matsumura M, Kyo S, Omoto R: Real-time color flow mapping of the carotid, femoral and tibial arteries by new 2-D Doppler with a convex transducer. Proceedings of the 30th meeting of the American Institute of Ultrasound in medicine. p 62, 1985.

9. Phillips DJ, Greene FM, Langlois Y, Roederer GO, Strandness DE. Flow velocity patterns in the carotid bifurcations of young, presumed normal subjects. Ultrasound Med Biol. 13: 19, 1983.

10. LoGerfor FW, Nowak MD, Quist WC. Structual details of boundary layer separation in a model human carotid bifurcation under steady and pulsatile flow conditions. J Vasc Surg 2: 263, 1985.

11. Langlois Y, Roederer GO, Chan A *et al:* Evaluating carotid artery disease. The concordance between pulsed Doppler spectrum analysis and arteriography. Ultrasound Med Biol. 9: 51, 1983.

Transcranial Doppler diagnosis

R. Aaslid

The transtemporal approach of the transcranial Doppler method [1, 4] is based on the existence of thin regions in the temporal or sphenoid bones just above the zygomatic arch. These 'ultrasonic windows' provide a Doppler view on the basal cerebral arteries including the circle of Willis. The transorbital [2] or transforamenal [3, 4] approaches also exploits gaps or thin regions in the cranial bone structures to obtain Doppler signals from intracranial arteries proximal to the circle of Willis. The purpose of this chapter is to describe the transcranial Doppler method and its use for diagnosis of cerebrovascular disease.

Methods

The basal cerebral arteries are located at an inaccessible site in the middle of the cranium. Furthermore, the bone structures both reflect and absorb ultrasonic energy. Sufficient penetration is achieved by using relatively low ultrasonic frequencies in the range from 1.5 to 2.5 MHz. To discriminate between signals from different depths the pulsed Doppler principle [5] is employed. The length of the sample volume is usually chosen between 5 and 10 mm. By careful transducer design and focusing it is possible to limit the sample volume laterally to a diameter of about 4 mm (in water). In subjects with good (thin) ultrasonic windows signal to noise ratios of 30 dB may be obtained with a power density of 100 mW/cm2. However, in many cases the signals are barely above the noise level, and in about 2 to 3% of the patients it was not possible to obtain signals through the transtemporal route.

Spectral analysis is the method of choice to evaluate the intracranial Doppler signals. The envelope or spectral outline is found either manually on a frozen display or automatically by an appropriate algorithm to quantify the signals.

The first step in the transcranial investigation is to locate the ultrasonic window(s). In the transtemporal approach the probe is placed in the temporal region just above the zygomatic arch and the depth of the sample volume is set between

50 and 55 mm. Ample amounts of ultrasonic gel are applied, and the area between the frontal process of the zygomatic bone and the ear is searched. Once Doppler signals have been found, the probe position is optimized with respect to signal-to-noise ratio. If the transorbital route is used, the power is reduced to 20 mW/cm2, and the transducer is placed on the closed eyelid and aimed towards the optic canal or the orbital fissure [2]. To use the transforamenal route, the patient is instructed to bend the head forward, and the vertebral/basilar arteries are insonated through the gap between the atlas and the skull [3, 4]. It is then usually possible to aim either directly from behind, in the median plane, or somewhat obliquely from the side parallel to the anatomical course of the vertebral artery.

For the identification of the various intracranial arteries there are basically two sources of information: 1) The depth setting and the aiming direction combined with the directional spectral display of the signal; and 2) the response of the Doppler signal to various compression tests.

As an aid to the spatial imaging skills of the operator it is possible to connect the transducer to a position sensing scanning arm and program a computer to display a flow map. This is similar to the principle described for use in extracranial arteries [6]. The various intracranial arteries can be shown in shades of grey (or color) depending upon the intensity of the Doppler signals. The contour of the skull is superimposed for ease of orientation. Figs. 1 and 2 show a representative collection of Doppler signals from a normal subject, using various routes to the different intracranial arteries. The maps were made in the horizontal plane (similar to scanning planes in computer assisted tomography of the head). The dotted line shows the direction of the ultrasonic beam and the ellipse at its end indicates the position of the sample volume.

Recently, this concept has been elaborated on to display the three-dimensional course of the intracranial arteries. The scanning arm sensor readings are transformed into an orthogonal coordinate system, color plate xx p.yy. X is the distance between the probe surface and the sample volume normal to the medial sagittal plane, Y and Z are sample volume distances from scull landmarks (normal to coronal and horizontal planes respectively). The three standard projections: horizontal, coronal (or A-P) and lateral are all shown on the display. For each cluster of dots on the screen, one spectral display is stored in computer memory. The size of the clusters is proportional to Doppler signal energy, and the color code shows Doppler velocity and direction. Warm/cold colors indicate direction towards/away the probe respectively. This principle can be regarded as an extension of the hand-held technique to allow precise documentation of sample volume position in space, and to give a reference for interpretation of the spectral display.

The following description of the 'free hand' Doppler signal identification procedure refers to the computer generated flow maps in Figs. 1 and 2 for convenience, basically, the free hand operator uses a similar 'mental map' for orientation.

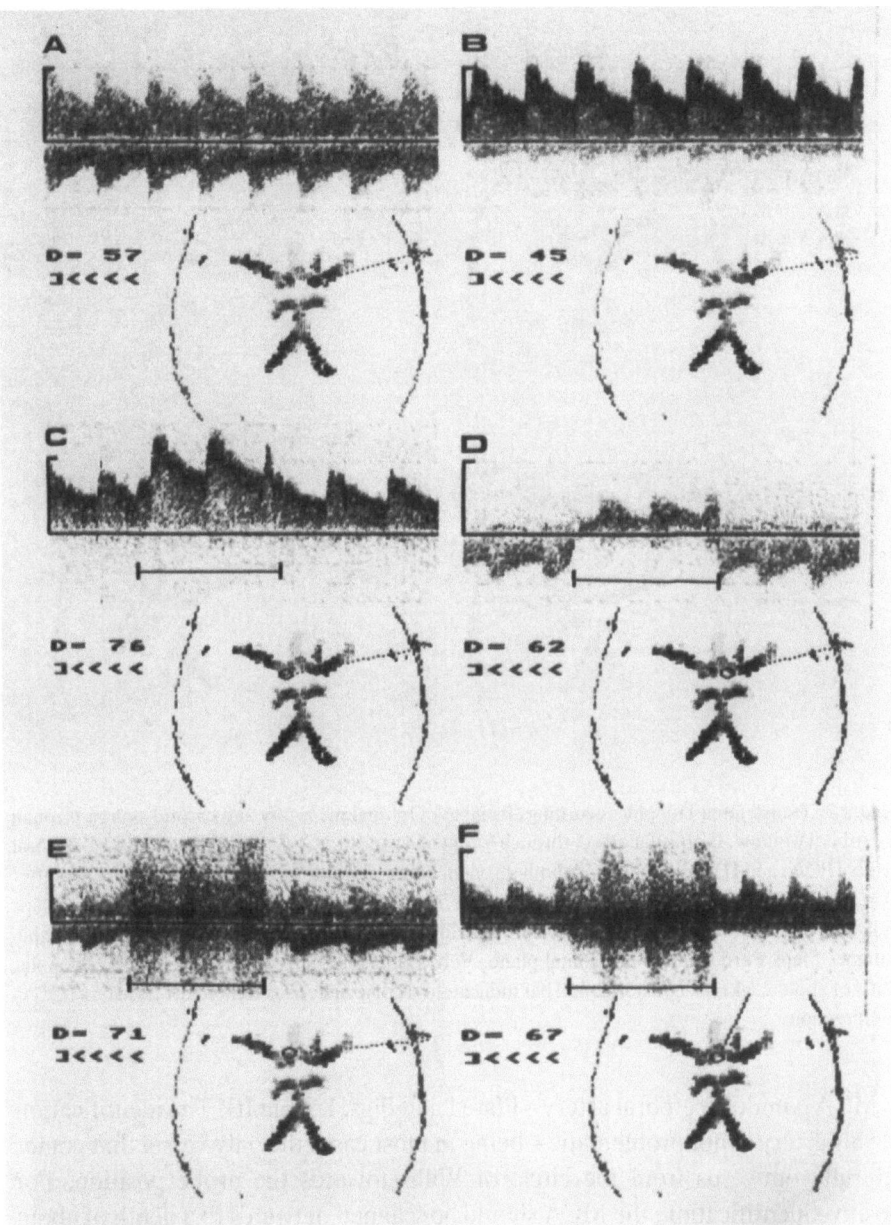

Figure 1. Transcranial Doppler recordings from: A) Bifurcation of internal carotid artery (ICA). B) Middle cerebral artery (MCA). C) Contralateral anterior cerebral artery (ACA). D) Ipsilateral ACA. E) Both ACA's and anterior communicating artery (ACoA). F) ACA(s) and ACoA through orbital window.

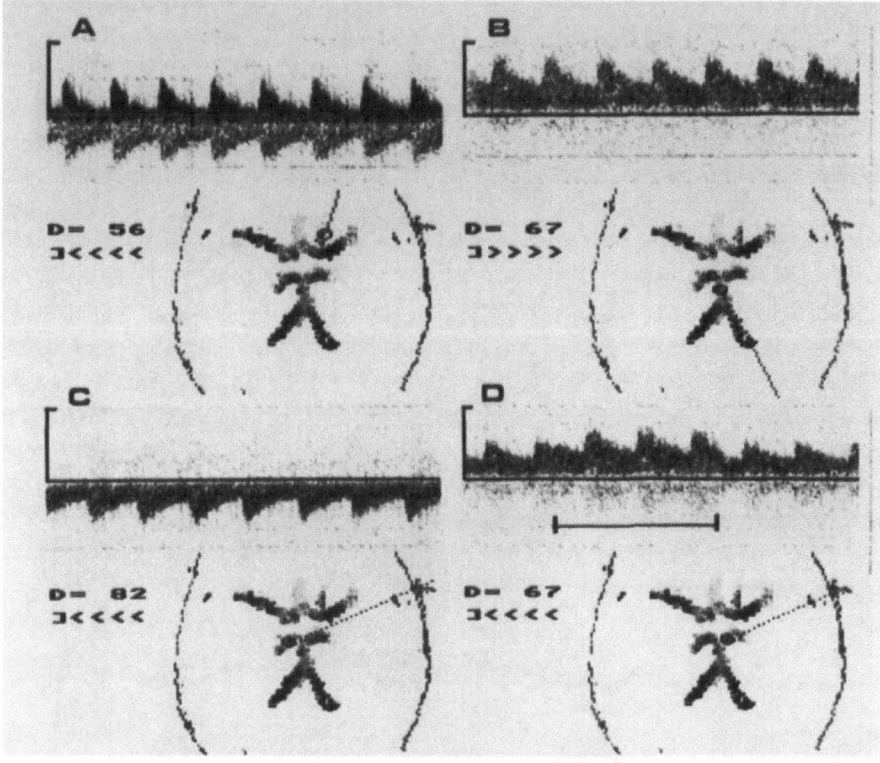

Figure 2. Transcranial Doppler recordings from: A) Ophthalmic artery and carotid siphon through the orbital window. B) Basilar artery through foramenal window. C) Contralateral posterior cerebral artery (PCA) and D) Ipsilateral PCA both through temporal window. Depth is indicated in mm after D =, the symbol below this indicates direction of flow shown as positive. Dotted line in flow maps indicates direction of ultrasonic beam, and the ellipse at its end shows the position of the sample volume. Maps were made in horizontal plane. Vertical bars indicate velocities of 1 m/sec (Doppler shifts of about 2.5 kHz), and horizontal bar indicates time of ipsilateral common carotid artery (CCA) compression.

MCA – middle cerebral artery – Plate 1 and Figs. 1A and 1B. The identification of this artery is not problematic – being in most cases the only vessel that comes laterally outwards from the circle of Willis towards the probe position. For positive identification, the MCA should be scanned outwards to a depth of about 35 mm to distinguish it from the ICA and the PCA both of which are located at considerably deeper levels. The negative low Doppler shift in Fig. 1B represent a small branch of the MCA running in the opposite direction. On compression of the ipsilateral common carotid artery (CCA), the flow velocity in the MCA is reduced and the pulsatile waveform becomes more damped (Fig. 1B). This compression test may be useful to determine the collateral capacity of the circle of Willis, however, the procedure is seldom necessary for MCA identification because of this artery's unique anatomical course. Some cases may show an early

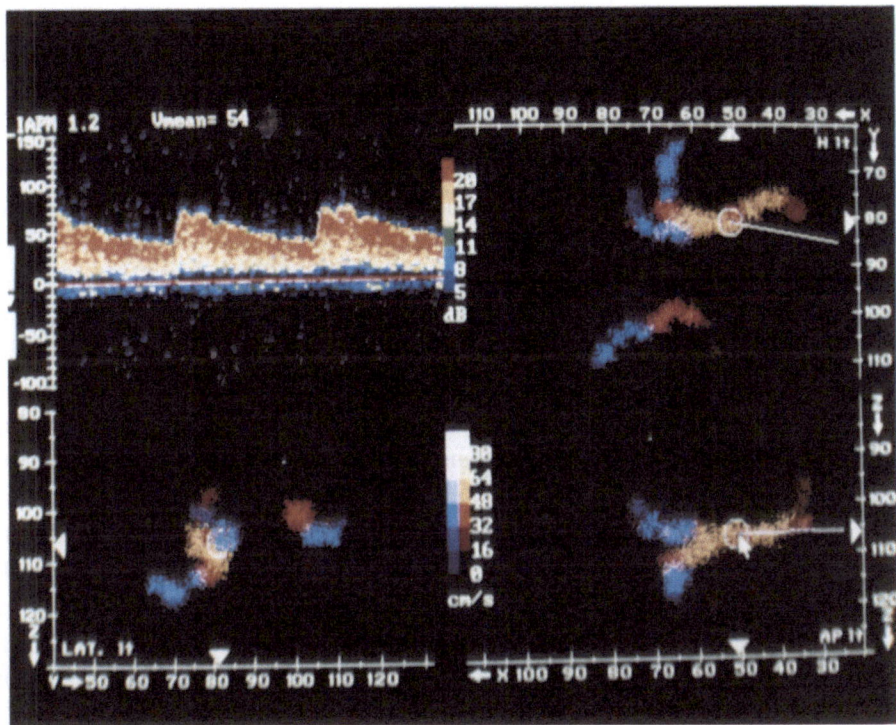

Plate 1. Three-dimensional scan of the basal cerebral arteries in a normal subject. *Upper right* shows horizontal projection, X is the sample volume distance from the probe, Y is sample volume distance from the surface of the forehead. The white circle represent the sample volume and the line shows the direction of the ultrasonic beam. The sample volume is placed on the main stem of the MCA, the recorded spectrum is shown *upper left*. The projectional displays are color coded for direction and velocity, the scale used is shown between the two lower panels. The column left (cold colors) represent negative Doppler shifts (away) while the warm colors (right) codes the positive Doppler shifts. The size of each cluster of dots represent signal strength.

The ACA runs medially from x = 60 mm (blue dots) in to the brain midline (x = 72 mm) where it curves anteriorly. The MCA runs laterally and curves superiorly at X = 35 mm. Note the decrease of Doppler shifts as the MCA branches curve superiorly, and the ACA curves anteriorly. Blunt angle insonation at these points may account for the decrease of observed velocities. The bifurcation of the basilar artery is shown at Y = 105 mm, the ipsi/contralateral PCA's have flows towards/away from the probe respectively.

Lower right shows coronal (or anterior posterior, A–P) projection, Z is the sample volume distance from the crown of the head. The PCA's are not shown for clarity because they superimpose on the MCA/ACA in this projection. The superclinoid ICA is seen running superiorly and laterally in this projection. The observed direction of flow in this segment changes due to probe angle: the color is blue (away) in lower segment and orange (toward) in terminal portion. The superclinoid ICA is also seen both in the lateral projection (*lower left*) as well as the horizontal view.

bifurcation of the MCA. It is then possible to scan and identify each of the two branches with the computer flow map.

ACA – anterior cerebral artery – Plate 1 and Figs. 1A, 1C, 1D, 1E and 1F. The MCA signal is used as the starting point. Scanning this progressively deeper (50–60 mm), a negative Doppler shift usually appears concomitantly with the MCA spectrum, Fig. 1A. When the sample volume is thus positioned at the bifurcation of the ICA, the spectra are broad with no 'systolic windows'. However, this is not a pathological sign as in examination of the carotid bifurcation. Because the sample volume is relatively large in relation to the intracranial vessels and therefore contains most of the very complex velocity distributions in the ICA bifurcation, a broadband spectrum would be expected at this location. Scanning the ACA signal deeper, the MCA signal disappears, Fig. 1D, then, coming towards the brain midline, the signal from the contralateral ACA appears as positive Doppler shift, Fig. 1E. The latter signal can also be recorded along, Fig. 1C, when the depth is advanced to between 75 and 85 mm. All recordings shown in Figs. 1A–E were made from an ultrasonic window located relatively anteriorly in the temporal region. This is an advantage when recording from the MCA and the contralateral ACA because the courses of both these vessels are usually directed somewhat anteriorly towards the position of the probe and they can therefore be insonated at acute angles. However, the ipsilateral ACA will then be insonated at a somewhat blunter angle, the effects of this are lower absolute Doppler shifts and lower signal strengths. (Compare panels C and D in Fig. 1). Clearly, in this case, it was preferable to insonate both ACA's contralaterally. If a posterior ultrasonic window (close to the ear) is used, it is the method of choice to insonate the ACA from the ipsilateral side. The ACA's may also be insonated via the transorbital route, Fig. 1F.

Compression tests of the CCA give rise to characteristic responses of the Doppler shifts in the ACA's. The case shown in Fig. 1 had a moderate to good collateral capacity of the anterior part of the circle of Willis. The ipsilateral ACA showed flow reversal during CCA compression, Fig. 1D, indicating flow supply to the MCA through this channel. This extra supply also showed up as a massive increase in the velocity of flow in the contralateral ACA, Fig. 1C. During compression, the anterior communicating artery (ACoA) had very high velocities which could not be recorded directly. However, their presence was indicated by the widening of the spectra in Fig. 1E and F. When evaluating Doppler recordings from the ACA's, the anatomical variation of one hypoplastic or missing ACA must be considered. Such variations as well as the absence of an ACoA with otherwise normal vessels can usually be assessed by compression tests.

ICA – intracranial internal carotid artery – Plate 1 and Fig. 2A. The terminal portion of this vessel can be found by moving the sample volume somewhat inferiorly from the position shown in Fig. 1A. It has a positive Doppler shift, but of lower absolute frequency than the MCA and ACA. This reflects the anatomical fact that the ICA usually is insonated at blunt angles via from the temporal window. Aiming the probe further inferiorly and anteriorly, it is possible to scan the ICA down into the siphon. (Plate 1, lower left). A better view on the intracranial part of the ICA can usually be obtained via the transorbital approach [2] as shown in Fig. 2A. The sample volume was directed to the site where the ophthalmic artery branches off the upper part of the carotid siphon. The positive Doppler shift came from the former artery, it can be recognized by the low Doppler shift in end-diastole signifying an extracranial supply component. In contrast, the ICA produces a Doppler shift below the zeroline with the typical cerebral artery pulsewave. Scanning deeper, the ophthalmic artery signal disappears and the ICA signal increases in strength. Tilting the probe and directing the sample volume inferiorly, the lower part of the siphon can be observed with positive Doppler shifts indicating flow direction towards the probe.

PCA – posterior cerebral artery – Plate 1 and Figs. 2C and 2D. This vessel can usually be observed by the transtemporal approach. Taking as a reference point the bifurcation of the ICA (Fig. 1A) or the ipsilateral ACA (Fig. 1D), the probe is tilted to aim somewhat posteriorly and inferiorly to this. If the patient has the normal anatomical configuration with both PCA's branching off the basilar artery, the signal from the proximal PCA then appears as shown in Fig. 2D. The identification should be checked by scanning inwards to the brain midline to observe the bifurcation of the basilar artery, with spectra similar to those shown in Fig. 1A (the absolute Doppler shifts are usually 25 to 40% lower in the basilar artery bifurcation). Scanning still further, signals from the contralateral PCA can be obtained, Fig. 2C. A further clue for identification is a CCA compression test, Fig. 2D, the proximal ipsilateral PCA showing increased volume flow due to the collateral supply through the posterior communicating artery (PCoA). If the sample volume was placed slightly more distally on the PCA (depths of 57 mm), there is no appreciable change in the Doppler recording during CCA compression.

A frequent anatomical variation of the posterior circulation is an enlarged PCoA with a hypoplastic proximal PCA, the supply coming mainly or even entirely from the ICA. In such cases, a PCA Doppler signal directed towards the probe will not be found, and the identification will be difficult without the mapping system. Moreover, the PCA will be intercepted at blunt angles. An oscillatory pulsewave has been found at the assumed location of the proximal PCA in some such subjects – probably reflecting transmission delays and interactions between the pulsewaves in the vertebral and carotid systems. The PCoA is usually not identifiable in the normal anatomical variation, however, in compression tests of the CCA, its presence becomes manifest as high frequency Doppler shifts and disturbed flow from the region between the ICA and the PCA.

BA – the basilar artery, Fig. 2B. Although the bifurcation of this vessel can be recorded transtemporally in many cases, the best route is through the major foramen [3, 4]. The signals from the vertebral arteries are scanned progressively deeper, and in most cases signals can be found down to 100 mm. The basilar artery is then insonated at an acute angle from behind. (The directionality of the signal is reversed on Fig. 2B compared to the other recordings; furthermore, the position of the probe is more lateral than commonly used. The best insonation is found close to the medial plane so that the aperture between the cranium and the atlas can be fully utilized.

Normal values: The time-mean of the spectral outlines in healthy adult subjects ranges from 20 to 85 cm/sec. In the MCA where the flow can be insonated at acute angles, we found a mean of 62 cm/sec with a standard deviation of 12 cm/sec [1]. The Doppler shifts from the ACA and PCA are practically always lower than those from the MCA.

The waveforms of the spectral outlines are normally very similar to the arterial pressure curve due to the low resistance component of the input impedance to the cerebral vascular bed. Furthermore, in the normal individual, the MCA velocities are symmetrical (left vs. right) within 20%.

Criteria for diagnosis

The transcranial Doppler method is new and only a few groups have reported results up to now. The criteria for diagnosis discussed in subsequent sections are based on this preliminary experience, and it is yet too early to report on specificity and sensitivity. There are three main types of findings which indicate pathology of the cerebral vascular system, and these will be listed before proceeding to discussion of specific diseases.

1) Higher than normal velocities. Arterial narrowing (stenosis, spasm) causes the flow to accelerate. However, such findings may also indicate an increased volume flow through a normal lumen size.

2) Intracranial vascular bruits or musical murmurs are associated with higher than normal velocities and flow disturbances [7]. The Doppler instrument then acts as a focused microphone. In some cases only the bruit effects will be observed because the high velocity Doppler shifts are below the noise level of the instrument.

3) Abnormal pulse waveforms – a damped waveform can be caused by a hemodynamically significant stenosis or occlusion proximal to the site of recording [8]. An increase in the pulsatility is found in patients with high intracranial pressure.

Carotid artery disease

In patients with angiographically verified slight stenosis of the extracranial ICA (diameter reduction less than 50%) we found no significant changes in the intracranial Doppler recordings when compared to a group of normal subjects.

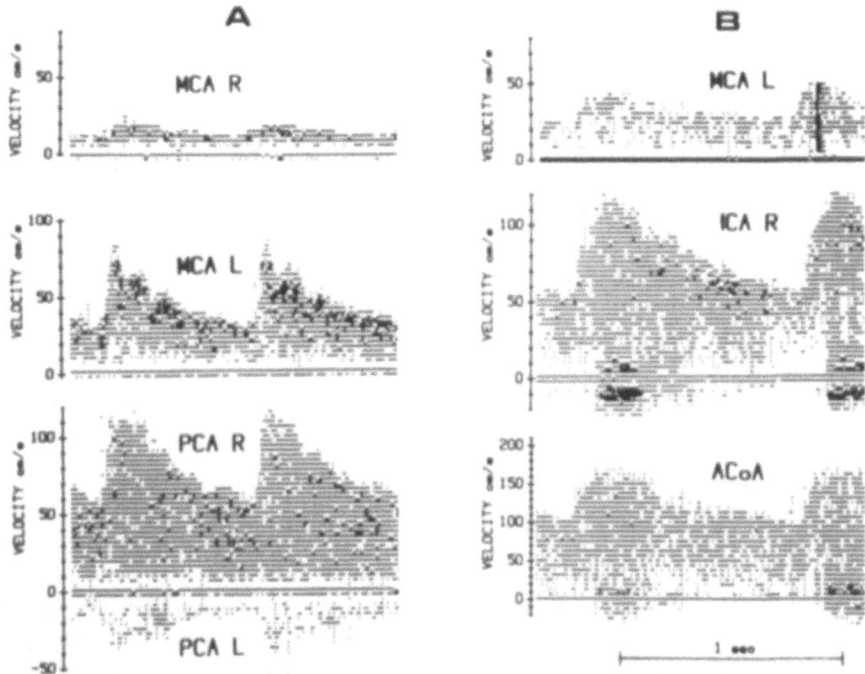

Figure 3A. Shows the transcranial Doppler recordings from a 58 year old man with recurring TIA's after occlusion of the right ICA. The flow in the right MCA was much slower than in the left, moreover, the waveform was heavily damped on the right side, indicating a critical loss of perfusion pressure. The ACA's had similar side differences (not shown), this was interpreted as a functionally missing ACoA. However, the right proximal PCA had markedly elevated velocities (over three times higher than in the left PCA), revealing its role in the collateral supply to the entire right hemisphere.

Figure 3B. Shows the transcranial recordings from a 58 year-old women with occlusion of the left ICA: The MCA on this side had a slow damped flow. The right ACA had reversed direction of flow, and in the region of the anterior communication artery, high velocities (140 cm/sec) were detected. On the right side the terminal ICA (middle trace of Fig. 3B) had a high flow velocity with bruits in systole. In this case, the anterior part of the circle of Willis served as the main collateral network and the right ICA had an increased volume flow.

Slight stenosis does not cause appreciable flow energy losses due to only moderate acceleration of the flow through the narrowed segment. Thus, the arterial pressure in the intracranial ICA distal to the stenosis will be practically equal to – or only slightly less than – the pressure in the nonaffected ICA or in the basilar artery. Therefore, flow through the collateral connections ACoA and PCoA will remain unspectacular.

If there is a significantly increased flow resistance of the carotid stenosis (diameter reduction of more than about 75%), changes in the distribution of flow in the basal cerebral arteries will be expected. However, the hemodynamics of the circle of Willis is complex – especially because there is a great divergence of the anatomy with many possible variants. Two of these are illustrated and described in Fig. 3 – the Doppler findings were verified by angiography.

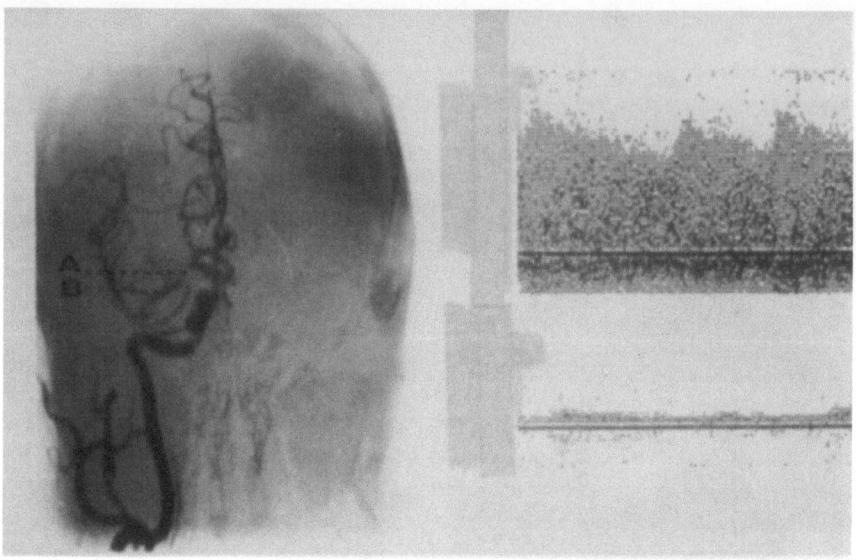

Figure 4. Angiograms and Doppler findings in a 65 year-old man (Doppler investigation by P. Grolimund of Bern) with severe stenosis of the right MCA. The patient had previously been investigated by conventional Doppler techniques in a reputable laboratory with no pathological findings. The transcranial technique revealed the cause of the patient's recurrent episodes of TIA's. High velocities and strong flow disturbances (high-amplitude low-frequency components of the spectra) were found in the proximal MCA. In the distal MCA the flow was very slow (panel B) and the pulsewave was heavily damped due to the flow energy loss through the stenosis.

By identification of the different vessels in the circle of Willis it is thus possible to evaluate the source and extent of collateral supply in patients with carotid stenosis and occlusion. However, identification by free hand scanning may be difficult in such cases because of pathological flow velocities and directions. The computer flow scanning system is intended to help in this respect.

Indirectly, the efficiency of the collateral system – or rather the total effect of the inflow system – can be evaluated by analysing the MCA velocity waveform by means of the Gosling pulsatility index PI and the pulsatility transmission index [8]: PTI = PI/PIref where PIref is the PI of a cerebral artery with unimpeded inflow. The case shown in Fig. 3A had a PTI of only 0.4 while the other case, Fig. 3B, had PTI = 0.81 indicating a much better collateral capacity. The former patient was a clear candidate for extra-intracranial bypass surgery.

Intracranial stenosis

Stenotic lesions of the intracranial arteries cannot be reliably diagnosed from extracranial Doppler investigations. This has been an important reason for advocating mandatory angiography in patients with carotid artery disease even if

B-mode realtime ultrasound scanners may image the lesion proper with equally good or even better resolution than angiography. This aspect may be viewed differently if the transcranial Doppler method turns out to be accurate in the diagnosis of intracranial lesions.

Both MCA, Fig. 4, and ACA stenoses can be evaluated through the transtemporal route. For diagnosis of siphon stenosis the transorbital approach should be used in addition [2]. Basilar artery stenosis can be diagnosed by using the transforamenal route (case to be published by Lindegaard and Aaslid).

Cerebral vasospasm

Vascular spasm of the cerebral arteries is a dreaded complication in patients with spontaneous subarachnoid hemorrhage (SAH). The hemodynamic effect of a spasm is similar to that of a stenosis, both causing flow energy losses. The main difference is the transient nature of spasm, seldom being endured more than one or two weeks. Before the introduction of transcranial Doppler there was no adequate method to monitor the onset and resolution of vasospasm. Angiography – besides being invasive and time consuming – is contraindicated in severe spasm because of its extra stress on the already marginal cerebral perfusion. A comparison study confirmed that there was an inverse relationship between velocity as found by transcranial Doppler and diameter of the cerebral artery as determined by angiography [9]. All patients with angiographic spasm of the MCA had significantly increased velocities (more than four standard deviations above a normal material) and the severity of the spasm evaluated by the two methods correlated well. Other studies [10, 11] have demonstrated the usefulness of the transcranial method to monitor vasospasm in neurosurgical practice.

Arteriovenous malformations

The most conspicious hemodynamical characteristic of AVM's is high flow velocity in the malformation feeders and the cerebral arteries involved in the supply [12, 14]. This is seen in transcranial Doppler recordings as high Doppler shifts (120–200 cm/sec) in the arteries involved. Furthermore, massive venous flows may be recorded in about 25% of the cases. If the AVM proper can be insonated, a very broad and 'disturbed' bidirectional spectrum is found. While the flow to a normal cerebral vascular bed reacts in a predictable and sensitive manner to changes in arterial pCO_2 [13], the flow to the AVM is not affected. Therefore, mild hyperventilation can be used to differentiate the high velocites caused by AVM's (and carotid-cavernous fistulae) from those caused by other types of pathology. A presumably normal cerebral artery in the same patient should be employed as control.

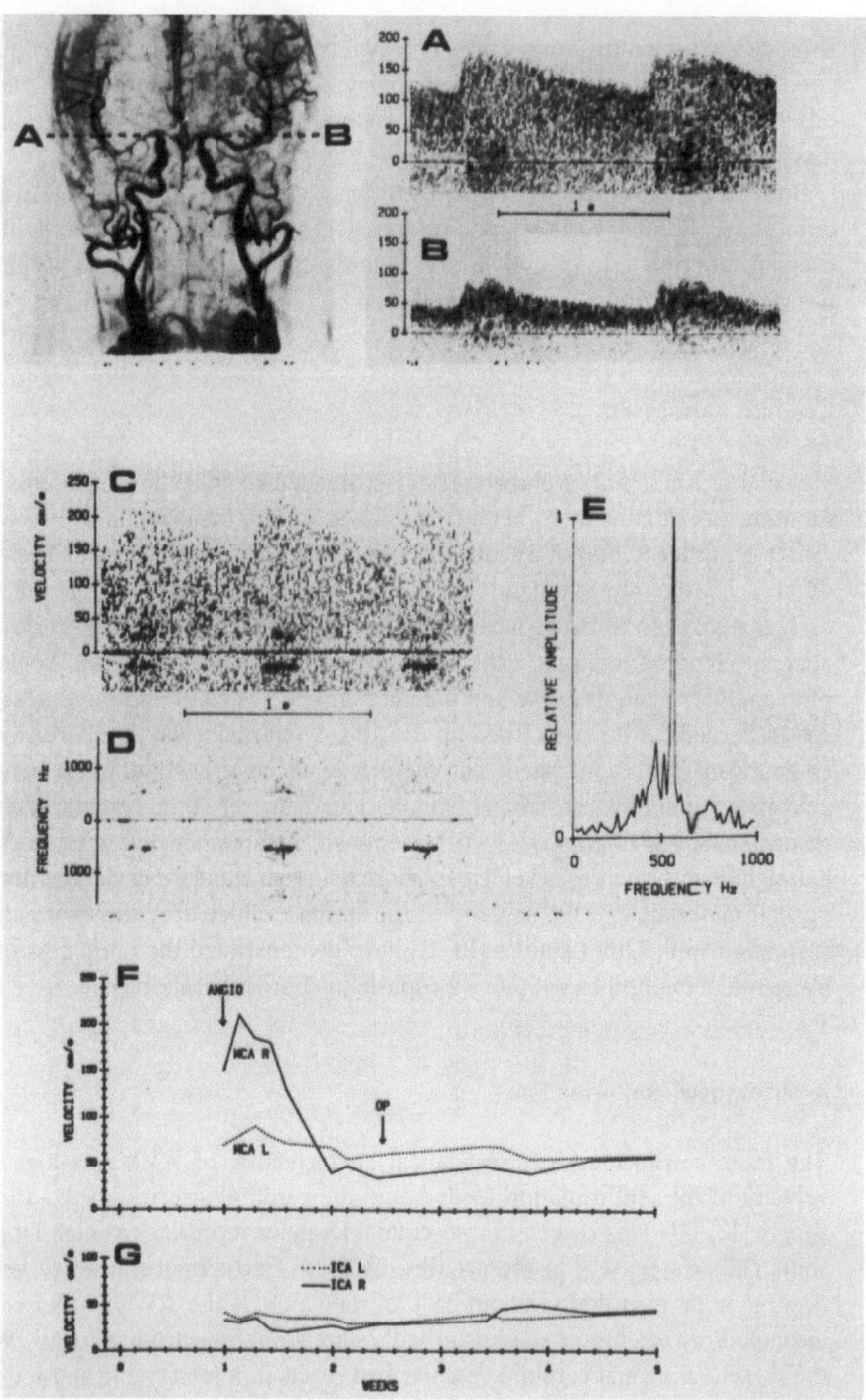

Figure 5. Shows angiograms and Doppler findings in a 47 year-old woman one week after SAH. The velocities were almost three times higher in the moderately spastic MCA on the right side than in the left. The velocity difference in the ACA's (not shown) was much smaller due to the excellent collateral capacity of the ACoA. Panels C, D and E show a musical murmur 8 hours later in the same patient. The MCA velocities had increased further, and the pure tone quality murmur was probably caused by periodic vortex formation in the narrowed arteries. The lower panels show the time course of the flow velocities in the MCA and the extracranial ICA during hospitalization and follow up of this patient. The peak MCA velocities were found between Days 8 and 10, and the patient had neurological symptoms on Day 10 and 11 corresponding to the decline in the right ICA velocity trend. Then the MCA velocities returned to normal parallel to an improvement in the neurological state, and the surgeon decided to operate on Day 17. Panels A, B, C, D and E were published previously (7, 9).

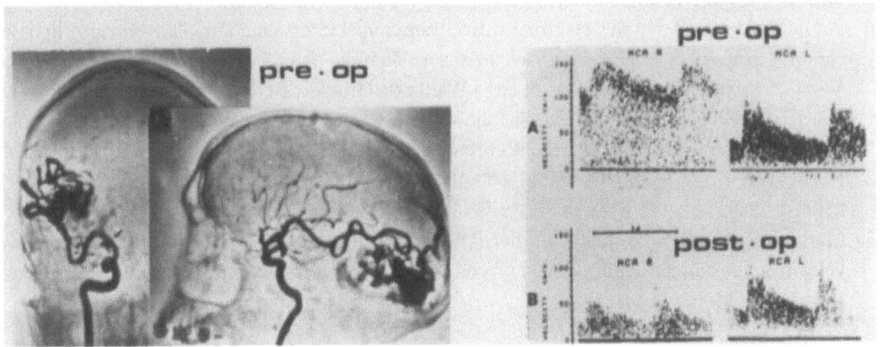

Figure 6. Shows angiography and Doppler recordings from a 45 year-old man with both an AVM and an aneurysm. The left MCA (panel A) had pathologically high velocities, while those from the right MCA were within the normal range. Postoperatively (panel B) the left side showed normal transcranial Doppler findings. The angiogram (not shown) also confirmed a successful operation. The transcranial Doppler method has a potential value for evaluation of such surgical procedures and the postoperative follow up of patients.

Acknowledgement

The angiograms shown in this chapter were performed at the Department of Neuroradiology, University of Berne by Prof. P. Huber.

References

1. Aaslid R, Markwalder T–M, Nornes H: Noninvasive transcranial Doppler ultrasound recording of flow velocity in basal cerebral arteries. J Neurosurg 57: 769, 1982.

2. Spencer MP: Intracranial carotid artery diagnosis with transorbital pulsed wave (PW) and continuous wave (CW) Doppler ultrasound. J of Ultrasound in Med Suppl 2(10): 61, 1983.

3. Arnolds B, von Reutern G–M: Transcranial Doppler sonography: Techniques of examination and normal reference values. Ultrasound in Medicine and Biology. – In Press, 1984.

4. Ringelstein EB, Korbmacher G, Zeumer H: Detection of intracranial arterial lesions by means of a new transcranial Doppler device. Proceedings of the International Congress: Applications of Doppler-Ultrasound in Medicine Duesseldorf 1984 – In press, 1984.

5. Baker DW: Pulsed ultrasonic Doppler blood-flow sensing. IEEE Trans Sonics Ultrasonics SU-17: 170, 1970.

6. Reid JM, Spencer MP: Ultrasonic Doppler technique for imaging blood vessels. Science 176: 1235, 1972.

7. Aaslid R, Nornes H: Musical murmurs in human cerebral arteries after subarachnoid hemorrhage. J Neurosurg 60: 32, 1984.

8. Lindegaard K–F, Aaslid R: Transcranial Doppler for assessing intracranial hemodynamic patterns in carotid artery disease. Proceedings of the International Congress: Applications of Doppler-Ultrasound in Medicine Duesseldorf 1984 – In press, 1984.

9. Aaslid R, Huber P, Nornes H: Evaluation of cerebrovascular spasm with transcranial Doppler ultrasound. J Neurosurg 60: 37, 1984.

10. Aaslid R, Huber P, Nornes H: Noninvasive transcranial ultrasound Doppler recording in basal cerebral arteries – A new approach to the evaluation of cerebrovascular spasm. Cerebral Vascular Spasm. (Voth D, Glees P, eds.) Walter de Gruyter, Berlin, 1984.

11. Harders A, Gilsbach JM: Angiospasm following early aneurysm operation – transcranial Doppler findings. In: Voth D, Glees P (eds.) Cerebral Vascular Spasm. Walter de Gruyter, Berlin, 1984.

12. Nornes H, Grip A: Hemodynamic aspects of cerebral arteriovenous malformations. J Neurosurg 53: 456, 1980.

13. Markwalder T–M, Grolimund P, Seiler RW, Roth F, Aaslid R: The dependence of blood flow velocity in the middle cerebral artery on end-tidal pCO_2 – A transcranial Doppler study. J Cereb Blood Flow Metab 4: 368, 1984.

Real-Time B-Mode imaging of the carotid bifurcation

J. Comerota, M.L. Katz and J.V. White*

Forty to fifty of all strokes are secondary to atherosclerotic disease of the cervical carotid arteries [1]. Techniques that image the carotid bifurcation have grown in popularity and are becoming an established part of the noninvasive cerebrovascular evaluation. Real-Time B-Mode ultrasonic imaging provides structural detail of the vessel wall and atherosclerotic plaque. Structures are visualized by sound wave reflection from the interfaces of tissues with different acoustic impedances, hence providing true anatomic detail. The Doppler imaging techniques diagrammatically recreate the vessel lumen on a storage oscilloscope when flow velocity exceeds a threshold values [2]. Doppler imaging also provides a direct evaluation but it is based upon the physiology of flow.

This chapter attempts to establish the place of Real-Time B-Mode imaging in the diagnosis of carotid artery disease. We were interested in determining whether scan quality influenced accuracy, whether experience influenced reliability, whether different testing centers could obtain similar results when common techniques and interpretation criteria were used and whether characteristics of atherosclerotic plaque could be prospectively identified. Data included in this report were obtained from three major vascular laboratories over a period including five years.

Materials

The imager used in these studies contains a 4 cm, 8 megahertz (biosound) transducer. The axial resolution is 0.3 mm at a 2 cm focal length (Fig. 1). To establish the sensitivity and specificity of this technique, a total of 1723 vessels were studied both noninvasively and arteriographically (Table 1). The noninvasive studies were performed by 11 technicians and interpreted by three physicians. Each patient was studied according to an established technique and the results

* In conjunction with: J.J. Cranley, W.G. Hayden.

242

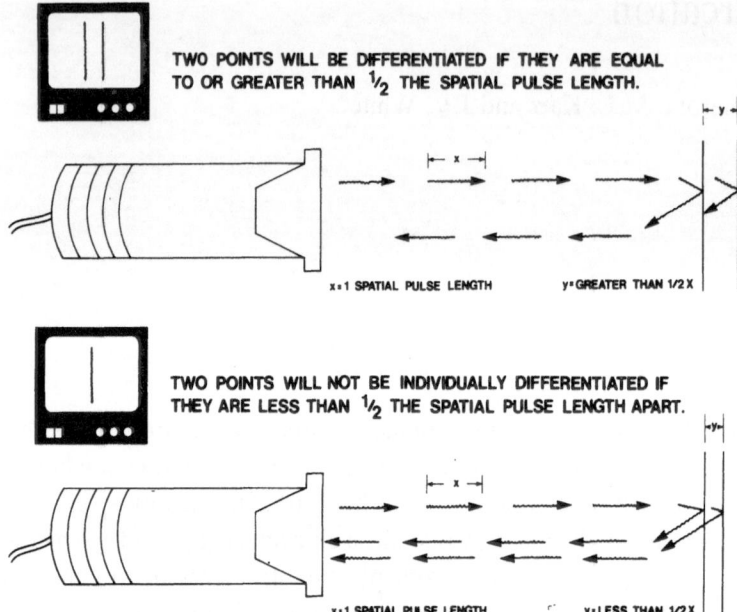

TWO POINTS WILL BE DIFFERENTIATED IF THEY ARE EQUAL
TO OR GREATER THAN ½ THE SPATIAL PULSE LENGTH.

x = 1 SPATIAL PULSE LENGTH   y = GREATER THAN 1/2 X

TWO POINTS WILL NOT BE INDIVIDUALLY DIFFERENTIATED IF
THEY ARE LESS THAN ½ THE SPATIAL PULSE LENGTH APART.

x = 1 SPATIAL PULSE LENGTH   y = LESS THAN 1/2 X

Figure 1. Schematic of the principle of axial resolution. (Reproduced with permission from Comerota, A.J. *et al.* Real-Time B-Mode Carotid Imaging in Diagnosis of Cerebovascular Disease. Surg., 1981, 89–6, 718–29.)

interpreted using standardized criteria [3]. During this analysis the influence of scan quality, technical experience and intracenter variability as well as the addition of indirect physiologic cerebrovascular studies were specifically evaluated.

Real-Time B-Mode ultrasound examines the majority of the vessel wall (Fig. 2). The method used for scanning as well as the interpretation of the tests have been previously reported [3] and will not be reviewed here. However, the importance of plaque orientation and plane of the ultrasound beam are illustrated in Fig. 3. Each ultrasonic scan and each arteriogram was divided into one of four grades of disease based on diameter reduction stenosis. The percentage of stenosis indicated by the scan and x-ray was determined by caliper measurement

Table 1. Real-Time B-Mode carotid imaging.

Patients		
7031	–	Patients studied noninvasively
877	–	Patients having carotid arteriography (8 pts. unilateral).
23	–	Vessels eliminated due to inadequate arteriographic visualization
1723	–	Total number vessels studied noninvasively and arteriographically

Patients studied.

SCHEMATIC OF RIGHT CAROTID EXAMINATION

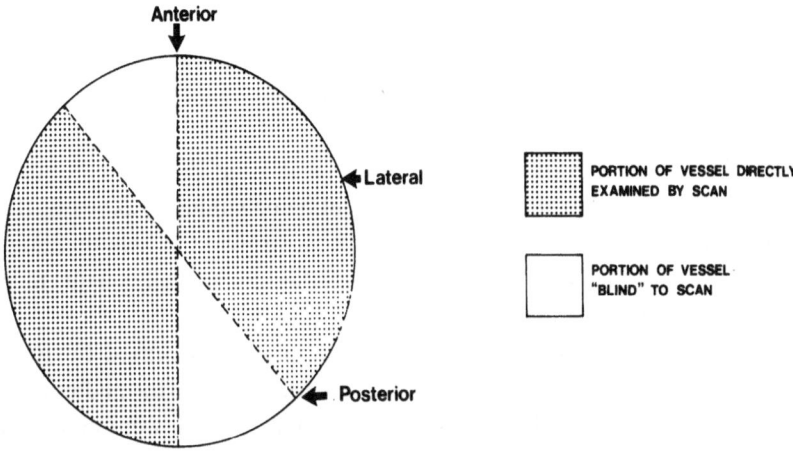

Figure 2. Shaded area represents circumference of vessel wall examined by Real-Time B-Mode carotid imaging technique. White area represents portion of vessel wall 'blind' to the scan in longitudinal section. (Reproduced with permission from Comerota, A.J. *et al.* Real-Time B-Mode Carotid Imaging in Diagnosis of Cerebrovascular Disease. Surg., 1981, 89–6, 718–29.)

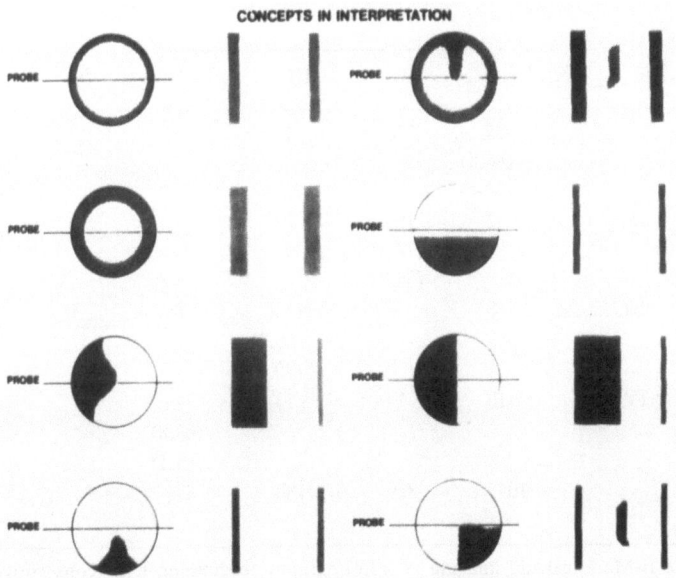

Figure 3. Various plaque configurations as they would appear in the longitudinal scan depending upon plane of transsection by ultrasound beam. (Reproduced with permission from Comerota, A.J. *et al.* Real-Time B-Mode Carotid Imaging in Diagnosis of Cerebrovascular Disease. Surg., 1981, 89:6, 718–29.)

of the narrowest portion of the lumen within the area of greatest disease compared with the most normal portion of the internal carotid distal to the stenosis. The four categories were Grade I (0–39% stenosis), Grade II (40–69% stenosis), Grade III (70–99% stenosis), and Grade IV (occlusion). The results of oculoplethysmography (OPG) were interpreted as positive or negative according to previously reported criteria.

Examination of the carotid arteries with Real-Time B-Mode carotid imaging provides direct structural detail of the vessel being studied. Likewise, the atheroma is directly visualized. Questions quickly arose as to whether important characteristics of the atheroma could be identified, specifically plaque ulceration and subintimal hemorrhage.

To evaluate whether ulceration could be reliably identified by Real-Time B-Mode carotid imaging a prospective evaluation was performed comparing it and standard arteriography to operative specimens which were considered the 'gold standard'. Ulcers were defined as sharp craters of 1 mm or more in diameter and 1 mm or more in depth. Scans and arteriograms were read independently prior to operation. Following endarterectomy and wound closure, the specimen was carefully inspected for the presence of ulceration.

Table 2. Real-Time B-Mode carotid imaging scan vs. arteriogram.

		Scan					
		I	II	III	IV	N.V.	Total
A-gram	I.	985 (86.5) (93.4)	113	18	3	20	1139
	II.	42	193 (72.3) (54.2)	24	2	6	267
	III.	18	39	133 (66.2) (70.7)	8	3	201
	IV	10	14	13	74 (63.8) (85.1)	5	116
Total		1055	359	188	87	34	1723

Real-Time B-Mode carotid imaging vs. arteriography, examining 1,723 consecutive vessels. The diagonal boxes represent the exact correlation of the scan with arteriogram. The numbers in parentheses represent specificity and negative predictive value for Grade I and sensitivities and positive preductive values for Grades II through IV. (Reprinted with permission from Comerota, A.J. *et al.* Real-Time B-Mode Carotid Imaging: A Three-Year Multicenter Experience. J. Vasc. Surg., 1984, 1:1, 84–95.)

Results

Accuracy

The complete distribution of scans compared with arteriograms is presented in Table 2. The diagonal four groups of numbers accompanied by footnote citations represent exact correlation of the scan with the arteriogram.

The specificity of the scan for detecting arteries with little or no stenosis was 86.5% (985/1139). The sensitivity for detecting Grade II disease was 72.3% (193/267); for Grade III disease, 66.2% (133/201); and for Grade IV disease, 63.8% (74/116). The negative predictive value of Grade I scans was 93.4% (985/1055). The positive predictive value (ppv) of Grade II scans was 54.2% (193/359); Grade III scans, 70.7% (133/188); and Grade IV scans, 85.1% (74/87).

There were 168 false positive scans, 136 false negative scans, and 34 internal carotid arteries were not visualized.

Image quality

The relationship of the quality and the predictive value of scans is presented in Table 3. A consistent relationship is observed; the better the quality of the scan the higher its predictive value. When relating quality and predictive value for each scan grade it was uniformly observed that the better the quality of the scan, the more reliable the result. The predictive values and the accompanying 95% confidence intervals for excellent or good quality scans are listed in Table 4. Larger 95% confidence intervals are noted with smaller patient groups.

Table 3. Quality vs. predictive value all scan grades.

	Correct	Incorrect	Total
Excellent	27 (100)	0	27
Good	747 (87.4)	107 (11.5)	854
Fair	556 (79.1)	147 (20.9)	703
Poor	55 (52.4)	50 (47.6)	105
Non-Viz	0	34 (100)	34
Total	1385 (80.4)	338 (19.6)	1723

( ) – Denote % predictive value.
Quality vs. predictive value for all scan and grades. The higher the quality of the scan the greater the predictive value. (Reprinted with permission from Comerota, A.J. *et al.* Real-Time B-Mode Carotid Imaging: A Three-Year Multicenter Experience. J. Vasc. Surg., 1984, 1:1, 84–95.)

Table 4. Real-Time B-Mode carotid imaging predictive value & 95% C.I. for each scan grade.

Scan grade	No. of scans	Predictive value	95% C.I.
I	585	97.3%	96–99%
II	155	61.3%	53–69%
III	103	75.7%	65–83%
IV	38	84.2%	68–95%

Real-Time B-Mode carotid imaging: predictive value and 95% confidence intervals for each scan grade (good and excellent quality scans). Note the 97% negative predictive value for Grade I scans of good quality and the narrow 95% confidence interval (96–99%). (Reprinted with permission from Comerota, A.J. *et al.* Real-Time B-Mode Carotid Imaging: A Three-Year Multicenter Experience. J. Vasc. Surg., 1984, 1:1, 84–95.)

Experience

The specificity and sensitivity per disease grade for each vascular laboratory participating in this study are represented by the graphs in Figure 4a–c. In each period there are consistent data shared by each vascular laboratory. There are no significant differences between laboratories for any disease grade or between either time period. Analyzing Figure 3 and 4, it is apparent that there is improvement in the diagnostic sensitivity for Grade III and Grade IV disease.

Figure 4c represents cumulative data obtained from three vascular laboratories comparing results of the first time period with the second time period. The improvement in the sensitivity for detecting Grade III disease is not statistically significant ($p = 0.12$). However there is a significant improvement in the ability to diagnose Grade IV disease (occlusion) ($p<0.002$). It is evident that experience did not improve the ability to detect a normal, mild or moderately diseased vessel.

→

Figure 4a. First period scan results comparing specificity and sensitivity per disease grade.

Figure 4b. Second period scan results for specificity and sensitivity.

Figure 4c. First period vs. second period specificity and sensitivity for each grade of disease. There is significantly improved sensitivity during second period for Grade IV disease. Although there is a trend toward improved sensitivity for Grade III disease, results do not achieve statistical significance ($P = 0.12$). (Reproduced with permission from Comerota, A.J. *et al.* Real-Time B-Mode Carotid Imaging: A Three-Year Multicenter Experience. J. Vasc. Surg., 1984, 1:1, 84–95.)

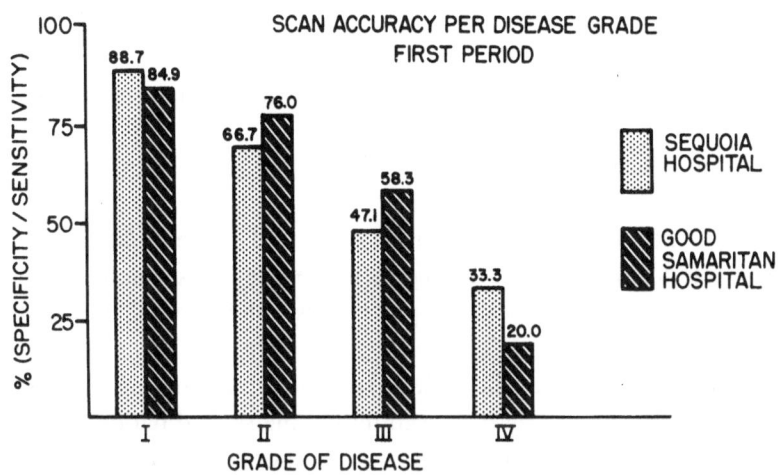

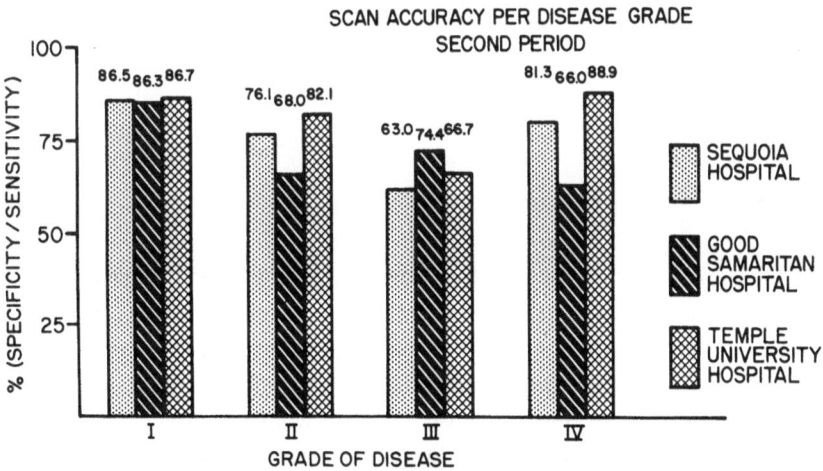

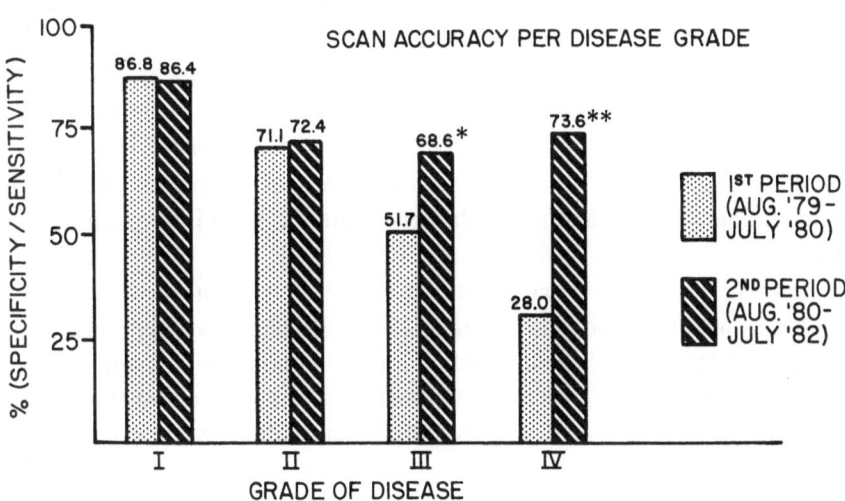

*P=0.12 **P<0.0002

Total occlusion

The criteria for the diagnosis of the completely occluded internal carotid artery are as follows:
(1) A technically good quality scan.
(2) Visualization of significant disease.
(3) The absence of radial wall pulsation distal to the area of disease.
(4) The absence of Doppler flow signals in the diseased segment and distally.
(5) Abnormal common carotid Doppler signals with loss of the normal diastolic flow pattern [4].

The sensitivity of diagnosing the occluded carotid was low during the first period; however, it was significantly improved during the second period of the study. Additionally, 47% (54/115) of patients with total occlusions were found to have greater than 50% stenosis of the contralateral carotid-artery; 70% (42/54) of the contralateral carotid arteries were accurately identified noninvasively.

Analysis of Errors

Stenosis

Each false positive and false negative scan was reviewed and the error placed into 1 of 11 categories (Table 5). Interpretation errors, scan/arteriogram mismatch and technically poor scans secondary to disease were responsible for the majority of the errors. In 7.4%, the internal carotid was not visualized high enough to see the stenosis. This was suspected in several instances when the direct carotid Doppler examination was abnormal and an OPG was positive. Misidentification of the external carotid for the internal carotid artery was responsible for 6.2% of the errors, and it appeared to be a more significant problem in the early part of the study. The inability of the B-mode carotid imager to detect red thrombus or soft plaque has been recognized as a major weakness of the technique and has contributed to diagnostic errors in over 1/3 of the patients in a previous report [5]. These problems were responsible for only 3.3% of the errors in this series. Artifact, anatomic variation and plaque orientation were infrequent causes of errors.

The good quality scan that identified more disease than the arteriogram is called a mismatch. When these false positive results were reviewed, no technical, anatomic or interpretive error could be found. Although it was our impression that these scans were representative of the existing disease and that the arteriogram underestimated the disease present, the mismatched scans are reported as false positive errors. Of the 79 mismatched vessels, 16 underwent carotid endarterectomy. In 14 the operative findings could be compared to the pre-operative studies. Twelve out of 14 (86%) demonstrated that the scan was more correct and in 2 of 14 (14%) the arteriogram more accurately represented the disease present. An additional interesting observation was that 70% of the OPG's in the mismatched group were positive, indicating a stenosis of >50% diameter reduction.

Ulceration

Fifty-six consecutive endarterectomy specimens were prospectively examined for ulceration. The scan and the arteriogram were evaluated preoperatively for the presence or absence of detectable ulceration. Fifty percent (28) of the patients had ulcers identified following endarterectomy. Ulceration was correctly identified in 61% (17/28) of the patients by B-Mode scan and 86% (24/28) of the patients by carotid arteriography (Table 6) (not significant p>0.14). Interestingly, the ma-

Table 5. Real-Time B-Mode carotid imaging frequency of errors overall.

	No. (%)
1) Interpretation error	90 (26.6)
2) Scan/Arteriogram mismatch	79 (23.4)
3) Technically poor/inaccurate scan disease	75 (22.2)
4) ICA not visualized high enough to see stenosis	25 (7.4)
5) ICA/Eca misidentification	21 (6.2)
6) Poor scan-cause uncertain	19 (5.6)
7) Red thrombus/soft plaque	11 (3.3)
8) Poor technique	8 (2.3)
9) Artifact	4 (1.2)
10) Anatomic variation	4 (1.2)
11) Plaque orientation	2 (0.6)
Total errors	338 (19.6)
No errors	1385 (80.4)
Total vessels	1723

Real-Time B-Mode carotid imaging: errors for all false positive and false negative scans in descending order according to frequency. (ICA = internal carotid artery; ECA = external carotid artery) (Reprinted with permission from Comerota, A.J. *et al.* Real-Time B-Mode Carotid Imaging: A Three-Year Multicenter Experience. J. Vasc. Surg., 1984, 1:1, 84–95.)

Table 6. B-Mode Carotid imaging Ulceration.

	Scan	X-Ray
Specificity	89% (25/28)	89% (25/28)
Neg. pred. value	69% (25/36)	86% (25/29)
Sensitivity	61% (17/28)*	86% (24/28)
Pos. pred. value	85% (17/20)	89% (24/27)

* Not significant.
Real-Time carotid imaging and arteriography and their ability to detect the ulcerated carotid plaque.

250

jority of the patients operated upon had high grade stenosis (Fig. 5a and b). Ninety-one percent of the arteries had >50% stenosis and 79% >70%. The overwhelming majority of the errors of B-Mode imaging occurred in highly diseased vessels. Seventy percent of the ulcers were correctly identified in vessels with <70% stenosis for both B-Mode ultrasound and arteriography.

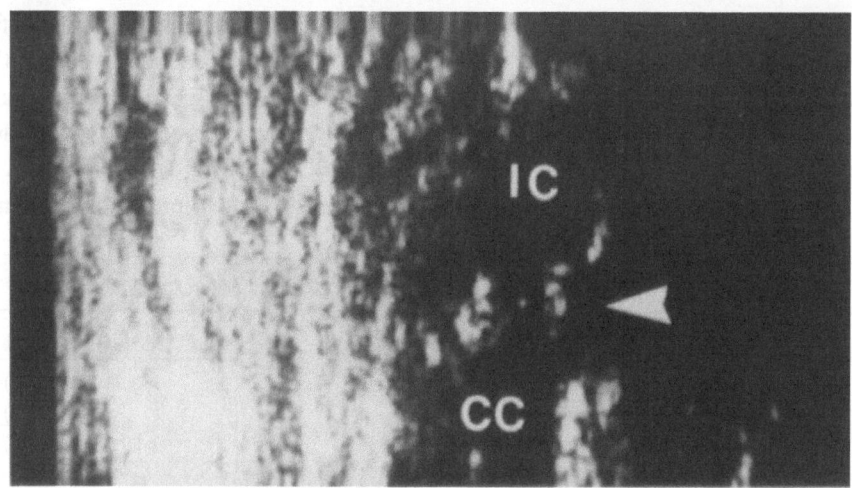

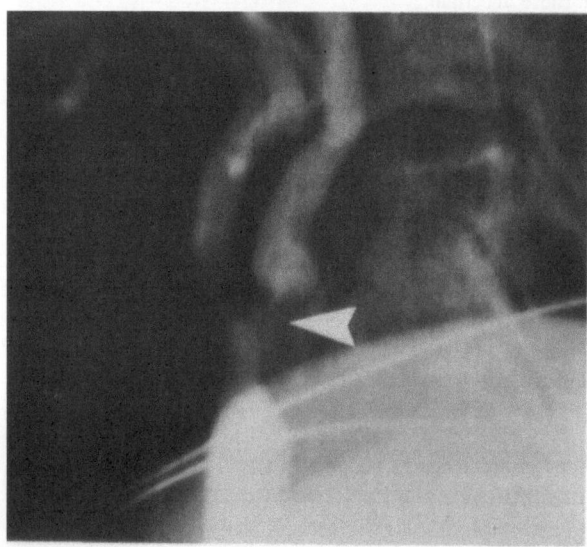

Figure 5a. B-Mode ultrasound of Grade III disease at origin of internal carotid artery. Note the irregularity of the plaque and intraplaque lucency.

Figure 5b. Corresponding arteriogram documenting high grade stenosis at origin of internal carotid artery.

Discussion

In determining sensitivity and specificity, arteriography was the standard used to judge the noninvasive study. As any noninvasive study approaches a 90% specificity or sensitivity, the reliability of arteriography may limit any further improvement by the noninvasive study because of the inconsistencies of arteriography. While it is well accepted that arteriograms can relatively reliably identify the normal and the highly diseased vessels, it has been clearly shown that arteriography does not reliably identify moderate disease [6]. The variability and inconsistency of carotid arteriographic interpretations have likewise been documented [7]. While it is not the intent of this report to evaluate arteriography, it is necessary to appreciate the shortcomings of the contrast arteriogram when the arteriogram is used as the standard for judging any noninvasive technique.

It seems appropriate that we should attempt to identify disease with more precision than the 'less than or greater than 50%' categories stenosis. Data suggest that symptomatic patients with hemodynamic lesions are at greater risk for stroke than symptomatic patients without hemodynamic stenosis [8, 9]. When compiling further data, it can be argued that selected asymptomatic patients with hemodynamically significant lesions have a higher risk of developing focal neurologic symptoms or stroke than symptomatic patients without a hemodynamic significant stenosis [8, 9, 10]. It has been further demonstrated that 50% of patients with an 80% stenosis or more are likely to develop TIA's or stroke [11].

The question of routine arteriography is raised when patients present with signs and symptoms suggestive of focal hemispheric ischemia. While angiography has been our routine in such patients, Ricotta et al. [12] have suggested that when noninvasive studies are clearly positive and lateralizing in patients with focal hemispheric ischemia, arteriography provides little, if any, additional information. Likewise, when patients present with a transient focal retinal or hemispheric symptom, and a technically good B-Mode scan fails to reveal any significant disease, the negative predictive value of that study is 97% with an extremely high 95% confidence interval. Therefore, the likelihood of documenting significant (surgically correctable) disease via arteriography is small. In this setting these patients might be appropriately treated with platelet inhibitors unless having recurrent and progressive symptoms, since the risk of a stroke is small in this patient population.

The consensus among vascular surgeons is that if a noninvasive technique could reliably identify an occluded internal carotid artery it would obviate the need for arteriography. During the initial experience with Real-Time B-Mode imaging, the sensitivity for diagnosing the occluded internal carotid was low (28%). However, with the integration and improvement of a pulsed Doppler system and establishing defined criteria for the ultrasonic diagnosis of occlusion, the sensitivity improved significantly during the next 24 month period to 74% (p<0.002). The positive predictive value of a good quality scan which diagnoses occlusion was 85%. It should be added that with continued experience the sensitivity for detecting the occluded internal carotid has further improved to 91%.

Difficulty in defining the degrees of stenosis often arises when evaluating scans and arteriograms showing disease in the carotid bifurcation. Since this is a bulbous area anatomically, a greater volume of atheroma will be required to produce a stenosis as previously defined. In selected instances, 50% of the bulb may be narrowed; however, relative to the distal internal carotid artery there may actually be minimal or no luminal narrowing. In such cases, does a stenosis truly exist? This was a major interpretative stumbling block in this analysis and remains a constant problem in all correlative studies of cerebrovascular diagnosis. Additionally, when one obtains a high resolution B-Mode image, there is an obvious difference in the diameter of the vessel during systole and diastole (Figs. 7 a–b). If one reads the study in diastole, a smaller luminal diameter would be calculated than if one were to read the study in systole.

Understanding the pathophysiology of atherosclerosis and the changes in vessel morphology as atheroma develop will also shed light on the reason for the large mismatch category and the low predictive value of the Grade II scans. In the formative stages of atheroma deposition degenerative changes occur in the elastic lamina with resultant dilatation of the vessel. Although the atheroma progresses, the lumen area is preserved, at least for a time. Since the B-Mode ultrasound technique is directed toward evaluation of the vessel wall, it will tend to draw attention to the disease contained within the wall. On the other hand, arteriography shows the residual lumen and does not address actual quantity of atherosclerosis present. When comparing these two techniques it becomes evident that the inherent nature of what is visualized by each image will prevent exact correlation.

Analysis of Real-Time B-Mode imaging for the detection of ulceration revealed that it was no better than arteriography. This is not truly surprising when one examines the specimens involved in this study. Since the majority of vessels evaluated contained extensive disease, it is reasonable to suspect that ultrasound will be unrealiable in detecting the nuances of surface plaque characteristics. The sensitivity of detecting ulceration improves substantially once the stenosis dropped < 70%. In evaluating these data with those reported by others, one must always consider the quantity of disease.

Attempts to evaluate for the presence of subintimal hemorrhage were discontinued because of the recognition that lucency within a plaque could represent much more than just blood. Calcification with drop out, dense and liquified atheroma, plaque of varying fat density and subintimal hematoma all have similar ultrasonic characteristics, i.e. intraplaque lucency. Rielly and colleagues [13] have most appropriately identified these plaques as 'heterogeneous'. That description might well represent the unstable plaque and such identification more realistically approaches the limits of B-Mode ultrasound. The findings that most

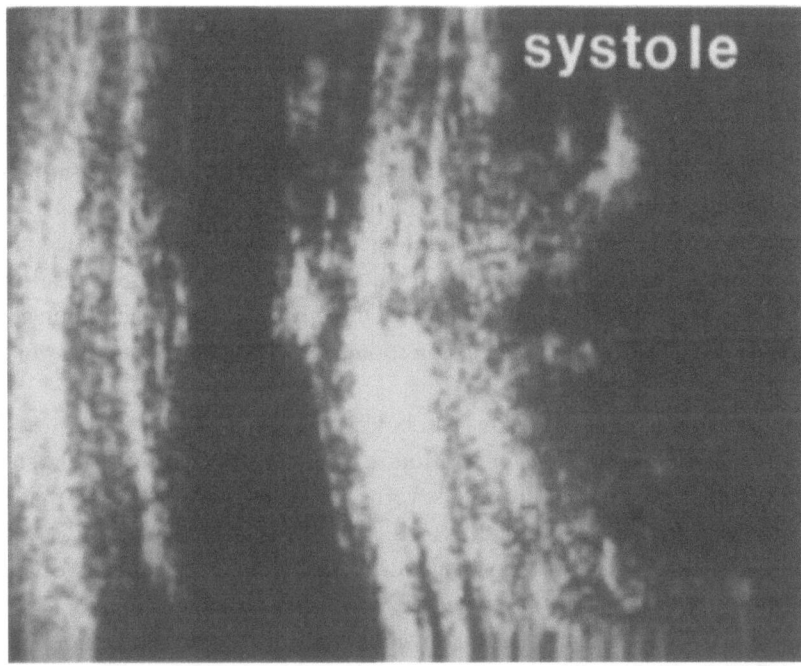

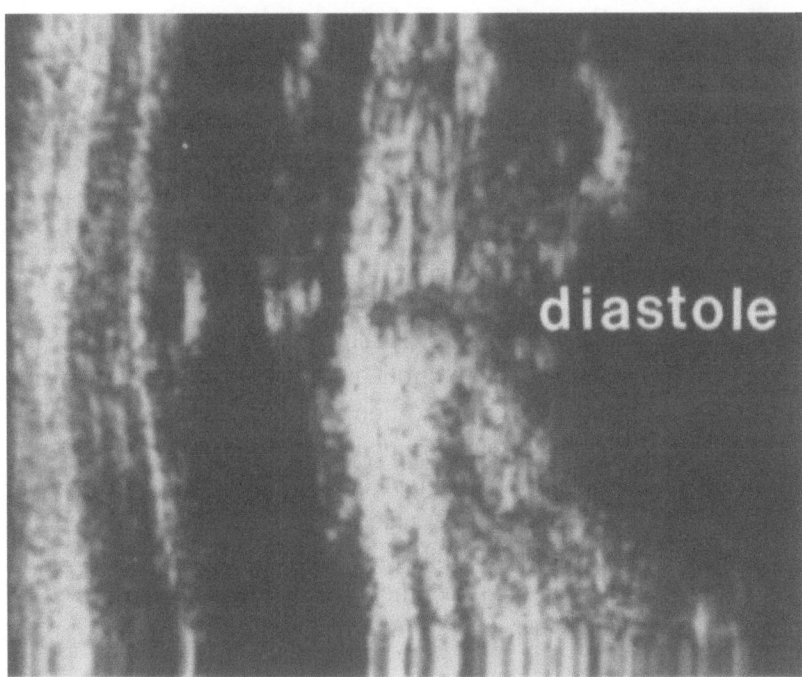

Figure 6a. en Figure 6b. Carotid artery examined with Real-Time B-Mode carotid ultrasound in systole and diastole. Note lumen size in systole vs. that of diastole is appreciably larger. This could contribute to errors when quantifying degrees of diameter reduction stenosis.

ulceration occurs in such heterogeneous plaque lends additional support to this approach.

To date we have no experience with spectrum analysis although we will have added spectrum analysis to our noninvasive cerebrovascular evaluation by the time of this printing. It is our contention that the addition of spectrum analysis will add to the reliability and reproducibility of the direct noninvasive carotid artery evaluation. Often it is difficult to determine the precise interface between the lumen and margin of atheroma in extensively diseased vessels, resulting in a judgment as to the degree of stenosis. Objective and reproducible physiologic parameters of flow through the lesion should assist in quantitating the stenosis in such cases.

Several important conclusions can be drawn from this study:

(1) The accuracy of Real-Time B-Mode carotid imaging is directly related to the quality of the image and the severity of disease. It was found that as the disease increases, the quality of the scan decreases. However, it was also demonstrated that a scan of good quality has a high predictive value no matter what the grade of disease.

(2) The normal vessel can be reliably identified within narrow confidence limits when a good quality scan is obtained.

(3) Significant improvement has been made in the diagnosis of a totally occluded carotid artery. Factors leading to the improved sensitivity include experience with the technique, defined diagnostic criteria, and an improved integrated pulse Doppler system.

(4) High carotid bifurcations and red thrombus within the vessel lumen may not be visualized.

(5) The resolution of the scan was better than that of the arteriogram in several cases with operative documentation. Therefore when a good quality scan shows disease not apparent on the arteriogram, the arteriogram is probably falsely negative.

(6) Indirect physiologic cerebrovascular studies are complementary to the direct anatomic study of Real-Time carotid imaging. Doppler spectrum analysis of flow through the carotid bifurcation will add detailed direct physiologic information and should significantly improve and refine these data.

(7) Comparable results can be obtained by other centers when similar techniques and interpretation criteria are used.

(8) The qualitative evaluation of atherosclerotic lesions may be possible, however, precise definition of ulceration and subintinal hemorrhage is difficult when significant disease is present.

References

1. Fields WS, *et al.*: Joint study of extracranial arterial occlusion as a cause of stroke. I. Organization of study and survey of patient population. JAMA 203: 153, 1968.
2. Sumner DS, Russel JB, Ramsey DE, Jajjar WM, Miles RD: Noninvasive diagnosis of extracranial carotid arterial disease, a prospective evaluation of pulsed-Doppler imaging and oculoplethysmoraphy. Arch Surg 114: 1222–9, 1979.
3. Comerota AJ, Cranley JJ, Katz ML, Cook SE, Sippel PJ, Hayden WG, Fogarty TJ, Tyson RR: Real-Time B-Mode carotid imaging, a three-year multicenter experience. J Vasc Surg 1:1, 84–95, 1984.
4. Breslau PJ, Fell G, Phillips DJ, Thiele BL, Strandness DE: The role of common carotid artery velocity patterns in the evaluation of carotid bifurcation disease. Arch Surg 117: 58–60, 1982.
5. Mercier LA, Greenleaf JF, Evans TC, Sandok BA, Hattery RR: High-resolution ultrasound arteriography: a comparison with carotid angiography. In: Bernstein EF, (ed.), Noninvasive Diagnostic Techniques in Vascular Disease, pp. 231–44, C.V. Mosby, St. Louis, 1978.
6. Croft RJ, Ellam LD, Harrison MG: Accuracy of carotid angiography in the assessment of atheroma of the internal carotid artery. Lancer 1: 997–1000, 1980.
7. Chikos PM, Fisher LD, Hirsch JH, Harley JD, Thiele BL, Strandness DE: Observer variability in evaluating extracranial carotid artery stenosis. Stroke 14: 6, 885–92, 1983.
8. Busuttil RW, Baker JD, Davidson RK, Machleder HI: Carotid artery stenosis-hemodynamic significance and clinical course. JAMA 245:14, 1438–41, 1981.
9. Mendelowitz DS, Limmins S, Evans WE: Prognosis of patients with transient ischemic attacks and normal angiograms. Arch Surg 116: 1587–91, 1981.
10. McRae LP, Crain V, Kartchner MM: In oculoplethysmography and carotid phonoangiography, Tucson. Tucson Medical Center, pp. 1–87, 1978.
11. Roederer GO, Langlois YE, Lusiani L, Jager KA, Primozich JF, Lawrence RJ, Phillips DJ, Strandness DE: Natural history of carotid artery disease on the side contralateral to endarterectomy. J Vasc Surg 1: 1, 62–72, 1984.
12. Ricotta JJ, Holen J, Schenk E, Plassche W, Green RM, Gramiak R, DeWeese JA: Is routine angiography necessary prior to carotid endarterectomy? J Vasc Surg 1: 1, 96–102, 1984.
13. Reilly LJ, Lusby RJ, Hughes L, Ferrell LD, Stoney RJ, Ehrenfeld WK: Carotid plaque histology using Real-Time ultrasonography. Clinical and therapeutic implications. Am J Surg 146: 188–93, 1983.

Clinical applications of high resolution B-scan imaging with pulsed Doppler profiles (10 MHz)

M. Hennerici

A variety of non-invasive techniques have been developed for the detection of extracranial arterial disease (EAD) in recent years [1–7]. Some of them assess the hemodynamics of the carotid system (e.g., continuous wave and pulsed Doppler, Doppler imaging, frequency spectrum analysis of bruits and Doppler signals), others attempt to visualize the morphology of the carotid system in the neck (high-resolution real-time ultrasound B-mode and duplex scanning). Since each of these techniques measures different parameters, the question arises as to what extent they provide similar or complementary information and how reliably they can diagnose the different stages of EAD. Although some of these non-invasive methods have been shown to be of high diagnostic value for the management and treatment of symptomatic patients with cerebrovascular disease, confusion still exists about medical strategies for asymptomatic subjects due to the considerable lack of knowledge on the natural history and the prognosis associated with EAD [8–10]. In particular, we often fail to predict the hemodynamic significance with regard to preservation or compensation of cerebral collateral circulation and hardly understand the mechanisms of progression and repair of small plaques and their risk of becoming sources of cerebral embolism. Thus, the major aim of research with recently developed highly sophisticated ultrasound imaging techniques, combined with new methods providing a more detailed analysis of intra-arterial flow characteristics, is to gain more accurate information about the interaction of alterations in morphology and flow disturbances, which are thought to reflect different hazards of extracranial carotid disease.

This chapter therefore concentrates on the advantages and limitations of both imaging and flow analysis systems by demonstrating selected examples from a series of investigations carried out during the last four years. A high resolution (10 MHz) imaging instrument with a specially designed 16-parallel-gated pulsed Doppler blood flow measuring device was used [5, 11–12], the reliability of which has been tested both in vitro and in vivo examinations [13].

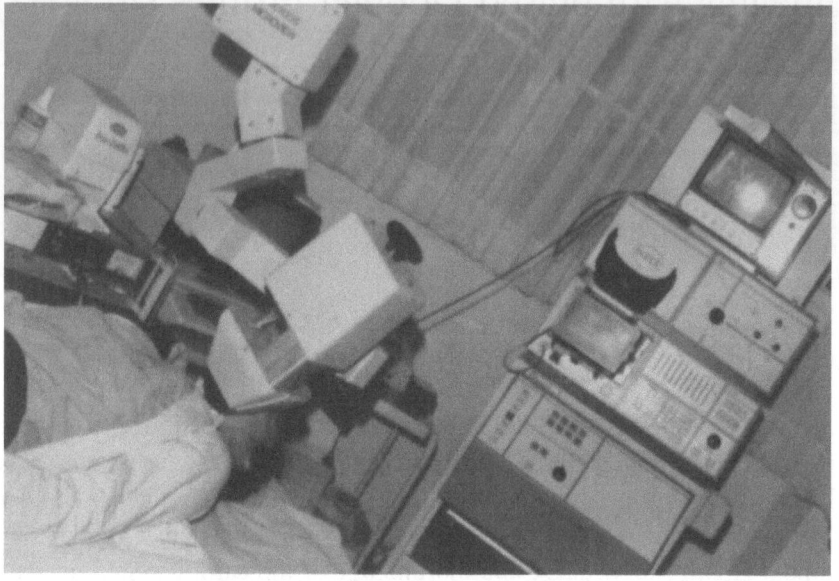

Figure 1. Duplex-system examination condition.

Materials and methods

A specially designed duplex system combining a high resolution B-scan with a multigated pulsed Doppler was used for ultrasonic imaging, as well as for the measurement of flow velocity profiles and flow volume of the extracranial carotid arteries (Fig. 1) [5].

The imaging component [11] (Picker Microview) consists of a linear mechanical, real-time B-scan operating at a nominal frequency of 10 MHz, covering a 3-cm × 4-cm area in either longitudinal- or cross-sections at 20 frames/sec. Lateral resolution is 0.5 mm, axial resolution 0.35 mm, thus providing instantaneous digitized display of the anatomical morphology under examination, giving 16 levels of grey. The probe of the 16 range-gated 5 MHz pulsed Doppler system is fixed laterally to the oscillating image transducer at an angle of 25°. Each of the 16 measurement volumes occupies 1 mm³.

As shown in Fig. 2, real-time B-mode images are generated on a TV-screen and used for adjustment of the Doppler-mode, which may be superimposed on any position in range and span within the center-scan line. Since simultaneous display of the B-mode and the Doppler-mode is not possible, the B-scan image and the flow velocity patterns across the arterial diameter, as well as the flow volume measurements for each cardiac cycle are displayed in correspondence with an A-scan recorded at the B-scan center line, where Doppler data are acquired.

This A-mode is superimposed on both displays and hence reflects small posi-

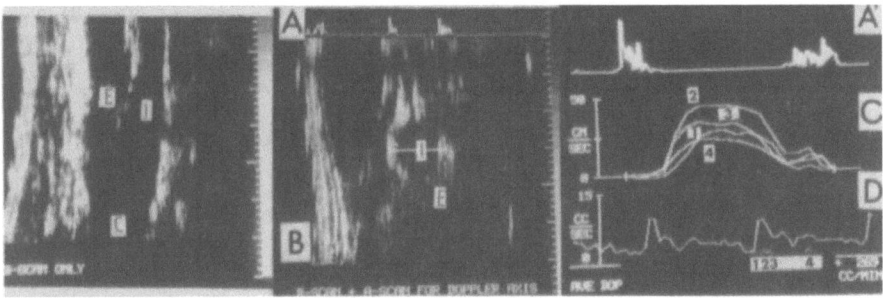

Figure 2. Duplex-system display. A longitudinal – (left) and a cross-sectional image (middle) of the neck with the common (C), internal (I) and external (E) carotid arteries is demonstrated. For correlation between these B-mode images and the Doppler-mode (right) and A-scan is superimposed in normal (A) and enlarged (A') size according to the B-scan center line. The multigated Doppler sampling line (white bar, middle) is adjustable in depth and width. The spatial distribution of flow velocity patterns (C) are indicated for selected sections of the cardiac cycle (1–4). Volume flow/time is indicated in D, the average flow rate (cc/min) is computed for 8 cardiac cycles in numerics.

tion changes of the probe, which is fixed in a tripod system to guarantee accurate and independent movements in all dimensions. The Doppler system generates about 30 profiles/sec leaving approximately 30 profiles/cardiac cycle. A fixed number of eight cardiac cycles may be averaged and the distribution of these velocity profiles then displayed at selected intervals of the cardiac cycle.

In addition, instantaneous quantitative volume flow measurements may be computed using a special algorithm for each 16-channel data set by assuming semicircular symmetry for the vessel examined. A numerical integration is performed by summing the product of each Doppler velocity sample and the corresponding semi-angular area. In addition, a flow estimate averaged over eight cardiac cycles is computed by summing the instantaneous volume flow values. However, since each measurements could only be taken on false assumption at the site of arterial obstructions, volume flow measurements could only be performed outside such areas. The reliability of the device to measure volume flow has been studied in a series of *in vitro* tests. In a model system, human blood (100–500 ml) was pumped through a teflon tube (4, 6, and 8 mm in diameter respectively) by a constant flow pump from one graded cylinder to another and the time required for transfer was measured. The ratios between the value of volume flow measurements and the actual flow are shown in Fig. 3.

In vivo flow volume measurements were restricted to the common carotid artery. 30 normal subjects of different age and sex were studied with particular attention to CO_2 reactivity, since initial examinations revealed a comparatively high intra- and intersession variability of results ($\pm 20\%$) [14]. Regular measurements of expired end-tidal percent CO_2 with an Engstroem analyzer stabilized the situation by reducing these variations to $\pm 10\%$.

Apart from a series of carotid arteries examined *in vitro* in a post-mortem study

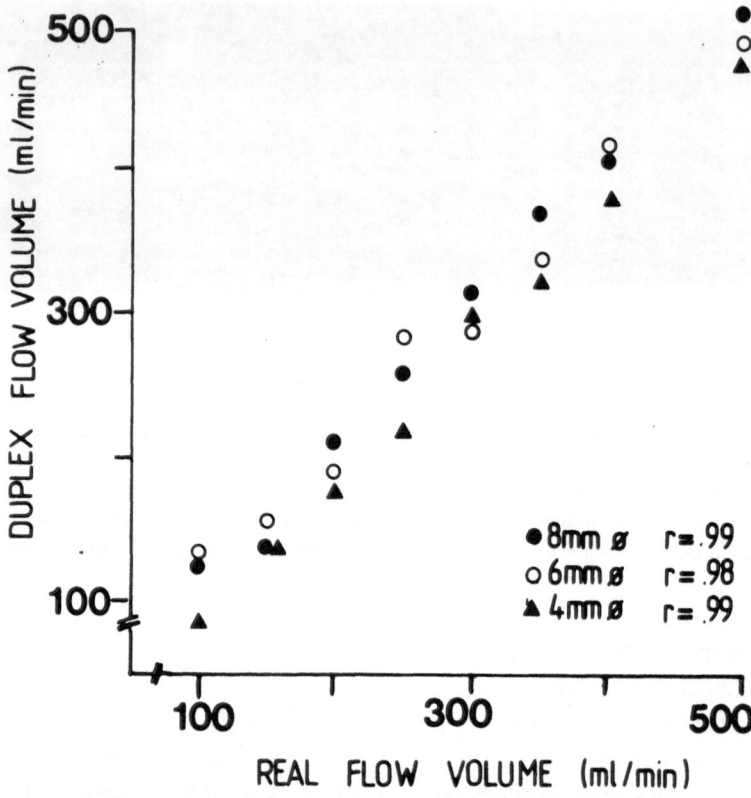

Figure 3. Doppler-mode volume flow readings and real-flow volume measurements for different tube diameters and constant flow conditions.

[13] approximately 2,500 patients have been examined in our department using this duplex-system. Patients considered for this manuscript showed a history and/ or signs of recent transient ischemic attacks or strokes, subarachnoid hemorrhages and migraine attacks, while others were neurologically asymptomatic but at high risk of having EAD because of coronary or peripheral atherosclerosis and/ or cervical bruits [15].

Results

In a series of both *in vitro* and *in vivo* examinations duplex-system analysis provided valuable information on various stages of carotid atherosclerosis. The system proved to be very useful in detecting and determining early, non-stenotic lesions and low grade stenosis rather than for evaluation of hemodynamically significant obstructions of the carotid artery as shown by a comparison of arteriographic and duplex system results performed in 134 patients (193 carotid arteries) in Table 1 [5]. Unfortunately, a technically unsatisfactory examination rate of 19%, the failure to differentiate total from sub-total carotid occlusion and

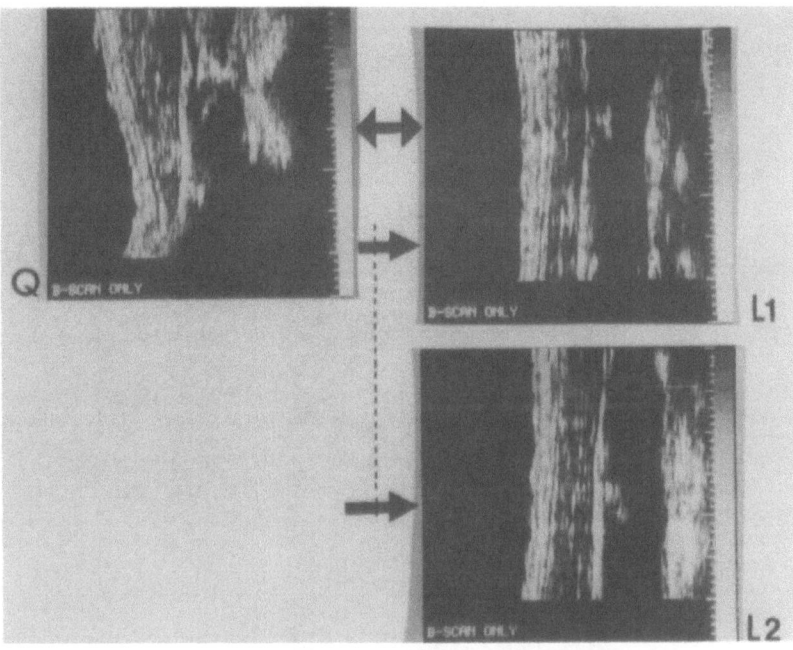

Figure 4. High-resolution images of soft carotid plaques in cross- (Q) and separate longitudinal-sections (L1/L2) indicating the need for multi-sectional examinations for accurate evaluation of the lesion's morphology.

underestimation of significant stenosis as well as impracticable vertebral flow studies were major disadvantages, while visualization of the morphology of small plaque in three dimensions (Fig. 4) and high accuracy in separating ulcerative from smooth surfaces made this technique favorable.

Despite these limitations, test-accuracy using duplex-system examinations versus angiography was 96% in detecting significant carotid obstructions (>50%); however, the more severe a stenosis, the poorer its morphological ultrasound

Table 1. Comparison of arteriographic and duplex-system results in 134 patients (193 carotid arteries) [5].

Arteriogram	Duplex-system				
	Normal	<50% stenosis	>50% stenosis	Occlusion	Equivocal
Equivocal (6)	6	–	–	–	–
Normal (59)	37	12	–	–	10
<50% S. (61)	6	45	–	–	10
>50% S. (57)	–	–	43	–	14
Occlusion (10)	–	–	2	5	3

262

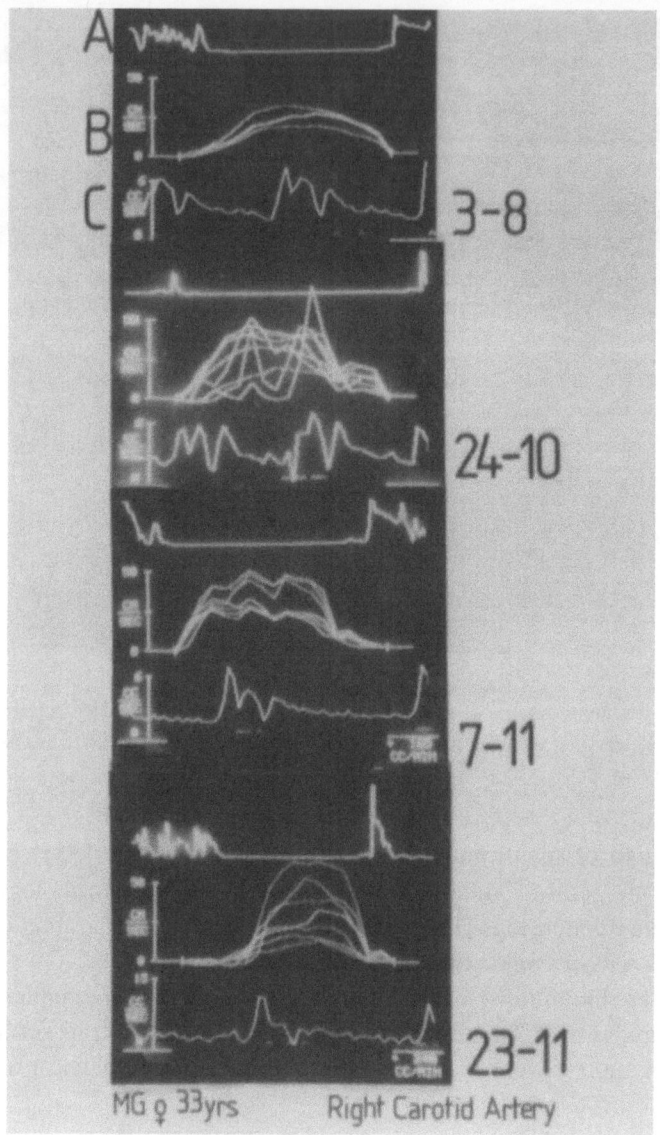

Figure 5. Sequential Doppler-mode displays (A: A-scan, B: flow-velocity pattern, and C: flow-volume measurements) of the common carotid artery of a 33-year-old female patient with left hemiplegic migraine attacks and right subtotal carotid stenosis at the onset of symptoms (3–8). Despite rapid clinical recovery within 2 days, the extensive extracranial spasm only gradually improved; repeated examinations showed severe (24–10) and moderate flow velocity pattern alterations with restoring flow volume (7–11) and normal conditions about 4 months later (23–11). Flow volume could not be measured initially due to the extent of the spasm involving the bifurcation and the distal common carotid artery similarly seen in the angiogram.

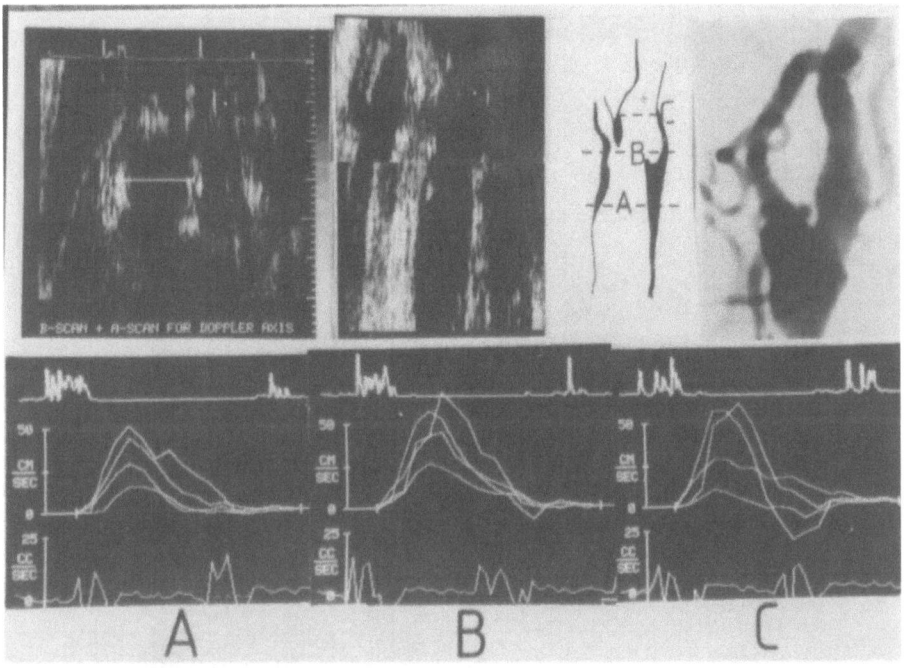

Figure 6. B-mode images, corresponding angiogram and Doppler-mode profiles (flow-velocity cm/sec; flow-volume cc/sec) from three sections of a mild carotid stenosis (A, B, C) as indicated in the schematic drawing (inset).

image. Consequently, correct estimation of the degree of stenosis was achieved in only 27 of 43 cases (63%) listed in Table 1. Loss of ultrasound energy beyond calcifications and sharp angulation of the vessels preventing perpendicular insonation were the major reasons for inadequate visualization of the arterial lesion.

In contrast, differentiation of the morphology of plaques was excellent with regard to extent, surface and structure: 'flat', 'soft' and 'hard plaques' as well as 'complicated plaques' with hemorrhages and ulcerations could be reliably separated as revealed by comparison with angiography and/or postendarterectomy histology [13]. In addition, the capacity of the system to detect initial stages of atherosclerosis was superior to angiography, providing reasonable ultrasonic visualization could be achieved in different longitudinal- and cross-sections.

The combination of the B-mode imaging device with a multigated pulsed Doppler system proved to be essential for a reliable diagnosis in order to avoid misinterpretation, as the latter compensated for some disadvantages of the B-mode, e.g. the distinction between intra-arterial flow and recent thrombus and the estimation of local flow alterations being diagnostic in the presence of sonolucent and shadowed plaques behind echodense lesions.

A few parameters characterizing various patterns of flow alterations could be established (Figs. 5 and 6) such as increasing peak velocity throughout a signifi-

264

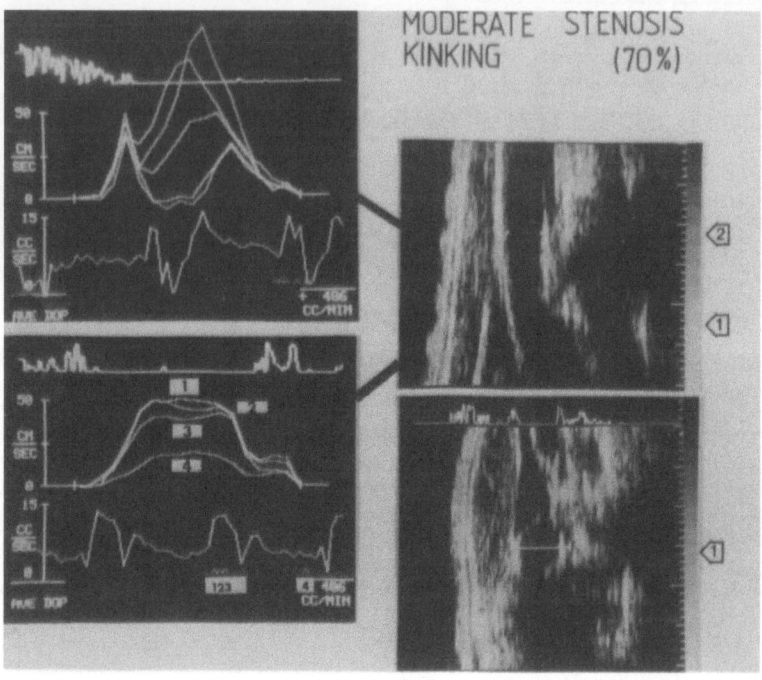

Figure 7. In the right hand panels: High-resolution B-mode display of a moderate stenosis within a kinking of the internal carotid artery in cross- and longitudinal-sections. In the left panels: Doppler-mode data was recorded as indicated by the numbered arrows. Proximal (1) and distal = (2) to the lesion normal-dichotomic velocity profiles occur at (1) nearby the bifurcation but considerably distal to the lesion (2), although the morphology of the vessel is normal at the distal site.

cant stenosis, decreasing flow velocity proximal to a severe obstruction, local flow decelerations, reversed flow and asymmetries of the normal laminar and/or dichotomic flow profiles [16] nearby the bifurcation in the presence of less obstructive lesions. However, the occurrence and degree of such parameters vary considerably and cannot be predicted or even suggested from the morphology of atherosclerosis as revealed by the B-scan image alone (Fig. 6): in this case small plaques are only slightly encroaching the lumen of the vessel at the anterior and posterior walls nearby the bifurcation and can hardly be seen at the slope of the internal carotid artery deep in the neck. Contrary to what one might have assumed, flow velocity profiles are quite similarly asymmetric with maximum values at the anterior wall throughout the area of the vessel affected and, in particular, show increasing velocity ratios (systole; diastole) until having passed beyond the extent of the lesion from proximal to distal sections, but reversed flow during the systole only nearby the distal, unaffected, contralateral wall.

Fig. 7 similarly illustrated the various alterations of flow, which are far more complex than has been suspected from FFT-analysis of single-gated Doppler systems [3]. Whereas, normal flow velocity profiles could be recorded from the common carotid artery nearby the bifurcation, distal to the stenosis, separation of the flow profiles and reversal of axial flow were most markedly pronounced in morphologically (B-mode) normal vessels. The separation (erratic) flow profiles downstream are presumably representing turbulent blood flow. Please see Chapter 9.

The profiles are even more complex if alterations of the flow velocity profiles are measured from different angles of insonation. *In vitro* experiments [17] have shown that the introduction of small, non-stenosis encroachments in a bifurcation model produce highly complex velocity profile alterations with separation and reversal of axial flow as well as the development of counter rotating helical trajectories. Further studies may reveal, whether atherosclerosis tends to progress in such areas rather more than in regions where unidirectional and laminar flow remains preserved.

Since no definite characterization has yet been established to differentiate normal flow disturbances from abnormal flow turbulences, the interpretation of the latter is questionable. This is especially true in cases of normal B-mode images, although they are more likely to be physiological in younger people than in elder ones.

In addition, flow abnormalities are not necessarily attached to morphologically B-mode detectable lesions but may well be observed in their absence (e.g. in the presence of 'sonolucent plaques' and vice versa. Fig. 8 illustrates some flow abnormalities in a large common carotid artery with only soft subintimal echogenicity seen.

Abnormalities sound in Migraine patients may, however, cause considerable flow changes in the absence of any detectable atherosclerotic lesions.

A typical example is given in Fig. 9, which relates to the case of a 28-year-old man who had repeated attacks of left hemiplegic migraine. Although carotid arteriography performed between attacks was fairly normal (as were flow-volume and flow-velocity measurements), a considerable asymmetry of flow volume and flow-velocity profiles could be demonstrated during the attack. This asymmetry persisted for a fortnight, despite the patient's relief of symptoms within one day suggesting the presence of functionally significant vascular spasms. Similar observations were made in 30 patients with migraine, as well as in patients with subarachnoid hemorrhages, who showed considerable changes of extracranial carotid volume-flow and velocity profiles even in the absence of clinical alterations.

Local flow alterations are not always due to pathological processes but may occur throughout the extracranial carotid system and at the bifurcation physiologically, as can commonly be observed in young people. They tend to reflect even minor sequential changes of the cardicac output from one cardiac cycle to the next and are hence most evident in patients with marked respiratory or absolute arrhythmia. They are commonly prominent at a particular interval either of the systole or the diastole but can vary within a cardiac cycle occasionally.

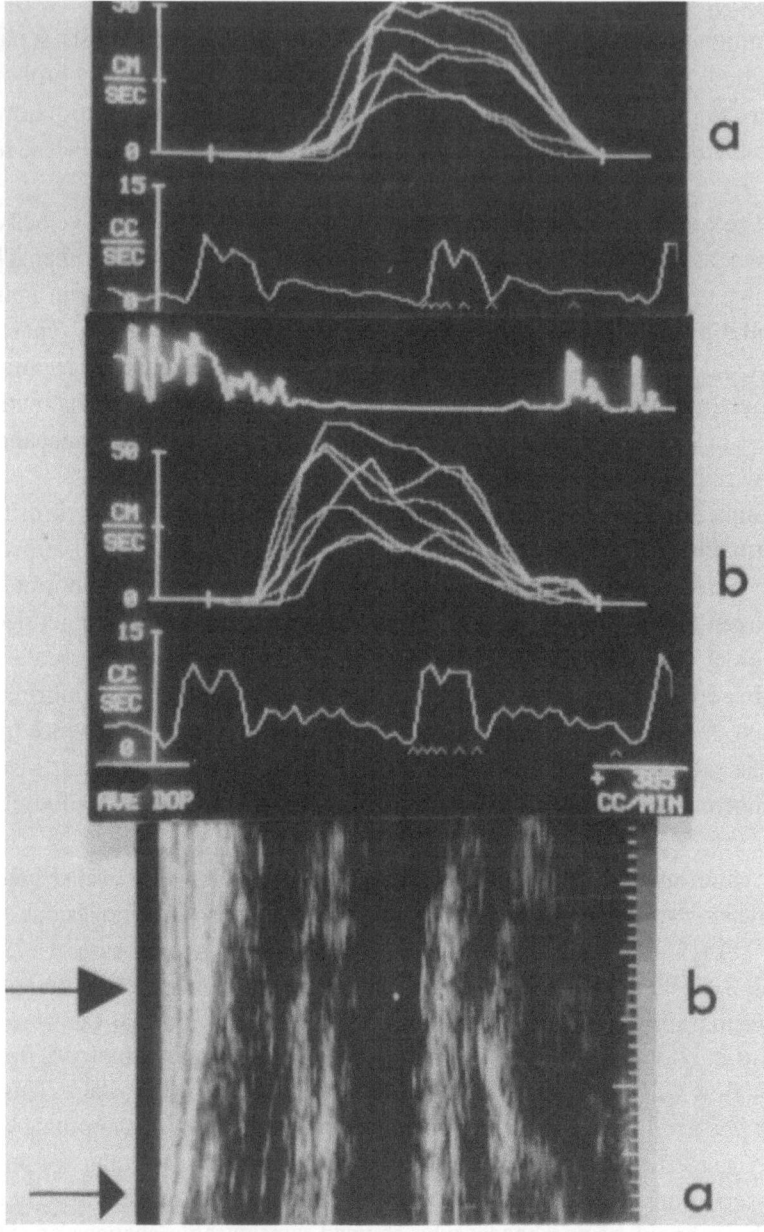

Figure 8. Comparison between Doppler-mode and B-mode displays in a common carotid artery with non-obstructive but severe dilative atherosclerosis. Normal (a) and only slightly asymmetric velocity profiles nearby the bifurcation (b) were recorded from cross-sections.

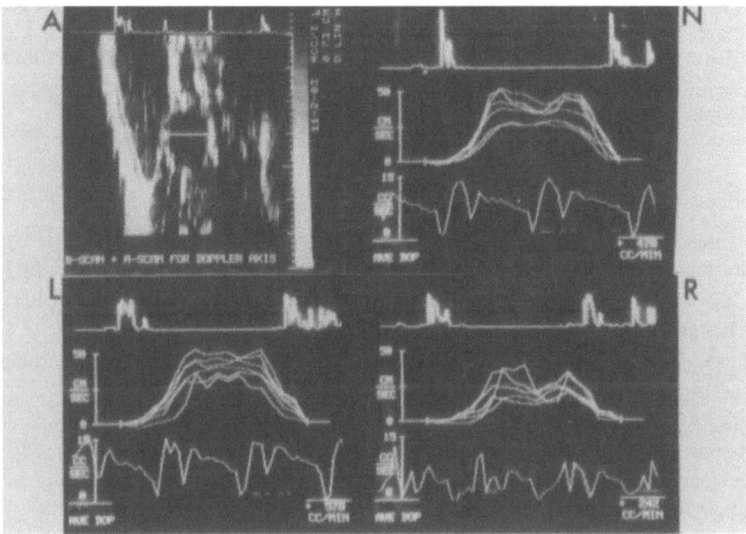

Figure 9. Flow-velocity and flow-volume measurements from the common carotid arteries of a 28-year-old man with focal migraine. During the attack, flow volume was asymmetrical with a considerable decrease on the right (R: 242 cc/min) and marked increase on the left (L: 578 cc/min), the latter causing considerable turbulence, as shown by the flow velocity undulations. During the interval between subsequent attacks, bilateral flow-volume and flow-velocity curves were symmetrical and normal (N:470 cc/min)[18].

Conclusion

High-resolution ultrasound imaging (10 MHz) represents a valuable method for the diagnosis of extracranial carotid disease if combined with a pulsed Doppler examination. The latter compensates for some disadvantages of the B-mode technique and particularly improves the detection rate for significant obstructive lesions. Visualization of the morphology of small plaques represents the main challenge for such a system and can usually be established with an accuracy higher than with angiography. The application of a multigated pulsed Doppler device in such a duplex system enables the investigation of interactions between hemo-dynamic parameters and the morphology of the lesion considered for the first time and is particularly necessary for an accurate estimation of volume-flow and velocity-pattern interaction. However, with the system used, this examination technique is highly time consuming and produces an enormous amount of data for further analysis with respect to its clinical and pathophysiological significance. We therefore mainly use this system for research follow-up studies of the natural history of initial stages of atherosclerosis, which may provide more information about the prognosis and risks associated with the disease.

Acknowledgements

The author gratefully acknowledges continuous support by the Deutsche Forschungsgemeinschaft SFB 200 (D2).

References

1. Pourcelot L: Continous wave Doppler techniques in cerebral vascular disturbances. In: Reneman RS, Hoeks APG (eds.) Doppler Ultrasound in the Diagnosis of Cerebrovascular Disease. Chichester, Research Studies Press, pp. 103–128, 1982.
2. Spencer MP, Reid JM: Cerebrovascular evaluation with Doppler ultrasound. Martinus Nijhoff Publ., The Hague, 1981.
3. Roederer GO, Langlois YE, Chan AW, Primozich J, Lawrence RA, Chikos PM, Strandness DE: Ultrasonic Duplex scanning of extracranial carotid arteries: Improved accuracy using new features from the common carotid artery. J Cardiovasc Ultrasound 1: 373, 1982.
4. Hoeks APG: On the development of a multi-gate pulsed Doppler system with serial data-processing. Thesis, University of Limburg, 1982.
5. Hennerici M, Freund HJ: Evaluation of the efficacy of different ultrasound methods for the detection of extracranial arterial disease. J Clin Ultrasound 12: 155, 1984.
6. McRae LP, Kartchner MM: Real-time B-mode ultrasonic carotid imaging with gated Doppler. In: Herskey FB, Barnes RW, Sumner DS (eds.) Noninvasive Diagnosis of Vascular Disease. pp. 281–298, 1984.
7. Zwiebel WJ: High-resolution B-mode and duplex carotid sonography. In: Zwiebel WJ (ed.) Introduction to Vascular Ultrasonography. pp. 103–149, Grune & Stratton, New York, 1982.
8. Mohr JP: Asymptomatic carotid artery disease. Stroke 13: 431, 1982.
9. Chambers BR, Norris NW: Stroke risk and asymptomatic carotid stenosis. Stroke 15: 189, 1984.
10. Hennerici M, Rautenberg W, Mohr S: Stroke risk from symptomless extracranial arterial disease. The Lancet II: 1180, 1982.
11. Green PS, Taenzer JC, Ramsay SD, Holzemer JF, Suarez JR, Marich KW, Evans TC, Sandok BA, Greenleaf JF: A real-time ultrasonic imaging system for carotid arteriography. Ultrasound Med Biol 3: 129, 1977.
12. Taenzer JC, Burch DJ: Real-time Doppler blood flow measurements: Qualitative and quantitative. Proceedings 6th International Symposium on Ultrasonic Imaging and Tissue Characterisation (Abstract), 1981.
13. Hennerici M, Reifschneider G, Trockel U, Aulich A: Detection early atherosclerotic lesions by duplex scanning of the carotid artery. J Clin Ultrasound 12: 455, 1984.
14. Uematsu S, Yang A, Preziosi TJ, Kouba R, Toung TJK: Measurement of carotid blood flow in man and its clinical application. Stroke 14: 256, 1983.
15. Hennerici M, Aulich A, Sandmann W, Freund HJ: Incidence of asymptomatic extracranial arterial disease. Stroke 12: 750, 1981.
16. Keller HM, Meier WE, Anliker M, Kumpe DA: Noninvasive measurement of velocity profiles and flow in the common carotid artery by pulsed Doppler ultrasound. Stroke 7: 370, 1976.
17. Zarins CK, Giddens DP, Bharadway BK, Sottiurai VS, Mabon RF, Glagov S: Carotid bifurcation atherosclerosis. Circ Res 53: 502, 1983.
18. Hennerici M, Trockel U: The clinical significance of blood flow measurements. Life Support Systems – in press, 1985.

Intraoperative Doppler sonography

J. Gilsbach and A. Harders

Intraoperative Doppler sonographic investigations on large vessels, e.g., on the carotid artery of the neck, can be carried out with commercially available continuous wave or pulsed systems having emitted frequencies between 4 and 10 MHz [1, 2, 3, 4, 5, 6, 7]. In some cases it is also possible to make recordings on microvessels. These systems do not allow further probe miniaturization and resolution increase, both of which are prerequisites for the intraoperative use of the Doppler ultrasound method on vessels with diameters of 1 mm or less.

Up to now, only two satisfactory microvascular Doppler systems have been developed [8] and tried in experimental and plastic microsurgery [9, 10, 11, 12, 13]. During the last 4 years, the Freiburg group has been studying the intraoperative application of one of these microvascular Doppler systems in neurosurgery. The method seemed ideal for atraumatic intraoperative control of the neurovascular procedures for aneurysms, angiomas, and bypass surgery. We expected to be able to check the surgical effects on the manipulated vessel itself, especially the (un)disturbed patency or (in)complete occlusion.

Materials and methods

Most recordings were done with a 3 mm standard probe, which is sufficient for superficial vessels. However, because of the narrow conditions at the circle of Willis at the base of the brain, 1 mm probes were preferable for recordings on this structures (Fig. 1). For direct intraoperative investigations, the probes could be sterilized by gas. The transcutaneous application was resticted to superficial vessels because of the limited penetration depth of the high frequency system (in clinical practice no deeper than 5 mm). The Doppler device used was a 20 MHz pulsed system (Fig. 2, Table I) with a built-in zero-crosser, automatic gate shift, adjustable pulse repetition frequencies, and adjustable pulse durations (pulse duration = duration of the receiving period). We exclusively used a pulse repetition frequency of 100 kHz, which offered the highest resolution. The theoretically

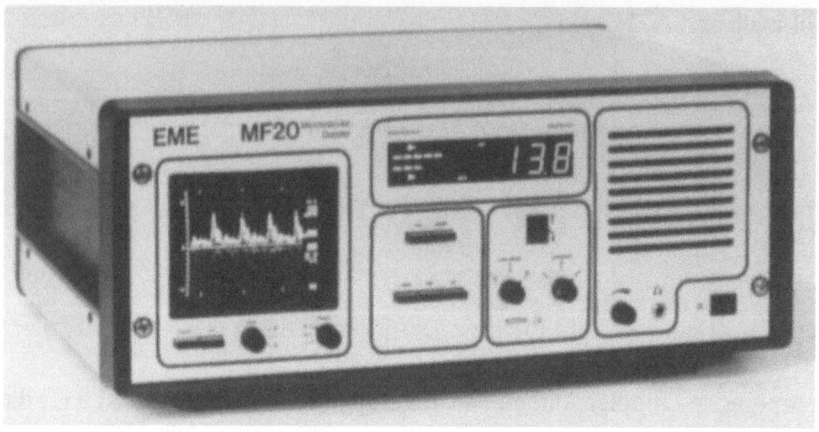

Figure 1. Microvascular Doppler device. 20 MHz pulsed system with miniaturized probes.

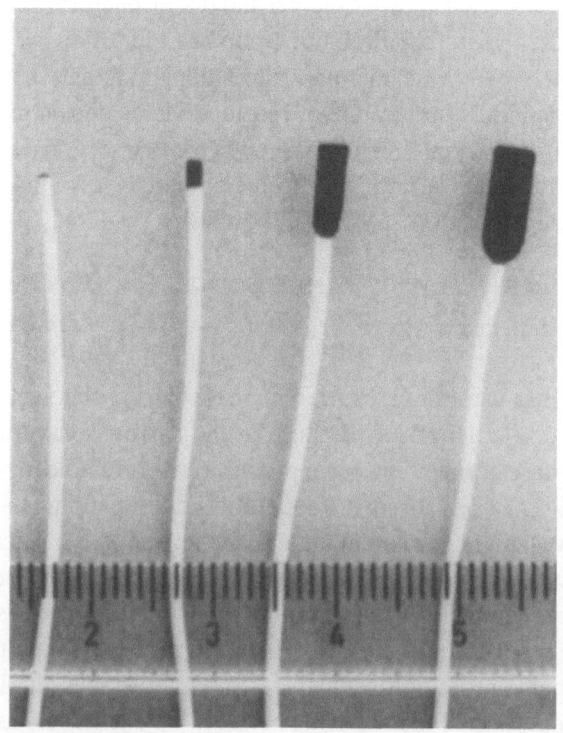

Figure 2. Different types of sterilizable probes for intraoperative use on arteries and veins with diameters larger than 0.1 mm.

possible detection of 50 kHz Doppler shift (1/2 of the pulse repetition frequency) was limited to about 10 kHz by the filter arrangement. But in neurosurgical clinical practice frequencies higher than 8 kHz were seldom found in cases of angioma and severe vasospasm.

Signal processing by the zero-crossing principle was abandoned in favor of the real time spectrum analysis (Angioscan I and II), which also in microvessels provided better and more complete information. More than 90% of the visible intracranial vessels with diameters greater than 0.15 mm could be recorded after coupling the probe with a drop of blood or saline. For recordings in the basal cisterns, the pulsed system proved useful because it helped to exclude other vessels commonly lying in the direction of the ultrasonic beam.

In some cases, the restricted working space, the anatomical properties, and the diameter of the probe posed hindrances to the investigation. Because of the relatively large sample volume, reliable flow profile measurements or recordings exclusively in the center stream could not be performed in vessels with diameters less than 1–2 mm [14]. We, therefore, chose to work with gates which were at least as large as the vessel itself and used the profiles only to estimate the diameter in comparison with neighboring vessels. For the microvascular Doppler system, as for many other Doppler systems, the ideal incident angle was found to be between 40 and 60 degrees with slight deviations. A reproducible angle adjustment [15] also proved favorable under open surgical conditions.

Results

Normal cases

In cases of small basal tumors or aneurysms in the asymptomatic stage, the flow pattern of normal cerebral vessels under open operative conditions could be studied. The flow pattern corresponded to those of the cervical internal carotid

Table 1. Technical datas of the Doppler device.

20 MHz Pulsed Ultrasonic Doppler Velocity Meter

transmitted frequency:	20 MHz
pulse durations:	250, 450, 850, 1500 ns
axial resolution:	0.4, 0.7, 1.3, 2.3 mm
lateral resolutions:	0.5, 1.1 mm
pulse repetition frequencies:	25, 50, 100 kHz
measuring depth:	7.5, 15, 30 mm
maximum detectable Doppler shift:	12.5 kHz
minimum detectable Doppler shift:	0.1 kHz

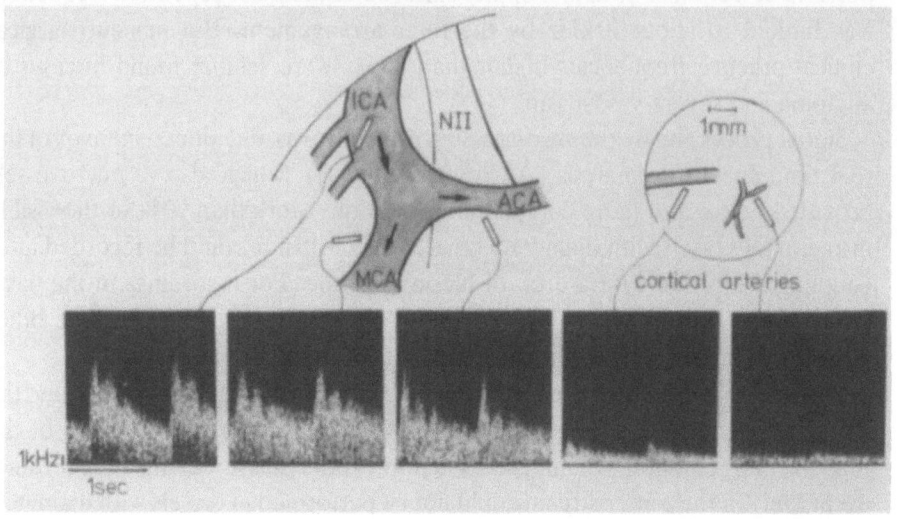

Figure 3. Intracranial vessel tree with typical flow pattern of a normal cerebral circulation. The flow velocities decrease depending on the decrease of the vessel diameters.

artery with a high diastolic flow component. With decreasing diameter the pulsations diminished and the diastolic flow increased relative to the systolic flow (Fig. 3).

The velocities in the internal carotid artery were equal to those in the trunk of the middle cerebral artery. The anterior system and the branches of the middle cerebral artery had slower velocities. The flow pattern changed, depending on the compliance and the peripheral resistance. Intraoperatively, we often found high flow velocities with a high diastolic component after releasing spatula pressure or a temporary clip or after discontinuing a sodium nitroprusside infusion. This velocity increase was taken to be a sign of reactive hyperemia with low resistance (Fig. 4). In contrast, in cases of hypercapnia or arteriosclerosis, there was increased resistance with a steep systolic amplitude and a low diastolic flow.

Aneurysm cases

Even under the operating microscope, sometimes uncertainties remained about the exclusion of the aneurysm and the patency of the parent artery, since we had to rely on the occasionally misleading outer aspect. To overcome the problems of not being able to look into the vessel after clipping, resection or suture, we needed an instrument to provide repeated, atraumatic, and direct control of the (un)disturbed patency from the outside. A striking discrepancy between a satisfactory outer aspect and a markedly reduced inner diameter after clip positioning was found in approximately 10% of our cases (Table 2). In the majority of cases,

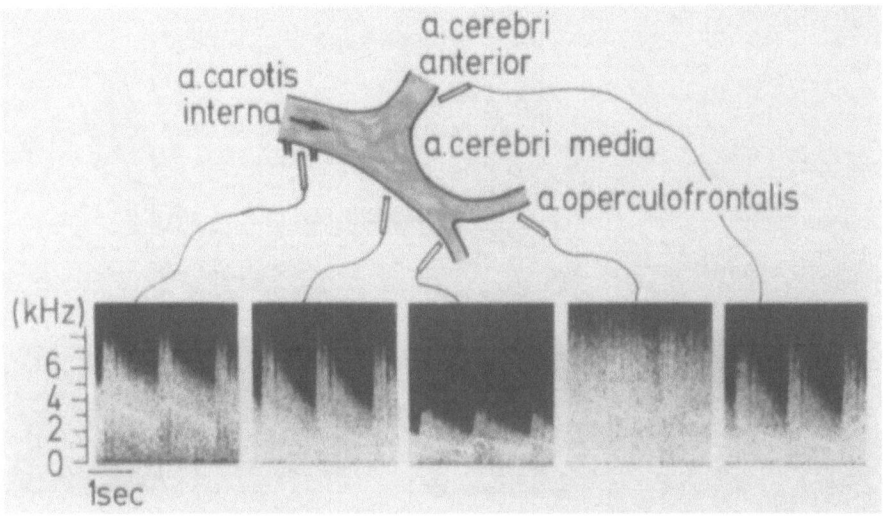

Figure 4. Internal carotid artery with its branches. In the territory of the middle cerebral artery there are accelerations with a high diastolic flow component. In this case they were a sign of a reactve hyperemia after the brain spatula pressure was released.

the patency could be restored without undue time loss by repositioning the clip or by resectioning and suturing the neck.

Hemodynamically effective stenoses due to a tight clip could easily be detected by flow velocity that was markedly reduced in comparison with the original findings (Fig. 5). The recordings of a local acceleration (important for recognizing a minor stenosis) was mostly restricted by the size of the probe, the spring of the clip, and the narrow conditions at the base of the brain. Due to the reaction of the intracranial vessel walls to manipulations, changes of the blood gas and blood pressure, and often changes of the flow pattern during the operation could be

Table 2. Doppler induced changes of the operative strategy in 8 cases out of 74 aneurysm operations (10.8%) (MCA: middle cerebral artery, ACA: anterior cerebral artery, ACoA: anterior communicating artery).

Aneurysm	Initial findings	Final procedure
MCA	stenosis of the parent artery	coating
MCA	occlusion of one MCA branch	aneurysm resection
ACA	occlusion of the distal ACA	and neck suture
MCA	occlusion of one MCA branch	aneurysm resection and neck clipping
MCA	occlusion of the MCA trunk	
MCA	stenosis of the MCA trunk	clip
MCA	stenosis of one MCA branch	repositioning
ACoA	stenosis of the distal ACA	

274

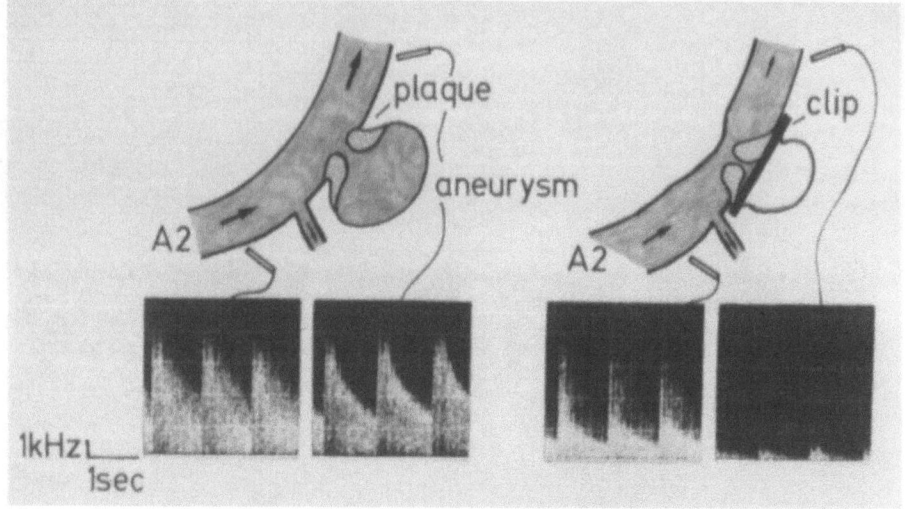

Figure 5. Distal anterior cerebral artery aneurysm. After an attempt to position the clip a marked reduction of the flow velocities in the distal segment occurred. In this case a definite exclusion was not possible (A2: distal anterior cerebral artery.

observed. This restricted the significance of the absolute value of frequencies or velocities, as do the anatomical properties which could not guarantee an optimal and reproducible incident angle.

Localized accelerations in one or more segments of the circle of Willis occurred in 65% of the patients who were operated on between day 4 and day 21 after the last hemorrhage (Figs. 6 and 7).

Vasospasms were also found in 9% of acute surgery cases. But a re-valuation of the patient's history revealed that there had been other recent bleedings.

The intraoperative Doppler findings of 140 individual vessels in 45 patients could be compared with the angiographically proven diameters (angiography under the same anesthesia). A good correlation between acceleration and vasospasm could be established (Table 3). In no case did the Doppler system fail to

Table 3. Comparison between intraoperative accelerations and direct postoperative angiographically proven diameters. Severe means a 60–80% stenosis and moderate 30–60%.

Doppler	Angiography		
	No/moderate stenosis	Severe stenosis	Occlusion
no/moderate stenosis	80%	0%	0%
severe stenosis	12%	5%	0%
occlusion	0%	0%	3%

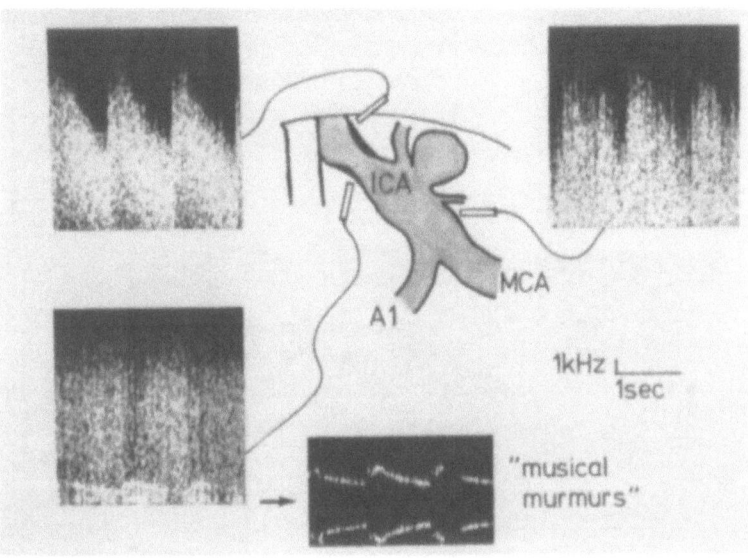

Figure 6. Internal carotid artery (ICA) aneurysm at the origin of the posterior communicating artery. Vasospasm and visible calcified plaque with a consequent lumen narrowing and accelerated flow velocities. Within the irregular flow pattern nearly pure sinus like tones ('musical murmurs') due to wall vibrations.

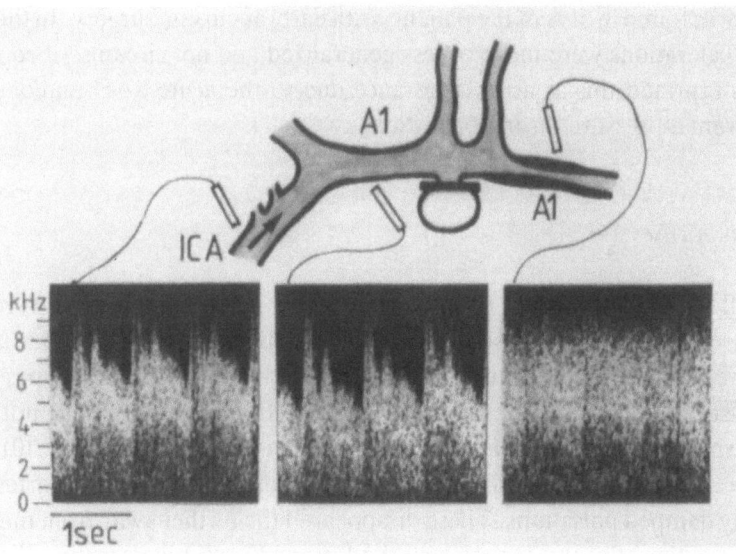

Figure 7. Anterior communicating artery aneurysm. Relatively high velocities in the internal carotid artery and the right anterior cerebral artery either due to a moderate lumen narrowing or reduced peripheral resistance. Marked localized acceleration with irregularities in the left anterior cerebral artery as a sign of a significant lumen narrowing (vasospasm).

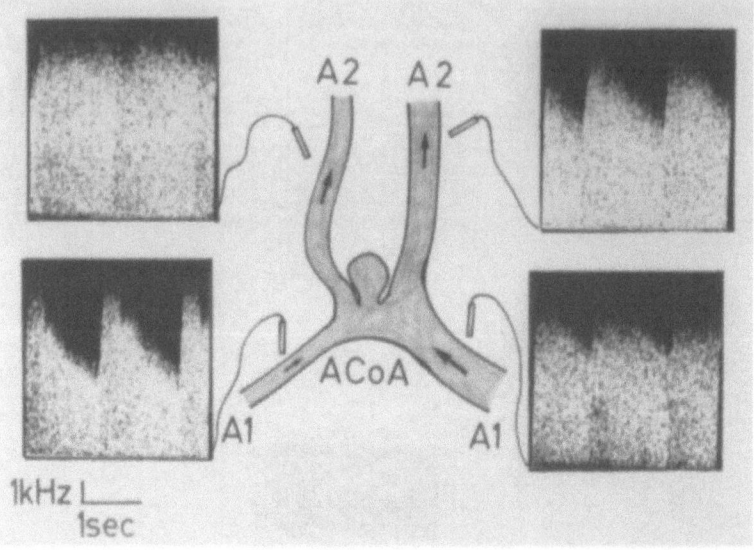

Figure 8. Anterior communicating artery aneurysm with generally high and irregular flow pattern as a sign of a reduced peripheral resistance, which is a common finding in early aneurysm surgery.

detect severe stenosis. In 12% the angiography showed normal diameters despite high velocities. In these cases the spasm had disappeared until the end of the operation or a reduction of the peripheral resistance caused the acceleration. The latter was found in 51% of the patients with early aneurysm surgery. In these cases the accelerations were more or less generalized and not circumscribed (Fig. 8). We interpreted this as a low resistance due to the acute SAH and/or lowered intracranial pressure during operation.

Angioma cases

High flow velocities with a relatively high diastolic flow component were typical in vessels feeding an angioma or a fistula. Depending on the caliber and flow volume, the flow pattern varied from accelerated forms to irregular types (Fig. 9). A vessel feeding both the angioma and the normal brain could not be distinguished from a purely pathological, angioma-feeding vessel (Fig. 10).

The venous flow pattern in the vicinity of the angioma looked like arteries with slightly damped pulsations. These disappeared the further away from the malformation. Clinically, the Doppler method proved useful in detecting, localizing, and tracing feeders of the angioma. The progressive exclusion of the shunt could be recognized by the decrease of the diastolic flow in the feeding arteries (Fig. 10). The method could detect remnants of the angioma in visible areas. But a Doppler control in the neighboring tissue was judged not considered reliable enough to rule out a residual fistula. This could be achieved only by angiography.

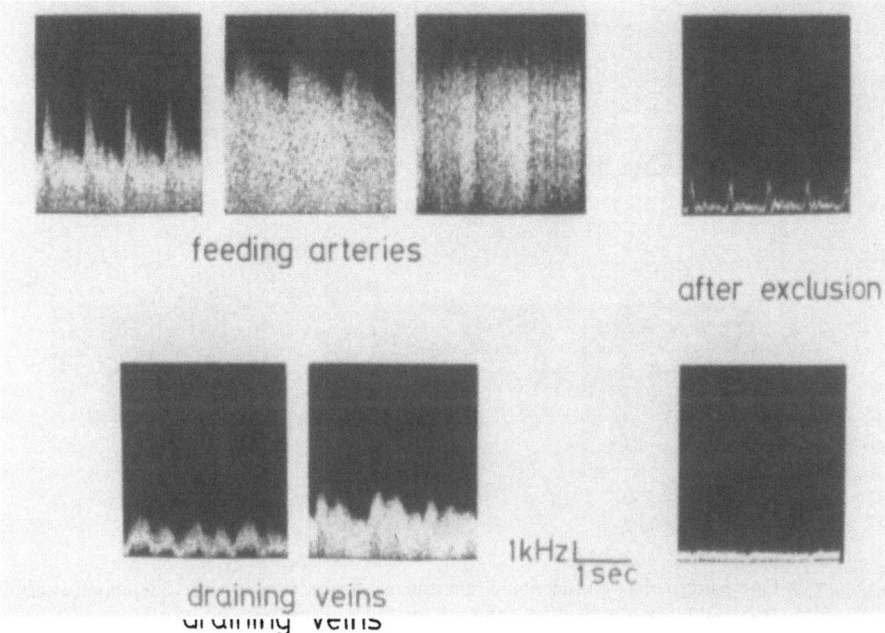

Figure 9. Intracerebral arteriovenous malformation. Depending on the diameter and flow volume in the arteries, an accelerated to irregular flow with high diastolic components are found. The veins show marked pulsations but with smooth peaks.

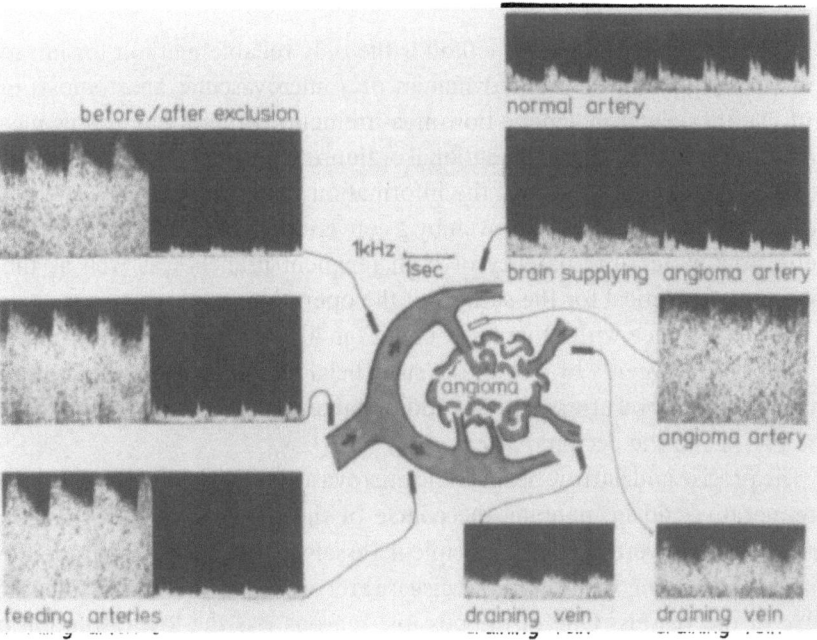

Figure 10. A-V malformation in the postcentral region. Note the very similar flow pattern of a vessel supplying the angioma exclusively and of a vessel supplying the brain and the angioma. It was not possible to distinguish between them. Note also the change of the pattern after exclusion of the shunt with signs of a slow flow and high resistance.

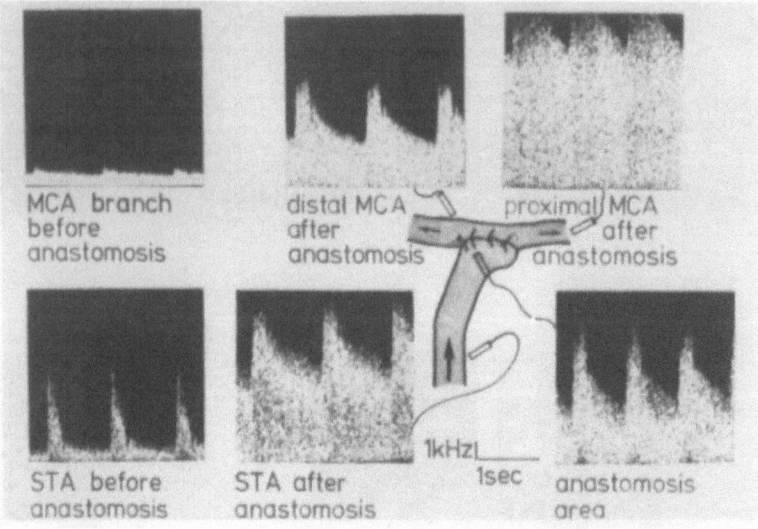

Figure 11. Flow pattern of a well-functioning anastomosis between the superficial temporal artery and a branch of the middle cerebral artery. Note the bidirectional flow in the recipient vessel and the increase of the velocities both in the recipient vessel and in the donor artery, in which a change from the external to internal type can be observed.

Extracranial-intracranial bypass cases

The microvascular Doppler method is the only reliable method for intraoperatively investigating the hemodynamics of a microvascular anastomosis in man [16]. Neither electromagnetic flow measurement, cerebral blood flow measurement, nor intraoperative conventional or fluorescein angiography proved acceptable for routine use. Besides the information about the patency of the donor artery, which can easily be proven by a conventional Doppler or an electromagnetic flow meter, the patency of both recipient branches as well as the flow direction are critical for the success of the operation.

Our experience with Doppler is based on 40 extracranial-intracranial bypass operations between a branch of the superficial temporal artery and a branch of the middle cerebral artery and two additional recordings of anastomoses between the PICA and the occipital artery.

The precise and narrow beam of the microvascular Doppler system was a useful preoperative aid in mapping the course of the donor artery on the skin. All arteries which were chosen as recipient vessels had had an orthograde flow. In one paper dealing with the same disease, recordings could be obtained in only 29% of the vessels. One of the possible reasons was the low resolution of the 4 MHz device used [4]. The pre-existing flow was pathologically slow as in a vein in cases with bilateral internal carotid artery occlusions. In cases with unilateral occlusion only two thirds of the patients had a pathologically slow flow. In cases

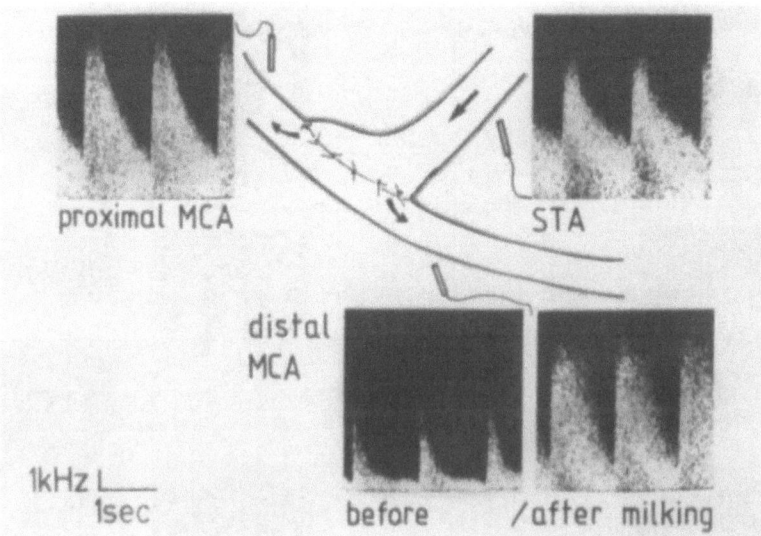

Figure 12. Flow pattern of an anastomosis with a stenosis of the distal acute angled part of the suture. After milking, a normal bypass flow could be restored.

with stenoses of the internal cervical artery, only one half of the velocities measured were too slow. All anastomoses were done as end-to-side sutures with a fishmouth incision of the donor artery. In all patients, recordings could be obtained from all parts of the anastomosis, including the suture area itself.

After the temporary clips were released, 90% of the anastomoses showed an undisturbed flow. They had no irregularities and no marked accelerations at the site of the temporary clip or in the suture region. With one exception, all recipient arteries had a postanastomotic bilateral flow. That means that in addition to the orthograde distal flow, there was a reversed flow towards the sylvian fissure in the proximal segment of the recipient vessel. The mean flow velocities in the recipient artery were on the average 3–5 times higher than before anastomosis. The flow velocities in the donor artery were also 3–4 times higher than before anastomosis and the flow pattern changed from the external type to the internal type (Fig. 11).

About 10% of the patients had stenosed or occluded anastomoses. The absence of the Doppler signal or a 'dead end' signal was a clear sign of an occlusion, which we observed almost exclusively in the donor artery between the site of the temporary clip and the suture area.

In cases of a hemodynamically effective stenosis, the typical increase of the flow velocities was not observed, the pulse waves were damped, and the amplitudes small (Fig. 12). In the case of a donor artery stenosis, the typical retograde flow in the recipient artery did not start. An immediate correction with lasting patency was possible in every case.

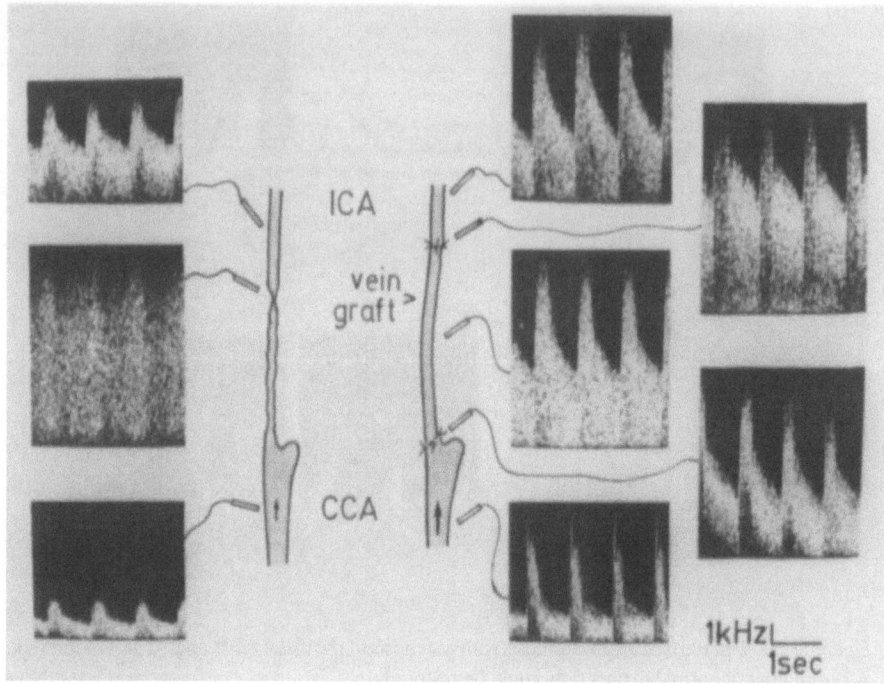

Figure 13. Flow pattern in a case of cervical carotid artery stenosis after a previous operation. Note the marked local acceleration with a pathological slow distal flow velocity as a sign of a hemodynamically effective stenosis. After a second operation with the interposition of a vein graft, the normal flow velocity in the internal carotid artery is restored. Note the only slight acceleration in the suture area as a sign of a perfect anastomosis.

Anastomoses

In microvessels (Fig. 14) as in larger vessels (Fig. 13), the (un)disturbed patency of any type of anastomosis could be judged with the microvascular Doppler system. Stenoses of more than 40–50% of the vessel diameter could be detected [16]. The quality of an anastomosis could be determined depending on the local accelerations and the change of the flow pattern. Severe hemodynamically effective narrowings could be corrected without any loss of time.

Final remarks

The microvascular Doppler system is a useful tool for simple and direct intra-operative control of neurovascular procedures. Due to the high emitted frequency, all manipulable vessels as small as 0.5 mm and less can be recorded. The system possesses all of the inadequacies found in the ultrasound Doppler flowmeter. But in clinical practice, neither the angle dependency, nor the problems with

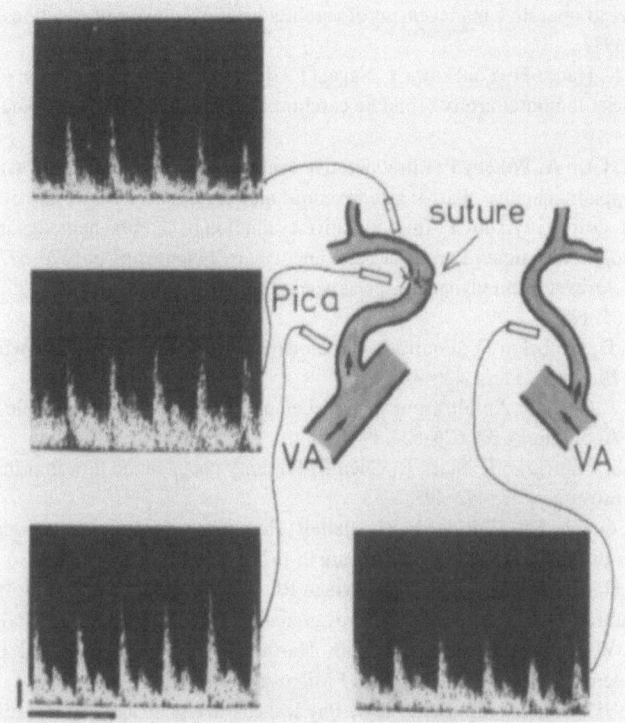

Figure 14. Flow pattern of both posterior inferior cerebellar arteries of which the left one was inadvertently cut and had to be reanastomized. Note the discrete acceleration in the suture area and the normal distal flow velocity as a sign of a well functioning anastomosis.

the frequency processing, nor the restrictions posed by the fact that only the flow velocity and not the flow is measured were important. The qualitative information provided by the flow pattern, the relative changes of the velocities, and the local accelerations and irregularities sufficed to give evidence of the unsatisfactory vascular operations which had to be corrected.

In the future, using double crystals and microcomputers it should be possible to obtain the absolute velocity. Furthermore, if the angle can be known and additional diameter measurements can be made possible, the flow volume can then be determined. That should eliminate the last criticism of the Doppler ultrasound method.

References

1. Meier WE, Keller H: Der Wert intraoperativer Carotis-Doppler-Sonographie im Hinblick auf Prognose bzw. postoperativen Verlauf. Helv Chir Acta 43: 107, 1976.
2. van Beek AL, Link WJ, Bennett JE: Ultrasound evaluation of microanastomoses. Arch Surg 110: 945–949, 1975.
3. Hitchon PW, Kassell NF, Carlstrom TA, McDonnell DE: The Doppler ultrasonic flowmeter as

an adjunct to operative management of cerebral arteriovenous malformations Surg Neurol 11: 345–347, 1979.

4. Moritake K, Handa H, Yonekawa Y, Nagata I: Ultrasonic Doppler assessment of hemodynamics in superficial temporal artery – middle cerebral artery anastomosis. Surg Neurol 13: 249–257, 1980.

5. Nornes H, Grip A, Wikeby P: Intraoperative evaluation of cerebral hemodynamics using directional Doppler technique. Part 1: arteriovenous malformations. J Neurosurg 50: 145–151, 1979.

6. Nornes H, Grip A, Wikeby P: Intraoperative evaluation of cerebral hemodynamics using directional Doppler technique. Part 2: saccular aneurysms. J Neurosurg 50: 570–577, 1979.

7. Nornes H, Grip A: Hemodynamic aspects of cerebral arterio-venous malformations. J Neurosurg 53: 456–464, 1980.

8. Cathignol D, Chapelon JY, Fourcade C: Velocimètre Doppler à l'usage des petits vaisseaux. Le Microflo. Biosigma, Paris, 426–429, 1978.

9. Hartley CJ, Cole JS: An ultrasonic pulsed Doppler system for measuring blood flow in small vessels. J Appl Physiol 37: 626–629, 1974.

10. Antunes JL, Muraszko K, Stark R, Chen R: Pituitary portal blood flow in primates: a Doppler study. Neurosurgery 12: 492–495, 1983.

11. Blair WF, Greene ER, Eldridge M, Cipoletti R: Hemodynamics after microsurgical anastomosis: the effects of topical lidocaine. J Microsurg 2: 157–164, 1981.

12. Freed D, Hartley CJ, Christman KD, Lyman RC, Agris J, Walker WF: High-frequency pulsed Doppler ultrasound: a new tool for microvascular surgery. J Microsurg 1: 148–153, 1979.

13. Pinnella JW, Spira M, Erk Y, Freed B, Hartley C: Direct microvascular monitoring with implantable ultrasonic Doppler probes. J Microsurg 3: 217–221, 1982.

14. Jorgensen JE, Campau DJ, Baker DW: Physical characteristic and mathematical modelling of pulsed ultrasonic flow meter. Med Biol Eng Comput 12: 404–429, 1973.

15. Eldridge MW, Greene ER, Berman WR, Hartley CJ, Yabek S: Ultrasonic pulsed Doppler characterization of the human neonatal peripheral circulation. Biomed Sci Instrum 15: 77–90, 1979.

16. Gilsbach J: Intraoperative Doppler Sonography in Neurosurgery. Springer Wien New York, 1983.

Perioperative transcranial Doppler sonography

A. Harders and J. Gilsbach

Introduction

In the last 2 years, transcutaneous Doppler investigations could be performed with a transcranial device [1]. Whereas, in neurovascular operations the intra-operative system was helpful in controlling the surgical procedure, the transcranial Doppler proved useful during the perioperative period for patency control of the main cerebral arteries, evaluation of the collateral circulation and diagnosis, and classification of vasospasm.

Materials and methods

The transcranial Doppler investigations were carried out pre-operatively through the orbit and a temporal bone window and postoperatively through burr holes when necessary. Routine recordings were made bilaterally of the flow velocities in the carotid syphon, the intracranial internal carotid artery (ICA), the trunk of the middle cerebral artery (MCA), the proximal branches of the middle cerebral artery (MCA), and the precommunicating part of the anterior cerebral artery (ACA, A1). Recordings of the posterior communicating system, the posterior circulation and individual vessels, e.g. in angioma cases, were also carried out. The frequency spectrum of the 2 MHz transcranial Doppler device was processed bidirectionally by a real time frequency analyzer (Angioscan I). The peak systolic and end diastolic frequencies of the maximum frequencies (envelope) as well as the time averaged maximum frequencies (time mean) were with a cursor determined on the screen of the analyzer and used for mathematical evaluation.

Results

Normal cases

Our flow velocity measurements on patients with normal cerebral vessels showed the same time averaged maximum frequencies (time mean) as those described by Aaslid [1], (1982), Arnolds, and v. Reutern [2] (1985).

Middle cerebral artery:	1.6 kHz +/− 0.3 kHz
Anterior cerebral artery, precommunicating segment (A1):	1.3 kHz +/− 0.3 kHz
Posterior cerebral artery:	1.1 kHz +/− 0.3 kHz
Internal carotid artery, intradurally	1.6 kHz +/− 0.3 kHz

To identify the individual vessels, not only the depth of the measuring gate, the

Table 1. Identification of segments of the circle of Willis with the depth of range gating, flow direction, and compression tests orthograde: flow direction towards the probe, retrograde: flow direction away from the probe.

Depth (cm) →	Flow direction →		Homolateral cervical ICA compression	→	Identified vessel
3–5 ↗ ↘	orthograde retrograde	↘ ↗	reduction of Doppler shift	→	MCA
5–6 ↗ ↘	orthograde	↗ →	reduction of Doppler shift increase of Doppler shift	→ →	ICA P1
	retrograde	→ ↘	no change in Doppler shift reduction of Doppler shift	→ →	P2 ICA
6–7 ↗ ↘	orthograde	↗ → ↘	increase of Doppler shift reduction of Doppler shift no change in Doppler shift	→ → →	P1 ICA A1 (occlusion of the opposite ICA?)
	retrograde	↗ → ↘	reversed flow no change in Doppler shift no change or increase	→ → →	A1 P2 P1
7–8 ↗ ↘	orthograde retrograde	→ ↗ →	increase of Doppler shift no Doppler shift no change in Doppler shift or increase of Doppler shift	→ → →	A1 contralat. A1 (ICA occlusion homolateral?) contralat.

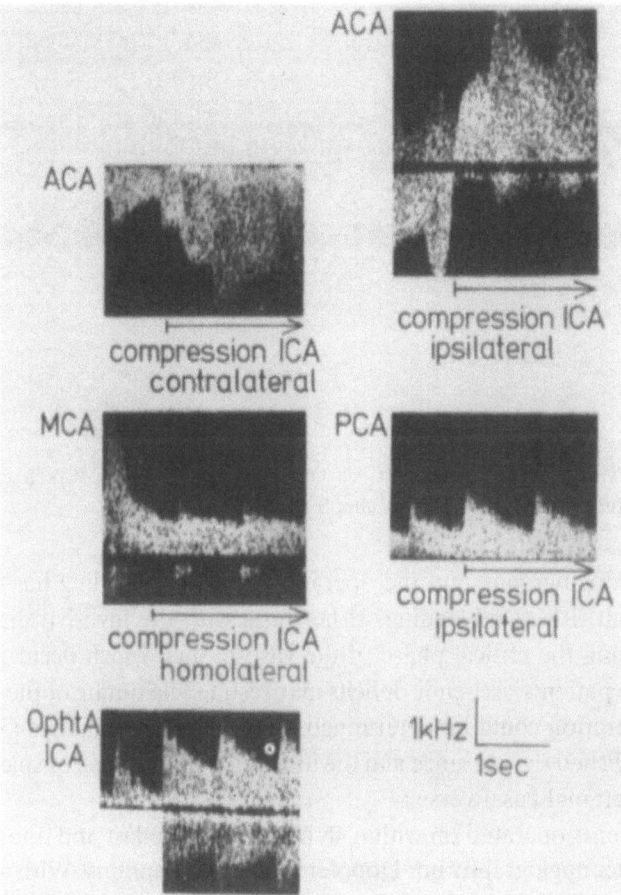

Figure 1. Compression test for identifying A1: Doppler shift increase by compressing of the contralateral ICA and change of flow direction by compression the ipsilateral ICA. Doppler shift decrease in MCA by compressing the homolateral ICA in a patient with unsufficient collaterals over the circle of Willis. Increase in Doppler shift in PCA by compressing the ipsilateral ICA shows increase in collateral flow in P1. Increased flow velocity in both directions near the origin of the ophthalmic artery in the carotid siphon.

direction of the beam, and the flow pattern were useful, but also the result of the different compression tests (Table 1). The reaction on the compression of the ipsilateral or contralateral cervical carotid artery could also be used to evaluate the collateral capacity of the anterior and posterior communicating system (Fig. 1).

Aneurysm cases

In patients with suspected aneurysms, it is difficult to decide when to perform angiography after a subarachnoid hemorrhage has occurred. If the surgeon waits

286

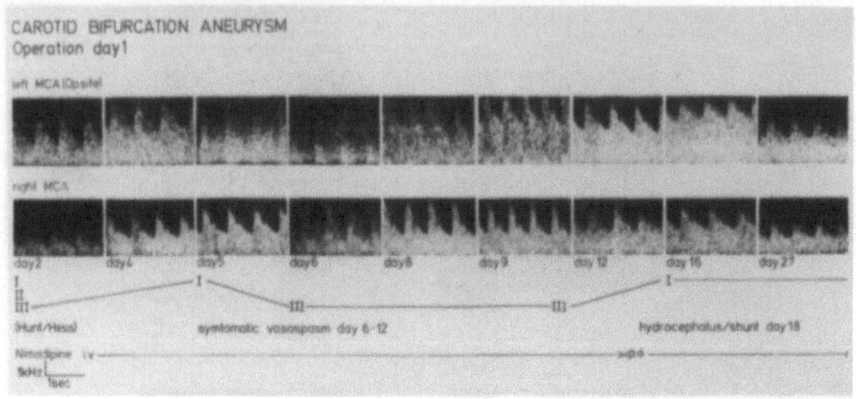

Figure 2. Time course of spasm in both MCA's. On the operated side (left MCA) a severe spasm with BRUITS and turbulences on the 6th day after SAH.

to perform angiography and the operation until the bleeding has subsided, he runs the high risk of rebleeding. If he starts with the invasive diagnostic procedures during the critical phase of the vasospasms, which occur in about two thirds of the patients, ischemic deficits may result. The timing of the angiography and the operation could be determined by the Doppler findings [3, 4, 5, 6, 7], which established the presence and the individual time course of spastic reactions of the intracranial basal vessels.

In 30 patients operated on within 48 hours after the last and one-time hemorrhage, neither angiography nor Doppler showed vasospasms. With the exception of two cases, all of the patients developed vasospasms within the following two weeks. Eight out of these 28 showed delayed ischemic dysfunctions between the 7th and 13th day after the subarachnoid hemorrhage. These patients showed a very rapid increase of the flow velocities within 4 days and a long period with extremely accelerated flow velocities and wall artefacts (Fig. 2). All of the patients with no neurological deficits had frequencies under 3 kHz (time mean) which did not increase very rapidly.

Based on these findings, 3 different velocity ranges were determined for clinical practice which helped to predict ischemic symptoms so that prophylactic medicamentous treatment could be initiated: 2 kHz and less was interpreted as normal, between 2 and 3 kHz was called subcritical spasm, because these patients developed no deficits, and more than 3 kHz, corresponding to a velocity of more than 120 cm/s, was defined as critical spasm, because these patients risked developing deficits. Patients admitted later than 3 days after the last subarachnoid hemorrhage underwent angiography only when the Doppler findings showed subcritical velocity values. In cases of critical velocities, angiography and surgery were postponed until the velocities showed a continuous decrease over a two-day period.

Postoperative Doppler control was also an aid in evaluating secondary clinical

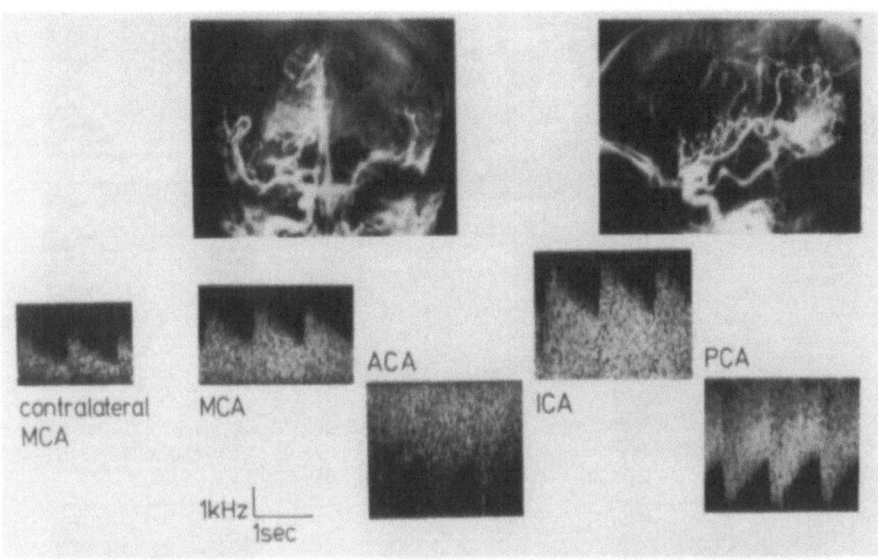

Figure 3. 32 year-old patient, increased flow velocities in the feeding arteries of ACA, PCA, ICA, and MCA.

deterioration. Flow patterns with signs of high peripheral resistance were typical for a hydrocephalus or a marked edema and no longer had to be differentiated from vasospasms by angiography.

Angioma cases

Depending on the shunt volume, the feeding arteries of cerebral angiomas showed more or less high flow velocities with a high diastolic flow component as a sign of low resistance. Postoperatively, in the prior angioma feeding vessels, the flow pattern resembled the externa type with a low diastolic flow as a sign that the resistance had increased after occlusion of the fistulas. The control investigation enabled us to follow the adaptation of the cerebral circulation and of the individual vessels to the changed hemodynamics (Fig. 3).

Extracranial-intracranial bypass cases

Pre-operatively, the transcranial Doppler method was useful in evaluating the functional change of the hemodynamics in occlusive diseases (Fig. 4). Moreover, the findings of pathologically decreased flow velocities were helpful in deciding whether bypass should be indicated in asymptomatic patients.

In cases with symptomatic occlusion of the internal cervical carotid artery, the pulse waves in the territory of the middle cerebral artery of the affected side were

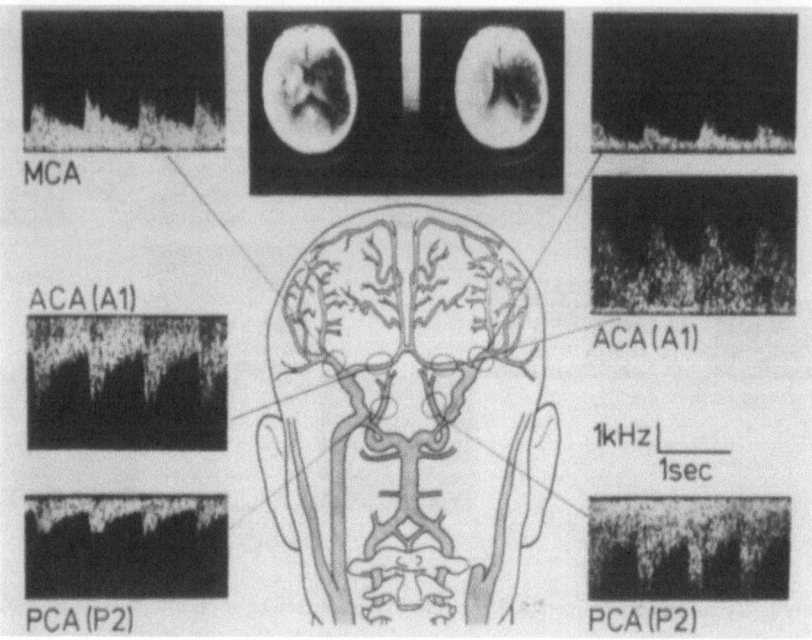

Figure 4. 52 year-old patient with severe hemiparesis on the left side and marked infarction in CT. In the right MCA the flow velocity is damped, there is a retrograde flow direction in the right ACA and an increased Doppler shift in the right PCA (P2). Good collateral flow from A1 and P2 on the right side but decreased Doppler shift in the right MCA.

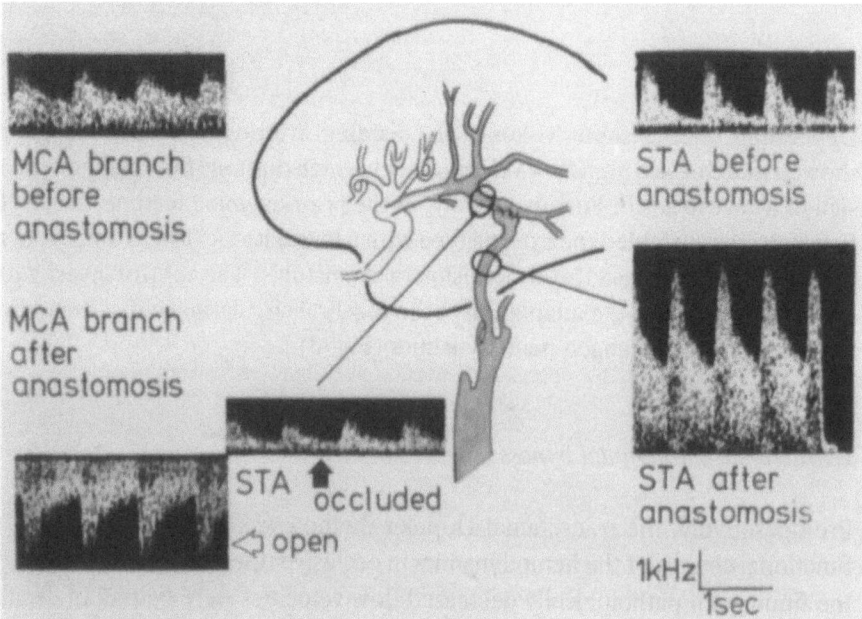

Figure 5. Hemodynamic changes after STA-MCA bypass operation. Increased and reversed flow direction in one branch of MCA. After the donor artery is compressed the reversed flow stops and the decreased flow velocity with orthograde flow direction is visible. The frequency spectrum of the donor artery changes after bypass operation from external type to internal type.

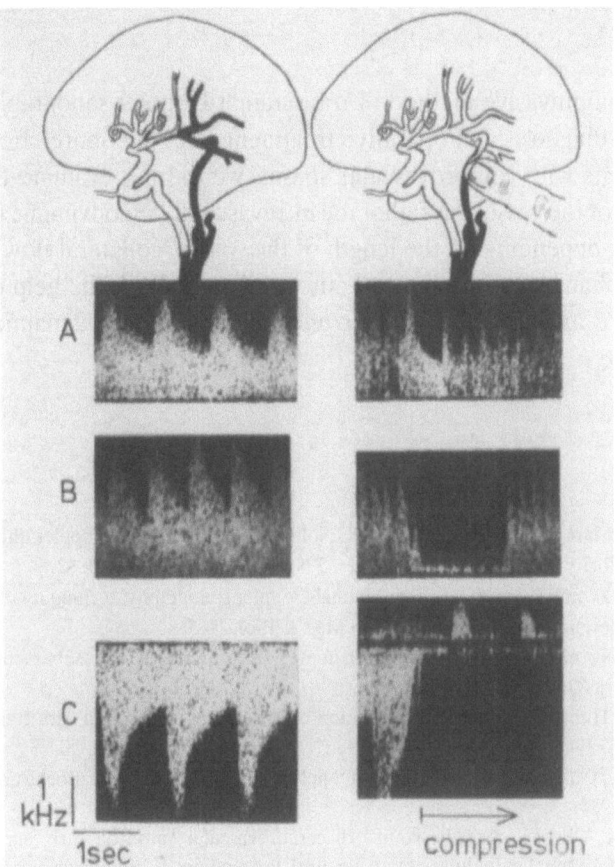

Figure 6. Compression test after extracranial-intracranial bypass operation: a) after bypass the flow contribution in a MCA branch with orthograde flow decreases after compression. b): the orthograde flow stops after compression – high dependence on bypass. c): the retrograde reversed flow in one branch of MCA stops and only a small Doppler shift with orthograde direction is visible.

damped and the total flow velocity fell below the normal range (Fig. 5). The velocities in vessels participating in the natural collateral flow were 2 to 3 times higher than in normal cases. In cases with collateral flow from the anterior and posterior communicating system, the ipsilateral precommunicating anterior cerebral artery (A1) and the posterior communicating artery had a high, reversed flow.

Postoperatively, the conventional Doppler systems only provide patency control of the donor artery. With the transcranial system additional information could be obtained on the changed hemodynamics in the area of the recipient artery and the collateral channels. A well functioning bypass showed high flow velocities with a high diastolic flow component in the donor artery and a reversed flow at a depth of 2.5–3 cm in the region of the recipient arteries [5]. This was typical for a bilateral flow distribution in technically well carried out bypasses [8]. Compression tests showed different reactions depending on the pressure gradient in the recipient artery (Fig. 6).

Conclusions

The new, noninvasive method of transcranial Doppler sonography makes neu-rovascular diagnosis and operative treatment safer and more effective.

In patients with cerebrovascular spasm, we did not evaluate the anatomical narrowing of the vessel but rather the intravascular hemodynamic reaction to this narrowing, depending on the length of the spasm, collateral flow, arterial pres-sure, compliance, resistance, and autoregulation. With the help of transcranial Doppler we are starting to better understand the hemodynamic principles in humans.

References

1. Aaslid R, Markwalder Th-M, Nornes H: Noninvasive transcranial Doppler ultrasound recording of flow velocity in basal cerebral arteries. J Neurosurg 57: 769–774, 1982.
2. Arnolds B, von Reutern G-M: Transcranial Doppler sonography: techniques of examination and normal reference values. Ultrasound in Med & Biol, 1985.
3. Aaslid R, Nornes H: Musical murmurs in human cerebral arteries after subarachnoid hemorrhage. J Neurosurg 60: 32–36, 1984.
4. Aaslid R, Huber P, Nornes H: Evaluation of cerebrovascular spasm with transcranial Doppler ultrasound. J Neurosurg 60: 37–41, 1984.
5. Harders A, Gilsbach J: Transkranielle Dopplersonographie in der Neurochirurgie. Ultraschall 5: 237–246, 1984.
6. Harders A, Gilsbach J: Time course of cerebrovascular spasm in early aneurysm operation. Transcranial Doppler findings. In: Auer (ed) Proceedings 'Cerebral Aneurysm Surgery in the Acute State' in press.
7. Harders A, Gilsbach J, Hassler W: Transcranial Doppler findings in extra-intracranial bypass surgery. In: Diresen W, Brock M, Klinger M (eds): Advances in Neurosurgery Vol. 13 in press.
8. Gilsbach J: Intraoperative Doppler sonography in neurosurgery. Springer Wien, New York, 1983.

Conclusion

M.P. Spencer, M.D.

The authors in this text have shown us that ultrasound imaging and Doppler are excellent modalities for evaluation of the cerebral circulation both extracranial and intracranial. It is also clear that considerable knowledge and skill is necessary before putting forth oneself as a diagnostician.

Choice of equipment

The choice of new equipment for the vascular laboratory is dependent on whether one is just beginning or what additions should be made to an existing laboratory. It seems necessary to combine in some fashion the capabilities of both Doppler with spectral analysis and real time 2-D B-mode. Which Doppler PW or CW, and whether 'stand-alone' or integrated with B-mode in one machine, is sometimes difficult to decide.

Both stand-alone Doppler and Duplex imaging instruments are capable of detecting with high accuracy stenosis >50 percent at the origin of the internal carotid artery. PW Doppler when integrated in the B-mode (Duplex) is often cumbersome to use but is helpful in separating the image of the external carotid from the internal and in deciding between patency or occlusion. Continuous wave Doppler alone is easy to use and excels in detection and grading higher degrees of stenosis on all the extracranial arteries with less costly equipment but lacks the B-mode image capabilities. Either Duplex B-mode or CW Doppler can be used to diagnose total occlusion of the carotid arteries but a combination is very helpful. Real time B-mode excels in detection of minor degrees of atherosclerotic plaquing but the hope of diagnosing ulceration with high accuracy has not yet been realized. B-mode equipment with mechanical scanning probes is especially costly compared to Doppler.

When equipment costs are paramount a cost-effective combination of equipment includes a CW Doppler with spectral analysis for detection of high blood velocities and a no frills linear array 2-D imager for full interrogation of the common and internal carotid arteries.

Table I

FIGURES OF MERIT - B-MODE EQUIPMENT

	BIOSOUND 2000 8MHz	TECHNICARE Autosector 7.5MHz	CAROLINA MEDICAL 1060 5MHz	ALOKA 260 7.5MHz
RESOLUTION	4	2	1	3
FIELD OF VIEW	1	2	3	4
DOPPLER	1	4	3	0
OPERATION	1	2.3	2.3	3.3
COST	1.5	1	3	4
OVERALL MERIT	1.7	2.3	2.7	2.8

OPERATIONAL FEATURES

EASE OF EXAMIN.	1	1	3	4
PORTABILITY	1	2	2	4
EXPANDABILITY	2	4	2	2
AVG.	1.3	2.3	2.3	3.3

DOPPLER FEATURES

QUALITY	1	4	3	0
SPECTRUM	1	4	3	0
PW-CW	1	4	3	0
AVG.	1	4	3	0

COSTS

INITIAL	2	1	3	4
MAINTENANCE	1	1	3	4
AVG.	1.5	1	3	4

Resolution in this Table refers to the ability to see intraplaque structural echogenicity variations. Field of view refers to the ability of the device to image the internal carotid artery all the way to the mandible. Doppler parameters are defined in the lower sections of the Table, the quality of the audio signal, the quality and flexibility of the spectral display and the availability of pulse and continuous wave Doppler. Operational features refer to the ease of the patient examination, portability of the equipment for bedside or intraoperative studies as well as an expandability of the system to other scanning probes. Cost is based on both the initial purchase price and maintenance cost contracts.

Table 1 presents the author's experience operating six laboratories in various hospitals around Seattle, Washington, where cost constraints were elected to keep the patient charges minimal yet sufficient to provide a high quality examination. A summarizing figure of merit integrating the scoring for these various features is shown. The Aloka 7.5 MHz linear array scored relatively high because of its low cost, good resolution and its ability to image the internal carotid further from the bifurcation than the sector scanner devices. All devices appeared to provide an adequate image in the center of the frame where sound beams are near normal to the axis of the blood vessels. Sector scanners, particularly wide-angle sector scanners, such as the Technicare encountered difficulties in imaging and following an artery to the edges of the sector. The CME 5 MHz B-mode improves on this problem but loses some resolution with the lower ultrasonic frequency.

The Doppler capability of Biosound Model 2000 was inadequate, barely able to assist in separating external from internal carotid artery. The Technicare Doppler system displayed excellent Doppler qualities and allowed the use of both pulse wave or continuous wave examination with an excellent frequency spectrum available. The Carolina Medical 5 MHz system lacks noticeably in resolution compared to the 7.5 and 8 MHz systems, however in most situations, the image was adequate to make a judgment concerning clinical management decisions. As a general rule all sector scanners combined with Doppler inherently have difficulty. Where the image is best the Doppler signal is poorest; where the Doppler signal is best, the image is poorest (Fig. 1A & B). The Diasonics' imager overcomes this difficulty by placing the Doppler crystal outboard to the echo imaging crystals to provide a better angle for the Doppler in the middle of the image. The author's experience with this equipment and that of Advanced Technology Laboratories equipment is limited.

The general consensus of physicians and technicians who operate the Seattle IAPM Vascular Laboratories concur that real time B-mode additions to a traditional CW Doppler laboratory are valuable.

1. The principal advantage of real-time B-mode imaging was to detect non-stenotic plaquing in minor grade that was not possible with continuous wave Doppler.

2. B-mode when no significant abnormal echogenicity is found eliminates the carotid bifurcation as a likely cause for the patient's cerebral symptoms.

3. B-mode is particularly helpful in confirming occlusion of a carotid artery

Institute of Applied Physiology and Medicine - Seattle, Washington
CEREBROVASCULAR EVALUATION

NAME _____ AGE____ SEX_____ DATE _____ TECH _____

INST #_____ HOSP.# _____ HOSPITA _____ REF. DR. _____

PREV. CVE_____ VIDEO TP #_____ POSITION _____

HISTORY

CHIEF COMPLAINT: PREVIOUS STROKE

APHASIA	WEAKNESS	PARESIS	NUMBNESS	TINGLING	VISUAL DISTURBANCE
DIZZINESS	IMBALANCE	FAINTING	CONTUSION	LOSS OF MEMORY	HEADACHE

Figure 1A.

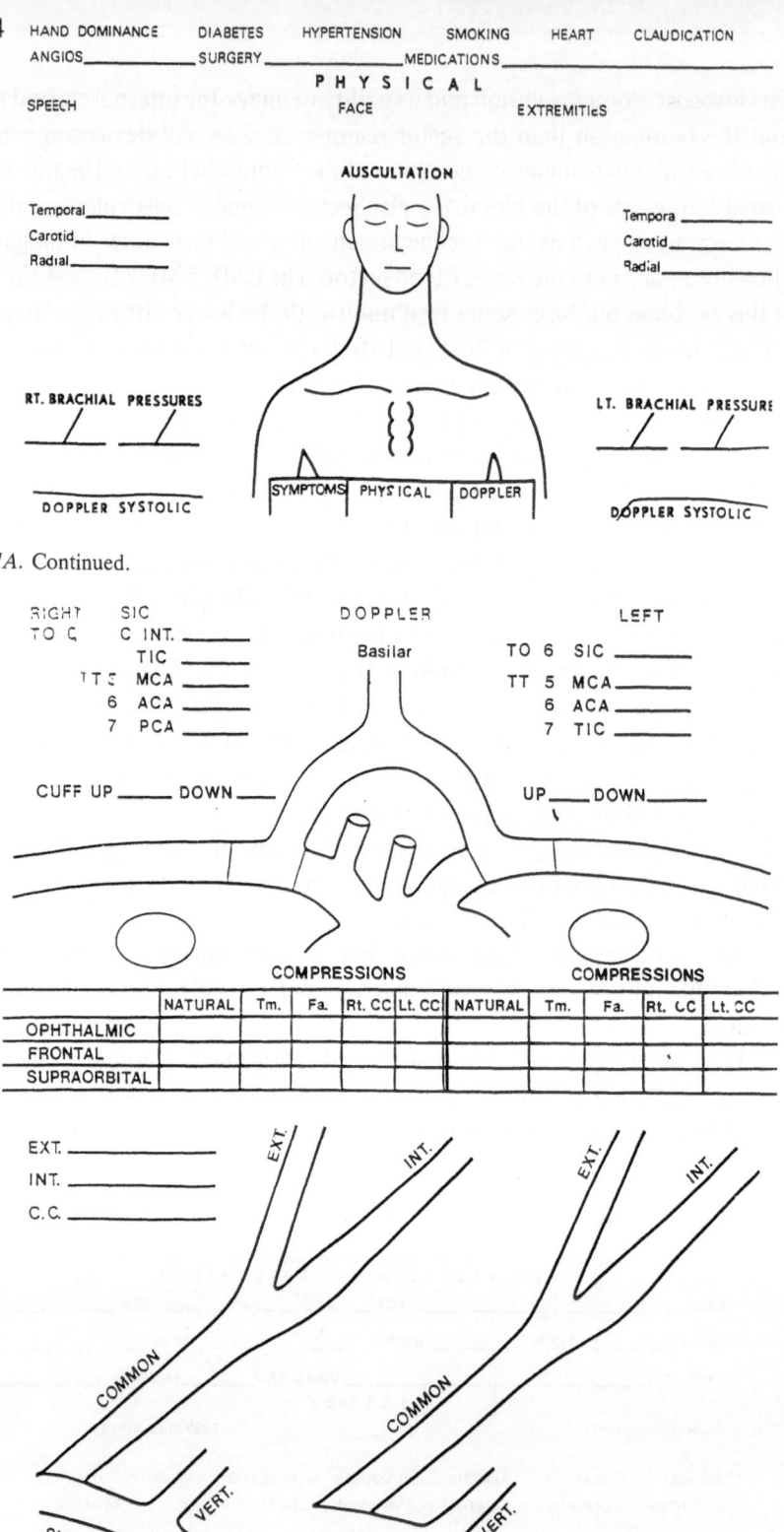

Figure 1A. Continued.

Figure 1B.

supplementing the information from stand-alone continuous wave Doppler examinations.

4. B-mode imaging had less clinical utility in patients who had Doppler evidence of >50 percent stenosis at the carotid bifurcation because the presence of stenotic plaque could be diagnosed by the Doppler signals alone with high accuracy.

5. When nonstenotic plaquing was identified with B-mode in TIA patients, a careful search for plaque surface irregularities often encouraged the use of X-ray contrast arteriography in the expectation that further evidence of ulceration might be found.

6. There is a need for a widely accepted system for grading extent and complexity of plaques from the B-mode image.

7. With sector scanning devices the availability of a good pulse Doppler signal is important to identify and separate the external from the internal carotid arteries in the image.

8. The linear array functions well without Doppler ability by skillful angling of the probe by the technician. The linear array, because it is considerably less costly than other systems, fits well with a stand-alone continuous wave Doppler instrument, and is considered the most cost effective device in our laboratories.

9. There is a need for a low-cost linear array in combination with either CW or PW Doppler.

10. The B-mode ultrasound capability of detection of ulceration or other features of atherosclerotic plaque such as intraplaque hemorrhage is interesting but accuracy must be established in each laboratory.

11. When a noninvasive vascular laboratory establishes a high positive predictive ability for stenosis of the cervical internal carotid artery endarterectomy, if indicated, can be performed without the use of invasive angiography. CT scan can be used to screen for major intracranial pathology.

The patient examination

A step-wise laboratory examination conducted in a consistent sequence should include the findings of pertinent history and physicals which focusses the ultrasound examination. In addition, an echocardiogram may be of value should it be available and when the source of the patient's symptoms is not found in the cervical and intracranial ultrasound examinations. A history should be taken beginning with the request for the patient's chief complaint followed by a series of leading questions which touch on each of the following symptom areas: speech difficulties, weakness, numbness, tingling, visual disturbances, dizziness, imbalance, fainting, confusion, loss of memory, and headache. Risk factors also may be recorded such as smoking, heart disease, prior surgery and medication.

The physical examination should include at least a summary of grossly deserved speech difficulties and any weaknesses of the face and extremities. The pulses should be palpated, including the radial, temporal and carotid arteries. Auscultation of the head and neck should be carried out to include the eyes, carotid artery bifurcation region, the supraclavicular region and the upper thorax. Brachial pressure should be recorded by auscultation using Korotkoff sounds and, if not available or should there be discrepancies, Doppler recording of the systolic pressures should be engaged. The results of the history and physical examination should be recorded by the examiner on a separate sheet to be made available to the interpreter of the complete test results. An example of the useful scratch sheet for the Cerebrovascular Laboratory is shown in Fig. 2.

The ultrasound examination should begin with continuous wave Doppler scanning of the vertebral and subclavian artery systems with free-hand techniques as explained by Dr. von Reutern in Chapter 11. Normally, the routine of this component occupies only five minutes of the examination time. Moving to the carotid bifurcation continuous wave Doppler screening or imaging of the common carotid, internal and external carotids, at the bifurcation should be carried out with care. Evidences of collateralization around the carotid arteries should be sought by examination of the periorbital arteries the ophthalmic arterial signals in the posterior orbit. Finally, using real-time B-scan imaging device the cervical carotid artery should be carefully interrogated from at least three different angles. The information from the B-scan primarily sought is that of the evidence of abnormal echogenicity, tortuosities and abnormal pulsations around the carotid bifurcation. The intracranial Doppler examination should, at a minimum, include transtemporal interrogation of the middle cerebral artery at a depth of 5 cm, an interrogation of the siphon of the internal carotid artery through the orbital pathway at 7 cm, and signals from the intracranial vertebrals and the basilar artery via the foramen magnum at a depth of 6–10 cm.

The laboratory report

The report to the referring physician from the Cerebrovascular Laboratory should provide the maximum decision-making information concerning the patient's problem. The laboratory report is preferably in the narrative form clearly separating in separate paragraphs the *history, physical examination, ultrasound, findings,* and the *interpretation* of those findings. A *conclusion* section then relates the interpretation to the patient's symptoms. The findings should be expressed in objective and definable terms reserving interpretive type of terminology for the interpretation section. The interpretation should be a projection from the findings using interpretive terms such as plaquing, stenosis, hemodynamic significance, possible embolic source, etc. Terminologies of findings such as kilohertz, abnormal echogenicity, abnormal pulsations, etc. should be confined to the 'findings' section of the report and not repeated in the interpreta-

INSTITUTE OF APPLIED PHYSIOLOGY AND MEDICINE
CARDIOVASCULAR LABORATORIES

NAME: PATIENT NUMBER: P-2344, 316040

AGE: 66   REFERRING PHYSICIAN: T. Jones

SEX: Male   DATE: 04-16-86

Dear Dr. Jones:

Thank you for the referral of the above named patient to the Vascular Laboratory for noninvasive
ULTRASOUND CEREBROVASCULAR EVALUATION.

PERTINENT HISTORY: This 66 year old man is referred to us because of bruits in his neck. He
denies, upon direct questioning, symptoms of cerebrovascular insufficiency.
The previous examination in the Cerebrovascular Laboratories on 10-11-85 was interpreted by Dr.
Thomas as 'no carotid or vertebral disease detected'.

PHYSICAL EXAMINATION at this time reveals no gross abnormality of speech, face, extremities,
or radial, temporal, and carotid pulses. There was a grade III bruit in the left supraclavicular region of
systolic and high frequency nature, with a slight whining quality. There were no carotid bifurcation
bruits, although this bruit did radiate widely. The blood pressure in the right arm, 194/100 mmHg; left
arm, 192/100 mmHg.

DOPPLER AND ULTRASOUND EXAMINATION:
POSTERIOR CIRCULATION: The left subclavian artery disclosed high frequencies at 16 kHz, with
grade III turbulence qualities, but downstream subclavian artery signals demonstrated a normal,
triphasic waveform. The right subclavian was normal, and both vertebrals were found with normal
velocities, both near their origin and at the base of the skull. Through the foramen magnum, we traced
with 2 MHz pulsed Doppler the vertebral-basilar system to 7.5–8 cm, with normal velocities represented by 2 kHz.

ANTERIOR CIRCULATION: Carotid bifurcation imaging with 5 MHz continuous wave Doppler
disclosed normal frequencies in the common-internal channels. On the left, there was a non-
visualizing origin to the internal carotid, and a slight fluttering in the distal internal signal.
B-mode ultrasound imaging on both sides disclosed some abnormal echogenicity, but particularly on
the left, where there was an area of echogenicity encroaching on the lumen slightly.
The posterior orbital and periorbital examinations were normal, without evidence of carotid collateralization. The siphon signals were normal by 2 MHz pulsed Doppler, represented by 1 kHz and
1.2 kHz. Through the left temporal bone, the middle cerebral artery signal was found through a small
anterior window, with normal velocities represented by 2.5 kHz. The right temporal bone did not
provide access.

INTERPRETATION: These findings represent approximately 50% stenosis on the origin of the left
subclavian artery, which is producing turbulence and a bruit at that point. This lesion is not affecting
arm flow or vertebral-basilar flow.
There is atherosclerosis in both common carotid bifurcations, particularly on the left, but not
producing stenosis.

MERRILL P. SPENCER, M.D.
MPS: aw

Figure 2.

tion. An example of such a well organized laboratory report follows.

In addition to the written report, immediate telephone communication with the referring physician following the examination is highly desirable by either a well qualified technician or the supervising physician. When clinically significant findings are present or when there is special urgency such as patients with TIAs or stroke the interpreting physician should report by telephone. By providing a careful and well organized report based upon a thorough and comprehensive examination the reputation of the laboratory will increase.

Surgery without angiography

It is generally agreed that stenosis greater than 50% at the origin of the internal carotid artery, when associated with transient ischemic attacks, justifies surgical intervention and endarterectomy. The basis of this general agreement is that TIAs, particularly upon their first occurrence, are highly associated with the future development of a stroke on the brain side of the carotid lesion. Standard medical practice has required arteriography by intravascular injection of radiopaque dye in all patients with TIAs and if a stenosis on the cervical internal carotid artery is found, to proceed with an endarterectomy. Where the local ultrasound laboratory has established a high accuracy level for stenosis of the carotid surgery, in certain cases, without arteriography has been advocated in certain cases. Carotid endarterectomy may be advised without the additional dangers and costs of angiography when 1) the local laboratory has a proven record of 90% accuracy on *all* carotid evaluations, and when criteria for 100% sensitivity for stenosis >50% in certain categories are validated.

For 5 MHz Doppler recordings the criteria for 100% positive predictive value of stenosis on the internal carotid are 1) clear evidence of a localized high frequency (>6 KHz when using 5 MHz Doppler ultrasound) with 2) associated turbulence, and 3) collateralization effects around the periorbital arteries and the ophthalmic artery. These criteria may be applied whether using duplex B-mode or freehand Doppler but, of course, the kilohertz threshhold must be adjusted if the ultrasound carrier frequency is other than 5 mmHz. Assurance that the stenosis is in the internal and not the external carotid include:

a) positive identification of the ECA signal and absence of response to temporal artery finger oscillations

b) collateral effects around the orbital arteries

c) waveform typical of ICA

Objection to the deletion of angiographic confirmation of carotid stenosis has been based on several arguments: 1) Angiography is necessary to determine if there are intracranial lesions which might contraindicate endarterectomy, and 2) Standard medical practice and therefore the medical malpractice liability advises against this action. Intracranial lesions which are considered to be contraindications include: a) tandem lesions in the syphon or other intracranial arteries, b) presence of an intracranial arterial aneurysm, and 3) presence of an intracranial tumor.

Regarding the question of possible tandem stenotic lesions in the intracranial internal or middle cerebral arteries, since it cannot presently be determined whether the cervical carotid stenosis or a tandem intracranial lesion is responsible for the symptoms the only prudent course we have is to proceed with cervical surgery as this is the only accessible artery lesion available. The cervical lesion may be the source of the patient's symptoms and may be the primary source of a future stroke in spite of the presence of intracranial lesions. To defer endarterectomy of a stenotic carotid lesion in the TIA patient because a tandem lesion is present is not reasonable.

In regard to the possibility of the presence of an unknown intracranial arterial aneurysm we submit the following: 1) Intracranial aneurysm in the general population is considered to be between 2 and 5% [1] in the neighborhood of 0.06% [1], 2) the possibility of a large aneurysm which might be prone to rupture upon the release of a significantly hemodynamic obstruction in the carotids is less frequent, and 3) the possibility that an aneurysm exists and will rupture producing stroke appears to be less likely than the possibilities of complications due to injection of iodinated contrast material into the arterial system.

Regarding the possibility of an intracranial tumor computerized tomography and other noninvasive brain scans which can minimize this possibility are available. In addition, it is certainly advisable that the classical symptoms of transient ischemic attack be well established in the patients whom we propose for surgical intervention without angiography. Even with the possibility that a small undetected tumor exists, it seems reasonable to operate on an existing carotid stenosis.

Regarding medical liability, it seems that the responsible physician should proceed with the primary objective of the welfare of his patient in mind. The patient deserves the opportunity of deciding for himself/herself if he/she wishes angiographic confirmaton after the situation is explained.

Some highly reputable and highly accurate noninvasive diagnosticians object to this argument on the basis that the local surgeon does not have a highly successful operation rate and low morbidity statistics. Others have objected to the concept on the basis that it is not totally proven that carotid endarterectomy does, in fact, prevent stroke and that the patient may die of coronary artery disease in spite of carotid surgery. This observer submits that these arguments are in the domain of surgical justification, not a question of diagnostic accuracy and should not be arguments to deny the patient the advantages of a more simple management course if, in fact, the local decision making group believes that carotid endarterectomy is indicated. If complications to carotid surgery arise, when angiography has not been performed these complications should not be necessarily blamed on the noninvasive diagnosis when, in fact, they are resultant to matters that do not regard the question of accurate diagnosis.

It is an unfortunate fact that the growth of the noninvasive vascular laboratories has preceded the qualifications and expertise of the operators in many laboratories. This state of affairs has led, in some areas, to disbelief and loss of creditability of ultrasonic diagnosis of carotid artery disease. Again we return to the original thesis that before such a procedure can be advocated in the local environment, the local laboratory must unequivocally document their high capability in Doppler ultrasonic diagnosis.

Reference

1. Heros RC, Kistler JP. Intracranial Aneurysm – An Update. Stroke 14, 628, 1983.

Credit and recognition list

The authors of this book wish to extend their appreciation and provide credit recognition to the following publishing organizations and authors for granting permission to use specific illustrations in order to enhance the contents of this book:

Chapter 1:
Fig. 2: By permission: American heart Association. Incidence. In: 'Stroke', Part II, Vol. 12, No. 2, Fig. 4–1, March/April 1981. Authors: Robbins Morton, Bau, Herbert N. Westat Research, Rochester, Minnesota, U.S.A.

Chapter 5:
Fig. 16: By permission: Permagon Press Inc., New York. Steady Flow in a model of the human carotid bifurcation, Part II, Laser Doppler anemometer measurements. Journal of Biomechanics, Vol. 15, No. 5. 1982. Fig. 8, p 371. Authors: Bharadvaj, BK; Mabon, RF; Giddens, DP. Editors-in-Chief, Verne L. Roberts and Rik Huiskes.

Chapter 9:
Fig. 1: By permission: Research Studies Press, England. Copyright 1982 by John Wiley & Sons, Ltd. All rights reserved. Using Carotid Imaging and Hand-Held Probing Doppler Evaluation of the Aortocranial Circulation. In: Doppler Ultrasound in the Diagnosis of Cerebrovascular Disease. Ch 7: p 191, Fig. 7–20.
Fig. 6A, B, C, D: Clinical Physiology (1985) 5, p 257–269. Prospective evaluation of the accuracy of duplex scanning with spectral analysis in carotid artery disease. Courtesy of Dr. Zbornikova, Vera, et al, Sweden.
Fig. 15B: By permission: Mosby Times Mirror. Continuous-wave Doppler imaging of the carotid bifurcation. In Noninvasive diagnostic techniques in vascular disease, ed. 3, 1985. Eugene F. Bernstein, ed. Fig. 35–10. Author: Spencer Merrill P.

302

Fig. 20: By permission: Mosby Times Mirror. Continuous-wave Doppler imaging of the carotid bifurcation. In: Noninvasive diagnostic techniques in vascular disease, ed. 3, 1985. Eugene F. Bernstein, ed. Fig. 35–6. Author: Spencer Merrill P.

Fig. 21: By permission: Reproduced with permission of copyright owner: Westminster Publications Inc., Roslyn, New York, USA 11576. All rights reserved. Research Studies Press, England. Doppler Measurement of the pressure drop caused by arterial stenosis: An experimental Study. In: Angiology, Vol. 36: 899, 1985. Authors: Faccenda, F., Usui Yoshiyuki, Spencer, M.P.

Fig. 22: By permission: Research Studies Press, England. Copyright 1982 by John Wiley & Sons Ltd. All rights reserved. Using Carotid Imaging and Hand-Held Probing Doppler Evaluation of the Aortocranial Circulation. In: Doppler ultrasound in the Diagnosis of Cerebrovascular Disease. 7: 205, Fig. 7–27.

Fig. 23: By permission: Mosby Times Mirror. Continuous-wave Doppler imaging of the carotid bifurcation. In: Noninvasive diagnostic techniques in vascular disease, ed. 3, 1985. Fig. 35–7. Author: Spencer Merrill P.

Chapter 14:

Fig. 3A and 3B: Courtesy of Quantum Medical Systems, Inc., Issaquah, Washington, USA.

Fig. 2: By permission: Research Studies Press, England. In Atherosclerosis Reviews, Vol. 10, edited by R. J. Hegyli. Raven Press, New York, 1983. Doppler Imaging. Fig. 19, Page 26, Courtesy of Dr. C. Wood.

Chapter 16:

Fig. 1, 2, 3: By permission: Journal of Vascular Surgery, 1981, 89: 6, 718–29. Author: Comerota A.J. et al.

Fig. 4: By permission. Journal of Vascular Surgery, 1984, 1: 1, 84–95. Real-time B-Mode Carotid Imaging: A Three-Year Multicenter Experience. Author: Comerota A.J. et al.

Table 2, 3, 4, 5: By permission: J. of Vascular Surgery, 1: 1, 1984, pg 84–95. Tables 1, 2, 4, 8. Real-Time B-Mode Imaging. A Three-Year Multicenter Experience. Author: Comerota A.J. et al.

Index

Acceleration, 57, 59, 275
Age evolution, 92
Aliasing 25, 26, 216
A-mode, 258
Analogy
  electrical, 62
Anastomosis, 28, 81, 279, 281
Aneurysm, 272, 286
Anatomy, 43
Angiographic data, 188
Angiographic evaluation, 173, 296
Angioma, 276, 287
Angle correction, 131
Aneurysm, 286
Anterior
  cerebral artery, 232, 273
  arterial circulation, 46
  communicating artery, 275–276
Aorta, 63
Aortic arch, 44
Auscultation Dynamic, 152
Autoregulation, 77
Arteriography, 251
Arterial 151
  compliance, 61
  compressions, 152
  models, 61
  occlusion, 168
  obstruction, 120
  pCO2, 78
  pressure, 67, 76, 136
  spasm, 286
Arteriovenous malformations, 84, 237, 277
Artery identification, 158
Atherosclerotic
  lesions, 105

plaque 4, 72, 223, 243, 252
Autoregulation, 76
Axial resolution, 242
Basal cerebral arteries, 129, 227
Basilar artery
  occlusions, 203
  stenoses, 193
Bernoulli effect, 130, 135

Blood
  density, 58, 130
  flow, 57, 66
    abnormalities, 265
    disturbances, 103, 110
    imaging, 175
    index, 94
    measurement, 87
    pulses, 63
    streams, 133
    velocities, 104, 108
    velocity patterns, 108
    waveform 67, 128
  pressure, 76
  velocity, 22, 66, 122, 124, 130, 235
  viscosity, 58, 129, 148
B-mode imaging, 35
  accuracy, 245, 246
  errors, 249
  images, 258
Boundary layer, 133
Brachiocephalic trunk, 45
Breathholding, 152
Bruits, 147, 150, 151, 154, 275, 286
Bypass
  EC/IC, 99, 278, 287

Carotid artery
  bifurcation, 241
  blood flow, 64
  bulb, 70, 108, 109, 111, 112, 160
  compression, 128, 153, 285, 289
  imaging, 242
  occlusion, 95, 141, 141, 260
  siphon, 149
  stenosis, 97, 105, 117, 122, 132, 137, 171, 179,
      223, 280
Cerebral
  artery aneurysm, 274
  blood flow, 75, 78
  circulation, 75
  vasospasm, 237
Cerebrovascular
  accidents, 2
  resistance, 76
Cervical arterial anatomy, 46
Cervival
  Collateral, 197, 198
  ICA, 164
Circle of Willis, 53, 54, 81, 230, 235, 269
Clinical experience, 143
Collateral, 126
  capacity, 230
  channels, 120
  circulation, 43, 142
  flow, 288
  pathways, 53, 127
  resistance, 136
  supply, 230, 236
  stenosis, 137
  system, 80
Color
  coding, 212
  flow mapping, 219, 221
Common carotid artery, 43, 87, 106, 107
  bifurcation, 70
  blood flow, 88, 89
Compliance, 60, 61
Compliant flow, 67
Compression maneuvers, 128, 153, 159, 161,
      285, 289
Computer simulations, 133
Costocervical trunk, 202
Cranial blood flow, 87
Curved artery, 169

Dampening, 125
Diagnostic Capabilities, 2

Diameter changes, 37
Diastolic velocities, 124
Distensibility, 60
Doppler
  continuous wave 19, 179, 291
  detection of turbulence, 155
  Doppler, 227
  effect, 9, 19, 20
  imaging, 211
  intraoperative, 269, 274
  microvascular, 270
  multichannel, 26, 36, 104
  perioperative, 283
  spectrum, 30, 67
  techniques, 157
  transducers, 14
  two-dimensional Doppler, 219
  ultrasound, 21, 29, 87
Duplex
  accuracy, 261
  Doppler, 258
  flow volume, 260
  imaging, 291

Embolism, 1, 3
Endarterectomy, 100, 186
Equipment, 214, 291
Experience, 246
External carotid artery, 162, 175
  lesions, 172

Filter, 26
  highpass, 27, 132
Fourier series, 24, 25
Frequency
  spectrum, 23, 107
  low, 26, 27, 132
  extimator, 39

Harmonic index, 69
Hemodynamic
  effects, 119
  significance, 118, 113
Hypercapnia, 78
Hypocapnia, 78
Hypoxia, 80
Hypertension, 72

Image quality, 245, 267
Inertance, 58
Infarctions, 3, 288

Internal carotid artery, 43, 65, 108, 160, 273
  blood flow, 139
  bypass, 99, 278, 287
  occlussion, 130, 248
  stenosis, 144
Intracranial
  arterial anatomy, 48
  internal carotid artery, 232, 273
  pressure, 82, 83
  stenosis, 166, 175, 236
  vertebral artery, 208
Intraoperative Doppler, 269, 274

Laminar flow, 58
Leptomeningeal anastomoses, 81
Liability
  medical, 297
Linear array, 18, 220

Microvascular Doppler, 270, 278
Middle cerebral artery, 230, 272
Modeling, 129, 133, 134
Multi-channel pulsed Doppler, 36, 37, 104
  imaging, 214
  pulsed Doppler, 26
Musical Murmurs, 275

Nonstenotic plaquing, 294
Normal
  cerebral arteries, 284
  cerebral circulation, 272
  laminar flow, 264
  spectra, 107
Nyquist frequency, 39

Occipital artery, 55
Occlusions internal
  carotid artery, 174
Ophthalmic
  artery, 128
  collateral, 94
Orifice equation, 129

Patient examination, 158, 180, 294
Perfusion luxury, 83
Perioperative Doppler, 283
Peripheral resistance, 66, 136
Positron emission scan, 83
Posterior
  arterial circulation, 49
  cerebral artery, 233, 284

circulation, 193
communicating artery, 49
inferior cerebellar
  arteries, 51, 281
Pressure drop, 59, 133, 134, 137, 141
Pressure
  flow, 65
  gradients, 126
Pulsatility indices, 68, 69
Pulsed
  Doppler, 23, 33, 35, 38, 106, 291
  Doppler imaging, 215
  echo ultrasound, 15
  Wave, 19

Real-time B-mode imaging, 241
Reactive hyperemia, 64
Recipient artery, 79
Resistance, 57
Resistive flow, 67
Report laboratory, 295
Resonant wave, 64
Retrograde, 279
Reynolds number, 147

Sample volume, 23, 24, 34, 107
Sector scan, 18, 292
Sound Waver, 7
Spasm, 286
Spectral
  analysis, 22, 23, 24, 154, 179, 180, 291
  broadening, 104, 124, 182
Stenosis, 24, 177, 248
  degree of, 118, 123, 181, 183, 188, 252
  effects, 120
  experimental, 140
  index, 183, 189
  length, 135
  quantitating, 184
  radius, 135
Steal, 128, 204
  intermittent, 207
Sterilized probes, 270
Stethoscopes, 148
Stroke, 1
Stump pressure, 142
Subarachnoid hemorrhage 1, 239, 285
Subclavian
  artery, 45, 196
  steal, 128, 204
Supratrochlear artery, 166

Surgery without angiography, 296
Superior cerebellar artery, 52
Symptom categories, 5
Systolic velocities, 124

Technique of examination, 198
Three-dimensional scan, 231
Thyroid artery, 164
TIA, 2
T-M mode, 212
Tortuosities, 165, 201
Transducers, 17, 18, 220
  sterilization, 270
Transcranial
  Criteria for diagnosis, 234
  Doppler, 227
  Mapping, 229
  Imaging, 229
Turbulence, 123, 132, 147, 201, 286
Turbulent flow, 182

Ulcer formation, 222
Ulceration, 244, 249
Ultrasound
  attenuation, 8
  examination, 295

focussing, 12
transmitter, 8
transducer, 10
Waves, 9–10

Vascular
  murmurs, 147
  resistance, 58
Vasodilatation, 80
Vasospasms, 84, 274
Velocity definition, 57
Velocity
  definition, 57
  of sound, 29
  profile, 34, 58, 111, 265
  waveforms, 64
Vertebral artery, 50, 128, 170, 194, 200
  occlusion, 201
Vertebrobasilar, 43
Vertebro-vertebral steal, 205
Viscosity of the blood, 148

Wall tensions, 72
  motion, 38

Zero-crossing meter, 31, 32